Essentials of
ORAL PHYSIOLOGY

Essentials of
ORAL PHYSIOLOGY

Robert M. Bradley

Professor of Dentistry and Physiology
University of Michigan
Ann Arbor, Michigan

with 110 illustrations

Mosby

St. Louis Baltimore Boston Carlsbad Chicago Naples New York Philadelphia Portland
London Madrid Mexico City Singapore Sydney Tokyo Toronto Wiesbaden

Mosby
Dedicated to Publishing Excellence

Editor: Linda Duncan
Developmental Editor: Melba Steube
Project Manager: Peggy Fagen
Manufacturing Supervisor: Betty Richmond
Electronic Production Coordinator: Pamela Merritt

Printed in the United States of America

Composition by Mosby Electronic Production
Printing/binding by Maple-Vail Book Manufacturing Group

Mosby–Year Book, Inc.
11830 Westline Industrial Drive
St. Louis, Missouri 63146

International Standard Book Number 0-8151-1183-5

95 96 97 98 99 / 9 8 7 6 5 4 3 2 1

For three special people in my life,

Charlotte, Anna, and Robin

Preface

This book is a successor to one I wrote in 1981 call *Basic Oral Physiology*. Since then there have been rapid advances in our understanding of the physiology of the orofacial region. Indeed the advances have been so rapid in some areas that it is difficult to keep abreast of the current knowledge. It is now time to put some of these advances in a textbook form so that students of the the function of the oral cavity have a suitable source of this material at a basic level. Although some of the material and contents are similar to the earlier text, this book is almost totally new.

In writing this book I have assumed that the student has already taken a course in general physiology and has a good background in neuroscience. Even with this caveat the student may be unfamiliar with some of the concepts and techniques of neuroscience. Because I did not want to interrupt the text to explain these techniques, I have used the device of incorporating these boxes into the text that provide the necessary explanation. The reader can then refer to these boxes whenever suitable. For students requiring additional information, I have included references at the end of each chapter that are a source of much additional reading on a particular subject. The credits in the figure legends are also a source of further reading material.

Many individuals have been influential in the preparation of this text, and I owe them a note of appreciation. My students, who over the years have listened to my lectures on the subject of orofacial function, have provided many helpful criticisms and comments that have helped refine and develop my approach to this complex subject. Drs. Robert D. Sweazey and Christian Stohler read an early manuscript of two chapters and gave valuable advice. Dr. Charlotte Mistretta's advice on many aspects of the text is much appreciated. I also wish to acknowledge the authors of review articles who have made my task much easier by sifting through the literature and providing a comprehensive overview of many of the topics covered in this book. In addition, I must thank numerous colleagues and scientific publishers for granting permission to reproduce many of the figures. Some of these authors kindly provided additional unpublished figures and suggested further sources of material when I wrote to them asking for permission. Although some of the figures have been reproduced exactly as in the original publication, most have been redrawn to make them suitable for the point I was trying to get across. All the artwork was done by Teryl Schessler, who deserves my thanks. I also want to thank Amy Steckel, who did a most efficient job of writing and obtaining permissions to use copyright material. Last but not least, I am grateful for the help and understanding shown by the editorial staff of Mosby.

Robert M. Bradley

Contents

1

Introduction

- *What is Oral Physiology?*
- *How the Functions of the Oral Cavity are Organized*
- *How This Book is Organized*
- *The Importance of the Study of Oral Physiology*

LEARNING OBJECTIVES:

At the end of this chapter you should be able to:
1. Name two important functions of the mouth.
2. Describe how oral functions are organized.

WHAT IS ORAL PHYSIOLOGY?

Physiology is the branch of biology that deals with the study of functions of living matter. Oral physiology, therefore, is the study of functions of the mouth and associated structures. For most organisms, beginning with those consisting of single cells, the fundamental function of the mouth is feeding. Because the oral cavity is the portal to the gastrointestinal tract, food materials are taken into the mouth, chewed, and swallowed. However, before these basic events occur, food has to be selected from potential sources in the environment, and when taken into the oral cavity it must be analyzed as suitable for entry into the gastrointestinal tract. A central focus of this book is to understand how the oral cavity performs the primary feeding functions of guiding food intake and preparing the food for swallowing and digestion.

A second important function of the human mouth is speech production. Although many animals use their mouths to produce various sounds, only humans use speech to communicate through language. This very important function involves sophisticated control of many oral, pharyngeal, and laryngeal structures to generate various sounds involved in speech production.

Other possible functions of the oral cavity could be suggested, such as holding objects; while this function is quite important in animals, it is trivial in humans; therefore, the role of the oral cavity as a prehensile organ and other more minor functions will not be considered in this book.

Many scientists and clinicians have studied feeding and speech production and produced a vast and complicated literature. These facts in themselves are interesting and important, but they need to be considered in relation to broad general principles of the functions of the mouth. Only then can an understanding of the physiology of the oral cavity have real relevance and provide the necessary information useful in designing better treatment of orofacial and dental disorders.

HOW THE FUNCTIONS OF THE ORAL CAVITY ARE ORGANIZED

A complex function like feeding involves many different body areas, and, at the level of the mouth, feeding consists of several basic levels of organization. First, food is selected and analyzed by a number of sensory systems including those involved in taste, smell, touch, and temperature perception of the food. This sensory information is then integrated by various centers in the central nervous system. Based on central integration, saliva is secreted, chewing movements begin, and swallowing eventually occurs. Each of these basic levels of organization involves additional phases of complexity. For example, additional sensory systems are needed in the control of muscle movements and protection of the oral structures from tissue damage while food is prepared for swallowing.

These basic levels of organization such as taste perception, neuromuscular control of mastication, and salivary secretion are themselves complex functions. To understand these behaviors requires an in-depth analysis of each system including receptor mechanisms, central pathways conveying information to the brain, neural connections used in integrating sensory information, neurotransmitters for synaptic transmission, motor integrating systems, and peripheral effector mechanisms. By analyzing these fundamental systems, we can understand the more complex behavior of the role of the oral cavity in feeding.

HOW THIS BOOK IS ORGANIZED

Initial chapters detail the physiology of the mouth's sensory systems involved in perception of the sensory quality of food, control of muscle movement, and protection of the oral cavity from tissue damage. In each of these chapters, receptor mechanism and central nervous system pathways are described. The later chapters discuss mechanisms for secretion of saliva, chewing, and swallowing. The final chapter presents an abbreviated discussion of the fascinating and complex function of language and speech production.

The material that serves as a background for these chapters is based on experiments in mammals and other animals such as salamanders and frogs. These animal models often provide favorable experimental conditions for studying a certain facet of physiology that cannot be investigated in humans. Moreover, when technical developments progress sufficiently that human experiments become possible, the results obtained from study of lower animals are often remarkably similar to those derived from human experiments. Therefore, facts obtained from animal experiments should not be considered less valuable than results of human experiments. Many basic physiologic functions are similar if not identical across species.

THE IMPORTANCE OF THE STUDY OF ORAL PHYSIOLOGY

Most of the information contained in this book derives from work of investigators interested in basic biologic mechanisms; their findings have resulted in remarkable progress in understanding orofacial function. These major advances are not only interesting in themselves, but also lead to explanations of orofacial dysfunctions and suggest better methods of diagnosis and treatment strategies. Many examples could be mentioned here, but one interesting study centered on the very familiar phenomenon commonly referred to as a "sweet tooth."

In more technical terms a "sweet tooth" is the exaggerated preference behavior resulting from stimulation of taste receptors with certain classes of chemicals. Sweet foods motivate consumption, so sweeteners are added to a broad variety of prepared foods to encourage purchase and consumption. Unfortunately, this behavior can lead to severe health problems including obesity and dental decay. It is therefore important to study the basic mechanisms of this phenomenon, and this has taken place at several levels. Neuroscientists have studied sweet taste receptor mechanisms and explored the coding of sweet taste by the central nervous system. Psychologists have designed experiments to explore the motivational aspects of sweet taste. As a result of these and other multidisciplinary studies, it has become possible to design sweeteners that have little or no caloric content, that do not act as a substrate for fermentation by oral bacteria, and that therefore do not result in tooth decay. In recent years, these alternative sweeteners have become common in many so-called diet foods. By fooling the taste system that evolved to select sweet-tasting, nutritious foods, we can experience the indulgence of sweet-tasting foods without some of the health-related consequences. In this example, scientists interested in how the taste system processes neural signals from chemicals placed on the tongue have contributed to major progress in controlling at least two serious health problems and have spawned a multimillion dollar artificial sweetener industry as well.

Other examples could be given to detail how basic research has contributed to the understanding of clinical problems. Until the elementary biology of the orofacial region and the central nervous system control of orofacial structures is better understood, progress in clinical diagnosis and treatment of many disorders will remain empirical. This is an introduction to the exciting work that has occurred in the study of the function of the mouth and associated structures.

2

Pain

- *Nociceptors*
  - *Cutaneous Nociceptors*
    - *Aδ Mechanical Nociceptors*
    - *C Polymodal Nociceptors*
    - *Other Cutaneous Nociceptors*
    - *Structure of Cutaneous Nociceptors*
  - *Trigeminal Nociceptors*
  - *Other Nociceptors*
  - *Receptor Mechanisms*
- *Central Terminations of Nociceptive Afferent Fibers*
  - *Dorsal Horn of the Spinal Cord*
  - *Medullary Dorsal Horn*
  - *Putative Neurotransmitters Released from Nociceptive Afferent Fibers*
- *Nociceptive Neurons in the Spinal and Medullary Dorsal Horns*
  - *Nociceptive-Specific Neurons*
  - *Wide-Dynamic-Range Neurons*
  - *Response Processing by Second-Order Nociceptive Neurons*
- *Ascending Nociceptive Tracts*
- *Nociceptive Mechanisms in Thalamus and Cortex*
- *Other Projections Important in Nociception*
- *Endogenous Pain Control*
  - *Endorphins*
  - *Opiate Receptors*
  - *Descending Nociceptive Control System*
- *Clinical Considerations*
  - *Measuring Pain Responses in Humans*
  - *Experimental Measurement of Pain Sensation*
  - *Measuring Pain Sensation in Humans with Pain*
- *Summary*

LEARNING OBJECTIVES

At the end of this chapter you should be able to:

1. Define the characteristics of a painful stimulus.
2. List the characteristics of a painful experience.
3. Describe the characteristics of a nociceptor.
4. List the functional characteristics of the various classes of cutaneous nociceptors.
5. Define the fundamental characteristics of noncutaneous nociceptors.
6. Describe the receptor mechanisms of a nociceptor.
7. Define the terminations of nociceptive afferent fibers in the dorsal horn of the spinal cord.
8. List the termination of nociceptive afferent fibers in the trigeminal sensory nucleus.
9. Name the neurotransmitters involved in synaptic transmission of nociceptive information in the dorsal horn of the spinal cord.
10. Describe the morphology and functional properties of nociceptive neurons in the spinal cord and trigeminal sensory nucleus.
11. Define the role of the substantia gelatinosa of the dorsal horn of the spinal cord in nociceptive mechanisms.
12. List the ascending neural pathways transmitting nociceptive information.
13. Describe the endogenous pain control system.
14. Name the three classes of endogenous opiates.
15. Define the functions of the endogenous opiates.
16. Name the three classes of opiate receptors.
17. List the relative distribution of the opiate receptors in the central nervous system.
18. Name the descending pathways in the central nervous system which control nociception.
19. List the experimental methods used to measure painful sensations.
20. Name methods used to measure pain in humans suffering pain.
21. Identify current theories of the mechanisms of pain sensation.

The experience of pain is often caused by a simple injury such as a skin cut, but it may also result from a complex set of circumstances like low back pain. The events leading to pain caused by injury are relatively well defined. A known stimulus excites cutaneous receptors connected by relatively well-characterized sensory pathways in the central nervous system. (However, for most individuals with low back pain are no obvious stimuli or sites of injury.)

When compared to other sensory systems, the experience of pain is unique because there are multiple forms of pain, all with potentially different physiologic bases. A further characteristic that demonstrates the uniqueness of the pain perception system is that for most individuals, pain is an uncommon occurrence, whereas sensations produced by most other sensory systems occur repeatedly during waking.

Because of the diversity of painful sensations and syndromes, pain is a complex, multifaceted experience. Pain can have classic sensory properties, such as intensity and quality, and usually has a temporal component. The site of the painful stimulus can frequently be localized. Pain often invokes vigorous reflex activity such as muscle withdrawal, vocalization, a startle response, and various autonomic responses like sweating, pupil dilation, and cardiovascular changes. The physiology underlying these characteristics of a painful experience is relatively well understood. However, the mechanisms of other aspects of a painful ordeal are less clear. For example, pain has strong motivational characteristics that require an individual to do something to stop the pain. In addition, the pain experience can be modified by various conditions such as individual tolerances to pain, history of other painful experiences, and the context of the pain. As an example, individuals can tolerate pain much more if they know that the painful sensation is only temporary.

The most frequent cause of pain is imminent or actual tissue damage. The potentially harmful stimulus produces a painful response that stops when the stimulus is removed and any necessary healing has occurred. This form of pain is usually classified as acute pain; it serves as an alarm system guarding the integrity of the organism. The mechanism of acute pain has been extensively studied in animals and humans, especially pain originating from stimulations of cutaneous receptors. Chronic pain—pain that is present almost continuously with no apparent site of injury—is not understood as well.

A further complication that has always hindered pain research and treatment is the lack of a single, reliable method to measure painful sensations. One of the most powerful tools to assess pain experiences and treatments in humans is verbal response. Nonverbal responses have also been employed, but because the input-output relationship of the central nervous system is not well understood, measures of reflex responses to painful stimuli have never been very successful. There are similar problems when other nonverbal measures of pain are used, such as with evoked brain potentials.

Because of the complexity of the painful experience, research on pain mechanisms has lagged behind that on other sensory systems. One major problem is that many investigators and clinicians have different basic assumptions regarding the nature of painful experiences. To introduce some conformity, a group of international experts defined pain as an unpleasant sensory and emotional experience associated with actual or potential tissue damage. They noted that pain is always subjective and that each person applies the word, "pain," in a personalized way, based on painful experiences early in life. They also noted that pain is unquestionably a sensation localized to a part of the body, is always unpleasant, and, therefore, has a pronounced emotional component. There is no way to distinguish between the pain derived from tissue damage and the reports of pain in the apparent absence of tissue damage. Therefore, both types of sensations should be accepted as pain, even when there is no apparent source. Finally, these experts stated that the neural activity induced in nociceptors and nociceptive pathways by noxious stimuli is not pain (which originates in the central nervous system), even though pain often results from an obvious stimulation of nociceptors.

NOCICEPTORS

On the basis of experiments conducted more than 100 years ago demonstrating that different points on the skin respond to different types of stimuli such as touch and temperature, it was suggested that specific receptors responding to distinctive types of stimuli are located under these points. It was further suggested that a population of skin receptors, called pain receptors, respond specifically to painful stimuli. However, as already mentioned, pain is a psychologic phenomenon resulting from the central processing of information, so the term "pain receptor" has been replaced by "nociceptor" to describe a nerve ending that responds to stimuli that actually or potentially produce tissue damage.

Applications to the skin of many different stimuli such as mechanical, thermal, chemical, and electrical results in a painful sensation. However, these same stimuli also excite other cutaneous receptors that give rise to touch and warm and cool sensations. Although these stimuli can excite both nociceptive and nonnociceptive receptor groups, each receptor group responds to different intensity ranges of these stimuli. For example, thermal nociceptors respond to high skin temperatures that would be described as hot or burning, while nonnociceptive thermal receptors respond to lower skin temperatures described as warm or cool.

Experiments in animals and humans have demonstrated that information originating in nociceptors travels over small-diameter afferent nerve fibers, specifically those that fall into the Aδ and C fibers groupings. The Aδ component is correlated with stinging pain and the C component with agonizing, intolerable pain. The existence of these two categories of fibers could explain the double nature of pain. A single, short-duration nociceptive stimulus applied to the skin gives rise to an initial, localized pricking pain followed by a second pain, usually more diffuse and burning. The faster-conducting Aδ group is responsible for the initial pain, and the slower conducting C fibers are responsible for the second pain.

Cutaneous Nociceptors

The existence of a set of receptors responding to noxious stimulation of the skin has only recently been accepted. As indicated by electrophysiologic recordings in animals, afferent fibers with defined receptive fields on the skin have shown a higher response threshold and a different intensity range than touch and thermal receptors. Based on systematic, neurophysiologic analysis of afferent fibers responding to noxious stimulation of the skin, two major groups of nociceptors have been described: the Aδ, high-threshold mechanoreceptors, activated by intense mechanical stimulation, and the C polymodal nociceptors, excited by intense mechanical, thermal, and chemical stimuli.

Aδ Mechanical Nociceptors

The Aδ nociceptors derive their name from the conduction velocity of their afferent fibers and the specific sensitivity to mechanical stimulation. Their receptive fields are large, consisting of 3 to 20 spots, each with an area of about 1 mm^2, distributed over a total area of 1 to 8 cm^2. The threshold of one of the sensitive spots is 5 to 1000 times higher than low-threshold mechanoreceptors innervated by large-diameter fibers (Fig. 2-1). Aδ mechanical nociceptors are not normally spontaneously active and initiate action potentials only when stimulated. The frequency of these action potentials increases with stimulus intensity. This type of nociceptor makes up about 20% of the cutaneous Aδ fibers.

C Polymodal Nociceptors

The C polymodal nociceptors are innervated by unmyelinated C fibers and respond to mechanical, thermal, and chemical stimuli. Their receptive fields are generally small, consisting of one or more spots with an area of 0.5 to 2 mm^2. In the absence of stimulation, the receptors do not produce any neural discharges. The threshold for mechanical stimuli is similar to that of Aδ mechanical nociceptors, and discharge frequency increases with stimulus intensity. Threshold for a response to heat is generally about 42° C. Response to a suprathreshold stimulus begins after a short latency and consists of an initial high frequency; it then adapts to a steady-state

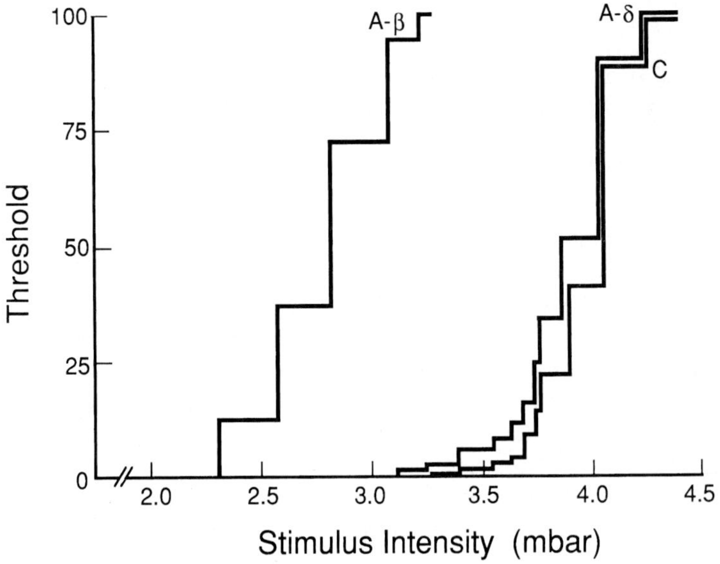

FIG. 2-1
Differences in thresholds to mechanical stimulation of mechanoreceptors supplied by Aβ, Aδ, and C fibers. (From Georgepoulos AP: *Journal of Neurophysiology* 39:71-83, 1976.)

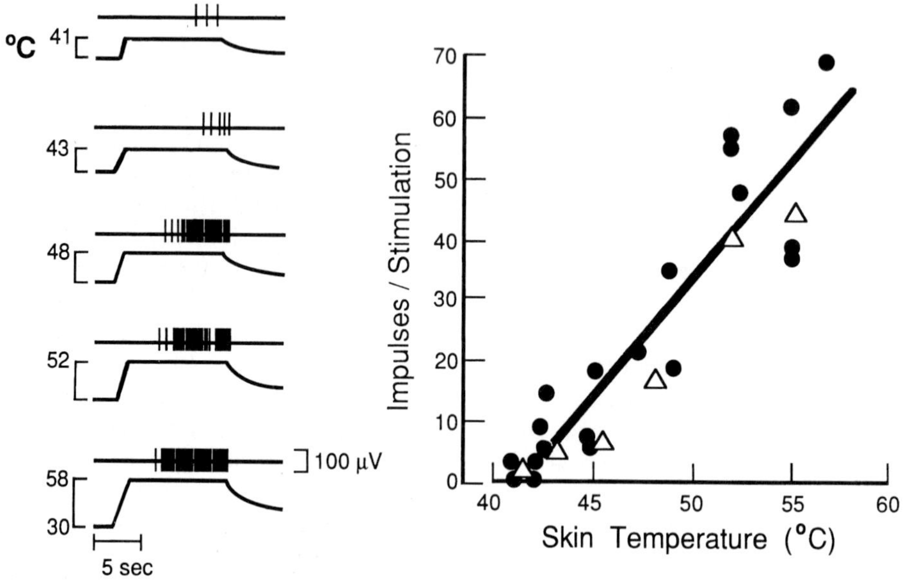

FIG. 2-2
A, Neurophysiologic recordings of responses by a C fiber supplying the skin of a cat to five different applied heating step stimuli. For each heating step, the skin is first adapted to 30° C and then the temperature is raised to 41°, 43°, 48°, 52°, or 58° C. For each heating step the neural discharge is the top trace and the heating step stimulus the bottom trace. Note that the stimulus steps vary in magnitude and the biggest step initiates the most action potentials. Note that the stimulus steps vary in magnitude and the biggest heating step results in the shortest response latency. **B**, Linear relationship between skin temperature and the number of action potentials initiated by the applied temperature. Symbols:• represents the total number of impulses per stimulus; Δ, the number of impulses in the last 4 seconds of stimulation. (From Beck PW, Handwerker HO, Zimmerman M: *Brain Research* 67:373-386, 1974.)

frequency that is maintained until the stimulus is removed (Fig. 2-2,A). Increasing the stimulus temperature decreases the response latency and increases the overall response frequency (Fig. 2-2, B). Many C polymodal nociceptors respond to cold stimuli as well. The response of C polymodal nociceptors to chemical stimuli is less studied. Locally applied bradykinin, histamine, acetylcholine, acids, and potassium salts have all been shown to activate C polymodal nociceptors. These nociceptors constitute 40% to 90% of the afferent unmyelinated cutaneous fibers.

In recent years the technique of microneurography (Box 2-1) has been used to study the response of C polymodal nociceptors with receptive fields on the human hand (Fig. 2-3, A). Human C polymodal nociceptors respond to heating of their receptive field with an increasing number of action potentials (Fig. 2-3, A and B). Subjective pain sensation is correlated with neural discharge frequency, providing direct confirmation that intensity of a stimulus is encoded by increasing frequency of neural discharges in peripheral sensory fibers. (Fig. 2-3, C). However, a certain

BOX 2-1

Microneurography

In this technique, pioneered by Hagbarth and Vallbo in 1968,[1,2] a sharpened tungsten needle, insulated except for a small area at the tip, is advanced through the skin under local surface anesthesia into a peripheral nerve. This procedure makes it possible to record the impulse activity of single afferent nerve fibers in human peripheral nerves, and, because no general anesthesia is used, to compare directly subjective sensations with primary afferent discharge patterns. The initial recordings were from single myelinated fibers, but, as experience was gained with the technique, recordings were obtained from single unmyelinated nerve fibers also. The recordings are similar to records obtained in animals by dissection of single axons. More recently, peripheral nerve fibers have been stimulated through the recording electrode, and activation of a single nerve fiber can create a sensation that corresponds to the receptive field properties of the fiber.

1. Hagbarth KE, Vallbo AB: *Experimental Neurology* 22:674-694, 1968.

2. Vallbo AB, Hagbarth KE: *Experimental Neurology* 21:270-289, 1968.

level of neural activity can be evoked in C polymodal nociceptors without any apparent sensation of pain. Furthermore, even if a level of activity induced by noxious heat stimulation is always accompanied by pain, the same level of activity produced by mechanical stimulation in the same fibers can produce a nonpainful sensation. Therefore, the relationship between sensation and neural discharge patterns is not a simple one; it demonstrates the importance of central nervous system processing in pain sensation.

A further important characteristic of nociceptors is the property of sensitization. Prior stimulation of both Aδ and C polymodal nociceptors changes their response characteristics. For example, response thresholds can be lowered, response latency can be reduced, and the fibers can become spontaneously active. This phenomenon is

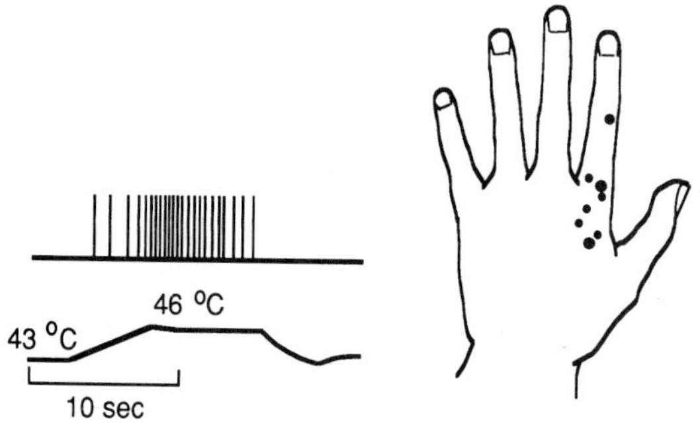

FIG. 2-3, A
Neurophysiologic recording from human C polymodal nociceptors with afferent fibers in the radial nerve to heat stimulation to the skin. **A**, Response of a C polymodal nociceptor to a heat stimulus of 46° C and the receptive fields of eight C polymodal nociceptors. Each dot represents the receptive field of a single C polymodal nociceptor. (From Gybels J, Handwerker HO. Van Hees J: *Journal of Physiology [Lond]* 292:193-206, 1979.)

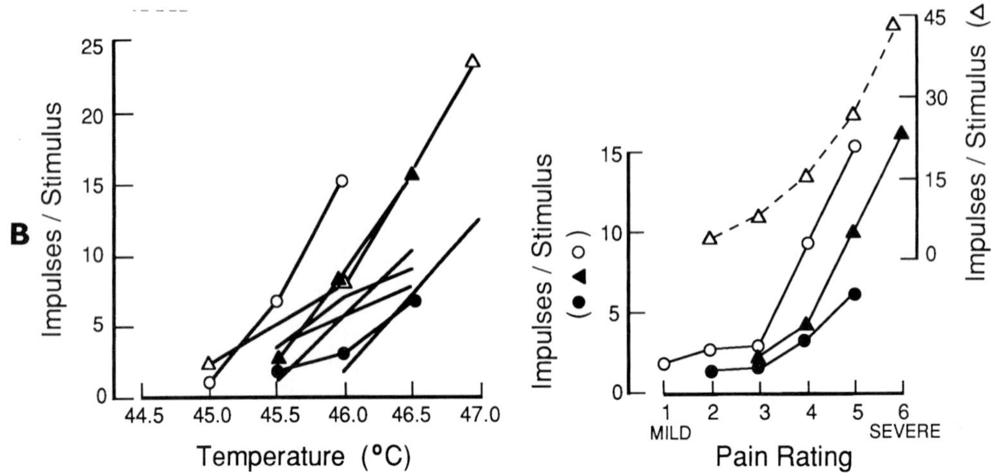

FIG. 2-3–CONT'D
Neurophysiologic recordings from human C polymodal nociceptors. **B**, Relationship between skin temperature and the number of action potentials initiated when the heat stimulus is applied to the receptive fields of the eight C polymodal nociceptors indicated in **A. C**, Relationship between number of action potentials initiated by temperature applied to four human C polymodal nociceptors and the verbal rating of the heat stimulus reported by the subjects. (From Gybels J, Handwerker HO, Van Hees J: *Journal of Physiology [Lond]* 292:193-206, 1979.)

thought to be responsible for hyperalgesia or the heightened sensitivity to pain that occurs in damaged tissue. Therefore, stimuli that were once innocuous may begin to excite nociceptors after tissue injury, and the receptive field of the nociceptor increases in size. Sensitization is a unique quality of nociceptors.

Other Cutaneous Nociceptors

Several other types of nociceptors have been described in addition to Aδ mechanical and C polymodal nociceptors. For example, some Aδ nociceptors appear to respond to noxious heat, but these could be Aδ mechanical nociceptors that have been sensitized. There are also nociceptors with unmyelinated afferent fibers that respond to mechanical noxious stimuli but not to noxious heat or to chemical stimuli. Therefore, there are C fiber mechanical nociceptors. Some receptors seem specifically responsive to extremely cold stimuli. These high-threshold cold nociceptors may have Aδ or C afferent fibers and are usually insensitive to mechanical stimulation (Fig. 2-4).

Structure of Cutaneous Nociceptors

Since the early studies on skin sensation it has been assumed that nociceptors are free nerve endings. This conclusion has been the subject of much debate, because it is difficult to correlate the structure and function of nociceptors. However, because pain can be elicited from areas of the skin devoid of all receptors

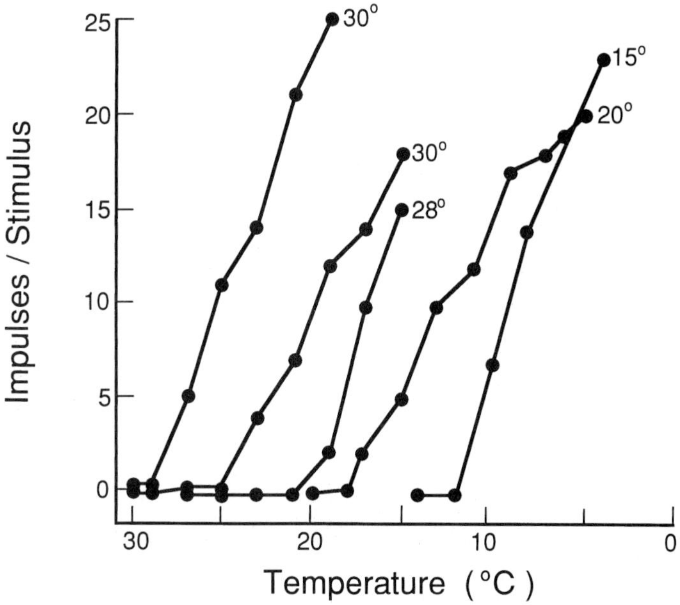

FIG. 2-4
Relationship between skin temperature and the number of action potentials initiated by the applied temperature for five high-threshold cold receptors. In this experiment the receptive field of the receptor was adapted to the temperature indicated at the top of each curve and then cooled to a lower stimulus temperature. For each cooling step the receptor initiated a number of action potentials. The receptive field was then returned to the adapting temperature and another cooling stimulus was applied. The points on each curve represent the number of impulses resulting from each cooling step. (From LaMotte RH, Thalhammer JG: *Brain Research* 244:279-287, 1982.)

except free nerve endings, it is generally agreed that some free nerve endings are in fact nociceptors. This conclusion is supported by anatomic studies in which the terminations of unmyelinated fibers are traced in serial sections and found to end in typical free nerve endings.

The structure of Aδ mechanical nociceptors has been studied with a combination of structural analysis and functional identification. First an Aδ fiber is isolated and the receptive field properties are determined. Once fully characterized, the receptive field area is removed and histologically examined, revealing the structure of the receptor (Fig. 2-5). The axon of the Aδ fiber loses its myelin sheath but remains ensheathed by the Schwann cell and the basal lamina. The Schwann cell–neurite complex branches beneath the basement layer of the epidermis and then terminates between or invaginates into cells of the basal layer. There are many similarities between the structure of this receptor and of cutaneous cold receptors (see Chapter 8), suggesting that response properties are determined not by the gross anatomic structure of the receptor but by biophysical specializations of the receptor endings.

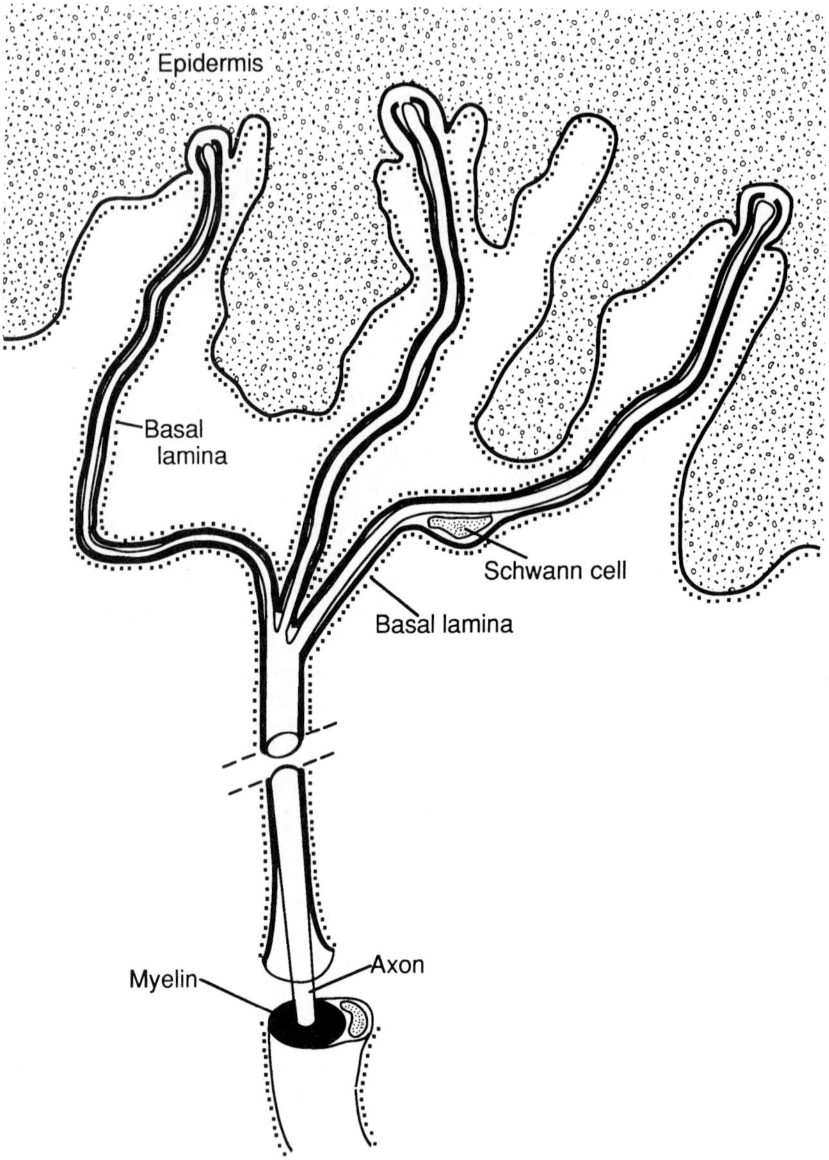

FIG. 2-5
Termination of an Aδ mechanical nociceptor. A single myelinated fiber (at bottom of diagram) branches, losing its myelin sheath to become covered by a Schwann cell and the basal lamina. The basal lamina surrounding the axon fuses with the basal lamina of the epidermis as the nerve endings penetrate the basal layer. The epidermal nerve terminal remains extensively or completely covered by extensions of the Schwann cell. (From Perle ER: Characterization of nociceptors and their activation of neurons in the superficial dorsal horn: first steps for the sensation of pain. In Kruger L, Liebeskind JC: *Advances in Pain Research and Therapy*, New York, 1984, pp 23-51, Raven Press.)

Trigeminal Nociceptors

With the notable exception of the dental pulp (see Chapter 3), nociceptive afferent fibers traveling in the trigeminal nerve are similar to cutaneous nociceptors. Both Aδ mechanical nociceptors and C polymodal nociceptors have been identified with receptive fields on the face. Trigeminal nociceptors have functional properties similar to those of cutaneous nociceptors.

Other Nociceptors

Afferent fibers are found in the innervation of muscles that are activated by intense mechanical stimulation, intramuscular injection of hypertonic saline, and thermal stimulation. On the basis of the response properties and fiber diameter, these muscle nociceptors resemble cutaneous polymodal nociceptors.

Small-diameter fibers have been found in the innervation of joints that respond to potentially painful and extreme joint rotation. Other small-diameter joint afferent fibers respond to infusion of bradykinin into the joint capsule and are sensitized by induced joint inflammation.

Although it cannot be confirmed that activation of these afferent fibers would produce a painful sensation, muscle and joint pain are familiar painful conditions. This is especially pertinent to dentistry because temporomandibular joint pain is a poorly understood and difficult condition to treat, and its sufferers are often referred to dentists.

Receptor Mechanisms

The difficulty in isolating a nociceptor has prevented direct analysis of the membrane properties of the receptors. Therefore, the process of transduction in nociceptors is not known, but because of the short response latency it is assumed that nociceptive stimuli directly activate the receptors. However, because it has been known for some time that certain chemicals such as histamine and bradykinin can activate nociceptors it has been hypothesized that these and other chemicals are released by tissue damage and stimulate the nociceptive endings. Moreover, chemicals applied to nociceptors can potentiate their responses to nociceptive stimuli. These and other observations suggest the role of chemicals in nociceptor activation, but more direct biophysical analysis of nociceptive endings is necessary to determine if nociceptors are directly activated by noxious stimuli, by way of chemicals released during tissue damage, or by both mechanisms.

CENTRAL TERMINATIONS OF NOCICEPTIVE AFFERENT FIBERS

Dorsal Horn of the Spinal Cord

Afferent fibers with cell bodies in the dorsal root ganglia enter the spinal cord by way of the dorsal roots. As nociceptive fibers approach the spinal cord, they become

BOX 2-2

Neural Tracing and Neuron Labeling

In the last 20 years investigators of central nervous system pathways have used an ever-increasing number of techniques to trace pathways and label individual neurons. Various compounds are injected into peripheral sites, placed on cut nerves, injected into the brain, or included in the microelectrode filling solution used for intracellular recordings. After a period of time to allow axoplasmic transport of the compound from the site of application, the brain is prepared for histology, and the labeled pathway and its terminations are visualized. Until recently neural tracing was accomplished in living animals, but it is now possible to trace pathways in fixed tissue which opens up this technique to study human central pathways. The method of transport is not always clear, but it is usually assumed that the tracer is incorporated into components of the neuron's axoplasmic transport system. Some of the past and current techniques used to trace neural pathways include:

- The oldest technique was to section peripheral nerve trunks, tracts, or nuclei, and examine the brain at a later time for signs of degeneration. Much of the basic understanding of central nervous system pathways is based on this methodology.
- The use of radioactive amino acids as tracers was an important step in the development of neural tracing. The amino acids were incorporated into the neuroplasm, which was then transported. The pathways could then be visualized with autoradiographic techniques in which the incorporated radioactive amino acids exposed a photographic emulsion placed on top of the tissue section. Although this technique was once widely used, it has problems associated with the use of radioactive materials and a relatively long time period required for the tissue radioactivity to expose the photographic emulsion
- The discovery that the plant enzyme horseradish peroxidase was transported by neural tissue was a major advance in neural tracing methods. The transported enzyme is revealed by a relatively simple histochemical technique and many neuroanatomical investigations used this methodology, providing important new insights into brain circuitry.
- Many fluorescent dyes are transported by nervous tissue. Since no histochemical methods are necessary to visualize the fluorescent label, the technique is simpler than horseradish peroxidase histochemistry. However, the fluorescence tends to fade, counterstaining is not possible, and it is not easy to make permanent specimens for later analysis. The labeled pathway is usually photographed. There are major advantages to the use of fluorescent tracing in that double labeling can be used with dyes having different fluorescent colors, and recently it has been discovered that fluorescent dyes will transport in fixed tissue.

BOX 2-2—CONT'D

- Most neural tracers do not cross synaptic junctions so that additional injections must be made to study chains of interconnected neurons. To overcome this problem live neurotropic viruses are being used as neural tracers. The viruses are replicated in the recipient neurons after transneuronal transfer. This replication produces a strong transneuronal labeling providing a powerful tool for demonstrating neuronal connections across synapses and thereby permitting the analysis of complete neural pathways.

Neural tracing techniques with fluorescent dyes have been used to label neuron populations, which can then be visualized and injected intracellularly with another fluorescent marker or other label to fill a neuron entirely. This technique can be combined with brain slice technology to fill electrophysiologically characterized neurons of a defined cell population and provide structure function correlations. The labeled neurons are subsequently reconstructed by use of a microscope equipped with drawing tube, or by the use of a computer three-dimensional reconstruction system. Examples of the use of this technique are shown in several chapters of this book.

segregated within the dorsal root, occupying the lateral part of the root. After they enter the spinal cord, the afferent fibers split into ascending and descending branches, both of which run in Lissauer's tract for a short distance before terminating in the dorsal horn of the spinal cord.

Based on cytoarchitectonic features the dorsal horn has been divided into 10 laminae. With a number of neural tracing techniques (Box 2-2), small-diameter afferent fibers have been demonstrated to terminate in the superficial laminae, particularly lamina I and the substantia gelatinosa or lamina II. Recently, intraaxonal recordings have been made from afferent fibers in the dorsal horn. This has allowed electrophysiologic characterization of the response properties and receptive field properties of single nociceptive afferent fibers. After functional characterization, horseradish peroxidase was used to fill the neuron by an intraaxonal injection through the recording electrode so that the precise morphology and termination of the nociceptive afferent fiber were revealed. This technique has helped show that Aδ mechanical nociceptors and C fiber nociceptors terminate mainly in lamina I and in the outer part of lamina II. Afferent fibers innervating nonnociceptive receptors terminate predominantly in laminae III to V, with extensions into II and VI, but the precise shape of the terminal arbors is related to the receptor type that is innervated by the fiber (Fig. 2-6).

Medullary Dorsal Horn

The most caudal extent of the trigeminal spinal nucleus is laminated like the dorsal horn of the spinal cord, and is in fact continuous with the most rostral extent

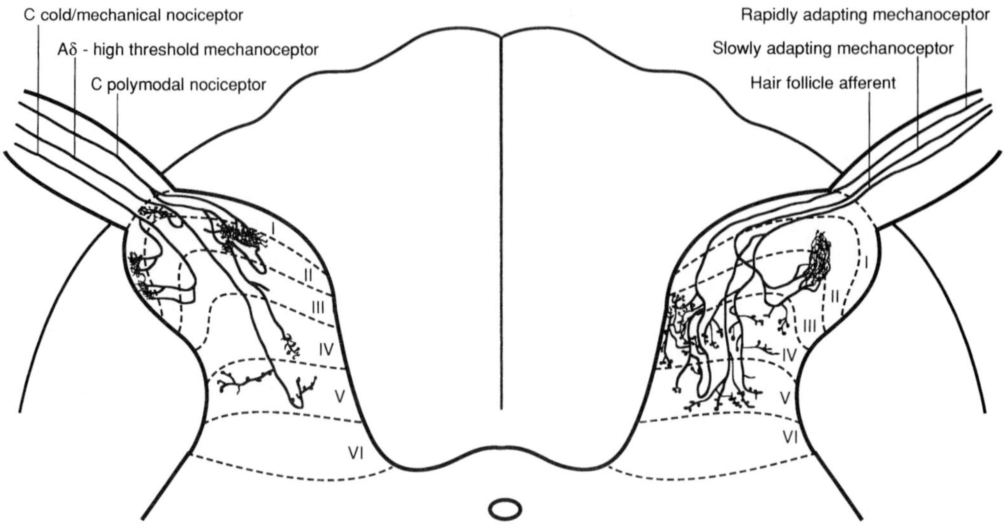

FIG. 2-6
Termination of afferent fibers in dorsal horn laminae of the spinal cord. *Left,* termination of nociceptive fibers. *Right,* Nonnociceptive fibers. Note that nociceptive fibers terminate in the superficial laminae and nonnociceptive fibers in the deeper laminae.

of the dorsal horn. Moreover, there is now considerable evidence of major functional similarities between the spinal dorsal horn and the caudal end of the trigeminal sensory nucleus. Trigeminal nociceptive fibers with cell bodies in the trigeminal ganglion enter the lateral border of the medulla and descend in the trigeminal tract to terminate heavily in the caudal extent of the trigeminal spinal nucleus. The pattern of termination of the Aδ and C nociceptive fibers appears similar to the terminations already described in the spinal cord. Because of the close structural and functional relationships between the spinal and trigeminal regions, the term medullary dorsal horn has superseded subnucleus caudalis for the caudal end of the trigeminal sensory nucleus.

Putative Neurotransmitters Released from Nociceptive Afferent Fibers

Numerous studies have implicated substance P, an 11-amino acid peptide, as a neurotransmitter associated with nociceptive transmission in the spinal and medullary dorsal horns. Evidence shows that substance P is present in regions known to be sites of transmission of nociceptive information. Immunocytochemical techniques, using an antibody to substance P, have shown a dense concentration of substance P containing fibers in the marginal layer (lamina I) of the spinal cord. Moreover, substance P is released from central terminals when afferent fibers are stimulated. When the dorsal roots are cut, resulting in degeneration of fibers entering the spinal cord, the amount of substance P in the dorsal horn is reduced.

Strong evidence implicating substance P in nociceptive transmission comes from studies using capsaicin. Capsaicin is the irritant compound contained in the fruit of a species of the capsium plant (for example, red peppers and chili peppers). When administered by subcutaneous injection to neonatal rats, capsaicin rapidly produces life-long insensitivity to noxious stimulations because it causes degeneration of nociceptive C fibers. Application of capsaicin in adult animals initially results in a violent irritation followed by a loss of sensitivity to noxious stimulation, but without loss of nociceptive fibers. However, there is a 50% reduction in substance P in the dorsal horn of the spinal cord. This suggests that insensitivity to noxious stimulation is caused by a depletion of neurotransmitter.

Substance P is not the only neurotransmitter found in small diameter–dorsal root afferent fibers. Somatostatin, cholecystokinin, and vasoactive intestinal peptide are also present and are depleted after capsaicin treatment. Although substance P is strongly implicated as the putative neurotransmitter in nociceptive terminals in the dorsal horn, other neuropeptides are involved as well.

NOCICEPTIVE NEURONS IN THE SPINAL AND MEDULLARY DORSAL HORNS

The medullary and spinal dorsal horns contain relay and local-circuit neurons excited by peripheral sensory stimulation. There are two major types of these neurons responding to noxious stimulation: nociceptive-specific neurons that respond exclusively to noxious stimulation of the skin, and wide-dynamic-range neurons that respond to both noxious and nonnoxious stimulation of broadly separated parts of the body. Intracellular recordings have been made from both types of neurons with subsequent filling of the neuron with a marker. Differences in response characteristics between the two neuron types are not reflected in morphology. The most consistent correlation between functional features and structural characteristics is that of the region of dendritic arborization with terminations of nociceptive afferent fibers. In general, morphologic types of neurons do not correlate with response properties.

Nociceptive-specific Neurons

These dorsal horn neurons are exclusively activated by nociceptive cutaneous mechanical or thermal stimulation and are found in lamina I. Two general types of nociceptive-specific neurons have been described: one responding to nociceptive mechanical stimulation and the other to intense thermal and mechanical stimulation. Presumably Aδ mechanical and C polymodal nociceptors synapse with these second-order neurons either directly or polysynaptically. The receptive fields of these neurons is small (one to several square centimeters), indicating that these neurons receive convergent input from several primary afferent nociceptive fibers with similar receptive field locations.

Wide-dynamic-range Neurons

Wide-dynamic-range neurons are so named because they respond to stimulus intensities in both the nonnoxious and noxious ranges, although other terms such as polymodal, multimodal, and multireceptive neurons have also been used. Therefore, as the intensity of the cutaneous stimulus is increased from light touch to noxious pinch, these neurons respond with increasing frequency of discharge. They also respond to nonnoxious and noxious thermal stimulation as well. Many wide-dynamic-range neurons, besides being excited by cutaneous stimulation, can be activated by visceral stimulation from the heart, gallbladder, testicles, and muscles, indicating widespread convergence of input to these neurons. Neurons receiving input from both cutaneous and visceral receptive fields may mediate the clinically important phenomenon of referred pain. Wide-dynamic-range neurons are found in laminae IV to VI, but are most frequently encountered in lamina V.

Cutaneous-receptive fields of wide-dynamic-range neurons vary in area from a single digit to a major portion of the leg and are frequently much larger than receptive fields of primary afferent fibers. The organization of the receptive fields of these neurons is often complex, consisting of a central excitatory zone surrounded by an inhibitory zone. The excitatory zone consists of a central area responding to nonnoxious and noxious, mechanical and thermal stimuli surrounded by less sensitive zones that respond only to noxious stimulation.

As would be predicted from the response properties of wide-dynamic-range neurons, the neurons receive input from both Aδ and C fibers and larger-diameter Aβ afferent fibers. Neurons receiving convergent input from large and small fibers are a critical component of the gate control hypothesis of pain (Box 2-3) in which they fulfill the role of the transmission, or T, cells.

Response Processing by Second-order Nociceptive Neurons

There is now evidence indicating that second-order nociceptive neurons are capable of considerable sensory processing. Moreover, with continued stimulation the response properties of these neurons change as demonstrated by alterations in excitability and receptive field properties. The mechanisms underlying these changes are not fully understood but involve increases in synaptic efficacy and modification of membrane excitability..

The substantia gelatinosa or lamina II of the dorsal horn contains mainly interneurons that project myelinated axons locally to other laminae. A number of different morphologic cell types have been described in lamina II, but the most common are the stalked cell and the islet cell. The soma of the stalked cell is situated at the

BOX 2-3
Pain Theories

Johannes Müller in 1842 published a treatise known as the Doctrine of Specific Nerve Energies, which stated that, "the nerve of each sense seems to be capable of one kind of sensation only, and not those belonging to the other sense organs; thus one sensory nerve cannot take the place and perform the function of the nerve of another sense." His statement led to the conclusion that each sensory system has its own receptors, sensory fibers, sensory pathways, and processing center in the central nervous system. However, for most of recorded history, pain was not recognized as one of the classic senses. When Blix[1] established that there were sensory spots on the skin sensitive to pressure, cold, and warmth, he could not identify spots responding to painful stimuli. His observations were taken one step further by the histologist Max von Frey[2], who suggested four specific skin modalities, including a specific pain modality, each with a specific sensory end organ. Subsequently, the notion of a specific end organ connected by a specific sensory pathway became known as the specificity theory of pain. Until recently, investigators could not identify specific nociceptors and pathways in the central nervous system. Much research in the last 25 years, however, has confirmed not only specific nociceptors in the skin and other body areas, but also specific pain pathways in relaying and integrating nociceptive information. Although these central nervous system relays process nociceptive information they also receive input from other sensory systems.

Twenty-five years ago, when the specificity theory had little neurobiologic basis and because of its inability to account for some clinical observations, Melzack and Wall[3] proposed an alternative theory know as the "gate control hypothesis." They suggested:

- The transmission of nerve impulses from afferent fibers to the spinal cord transmission cells (T) is modulated by a spinal gating mechanism (SG) in the dorsal horns.
- The spinal gating mechanism is influenced by the relative amount of activity in large-diameter (L) and small-diameter (S) fibers: activity in large fibers tends to inhibit transmission (close the gate), whereas activity in small fibers tends to facilitate transmission (open the gate).
- The spinal gating mechanism is also influenced by nerve impulses that descend from the brain.
- When the output of the spinal cord transmission cells exceeds a critical level, it activates the action system—those neural areas that underlie the complex, sequential patterns of behavior and experience that are characteristic of pain.

BOX 2-3–CONT'D

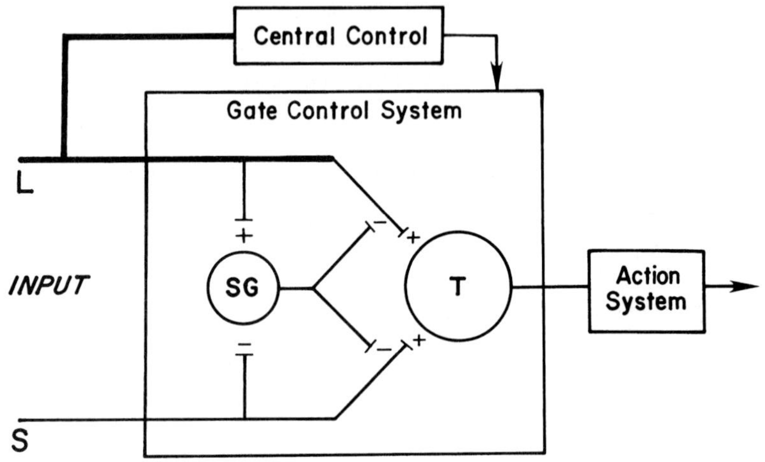

The gate control hypothesis of pain. Large-diameter fibers (*L*) excite spinal gating neurons transmitting (*T*) impulses to higher centers (*action system*). *S*, Small diameter fibers. Note opposite action of large and small fibers on the activity of the interneuron (*SG*), which presynaptically inhibits synaptic transmission by the T cell. Symbols: + represents excitation; −, inhibition. An ascending system that bypasses the gate control system can influence the activity of the spinal gate through a central control and a descending pain pathway. (From Melzak R, Wall PD: *Science* 150:971-979, 1965.)

At the time this hypothesis was proposed much regarding the underlying mechanisms was highly speculative. The hypothesis opened up a new era of pain research and most of the fundamental mechanisms proposed in the hypothesis have been shown to have a firm physiologic basis. This is especially true for the proposed descending pain control system, the sophistication of which could hardly have been imagined when the "gate control hypothesis" was first published.

Because of the advances made in understanding pain mechanisms, both the specificity theory and gate control hypothesis have been modified to incorporate new findings. The concept of interaction between sensory systems and modulation of nociceptive transmission by interneurons has been incorporated into both theories so that there is now less divergence between the two theories.

1. Blix M: *Zeitschrift fur Biologie* 20:141-156, 1884.

2. von Frey M: Beriechte uber die Verhandlung der Koniglichen Sachsischen Gesellschaft der Wissenschaften zu Leipzig, *Mathematisch-Physische Klasse* 47:166-184, 1895.

3. Melzack R, Wall PD: *Science* 150:971-979, 1965.

border between laminae I and II with an asymmetric dendritic tree oriented ventrally into lamina II and sometimes into laminae II to IV (Fig. 2-7). The unmyelinated axon of the stalked cell arborizes extensively with many synaptic boutons in lamina I. Islet cell soma are distributed throughout lamina II with dendrites oriented rostrocaudally, parallel to the laminar borders.

The substantia gelatinosa actually consists of two sublaminae called lamina IIa and lamina IIb. Substantia gelatinosa neurons situated in lamina IIa respond to input from nociceptive primary afferent fibers, while neurons in IIb respond primarily to nonnociceptive input. Other differences in descending termination and content of neuropeptides indicate that the two subdivisions of the substantia gelatinosa are both functionally and structurally different.

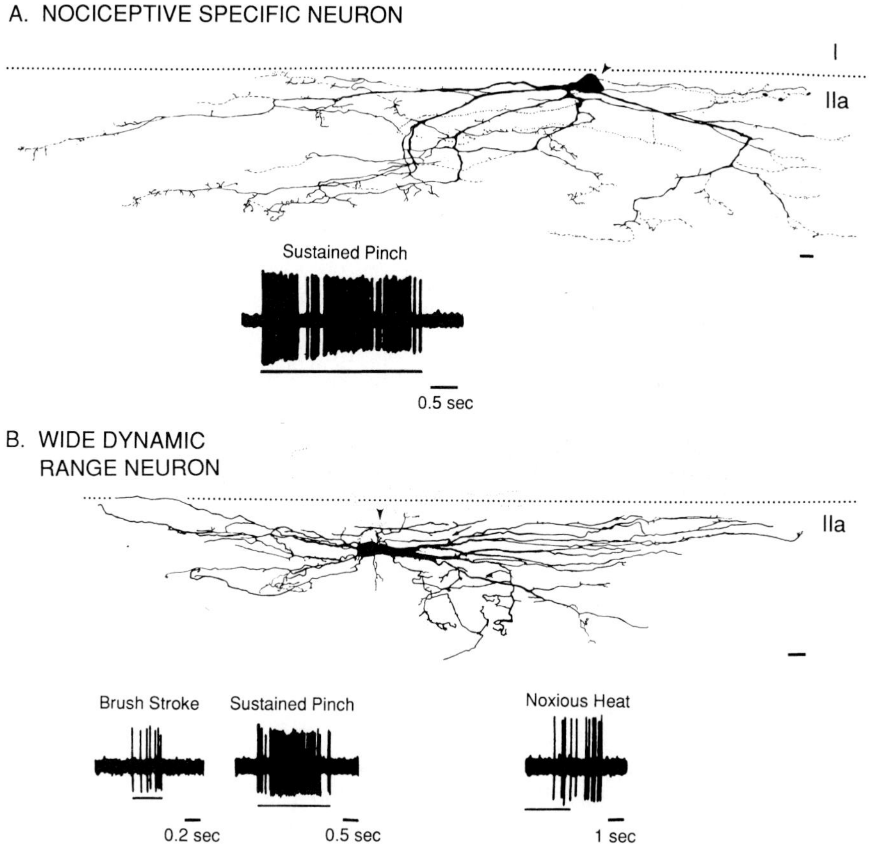

FIG. 2-7
Functionally characterized substantia gelatinosa cells intracellularly injected with horseradish peroxidase. **A**, Nociceptive specific stalked cell. **B**, Wide dynamic range islet cell. Below the drawing of each reconstructed neuron is an electrophysiologic recording of its response to stimulation of its receptive field. (From Bennett GJ, Abdelmoumene M, Hayashi H, Dubner R: *Journal of Comparative Neurology* 194:809-827, 1908. Reprinted by permission of Wiley-Liss, a division of John Wiley & Sons, Inc.)

Based on structure-function studies of substantia gelatinosa neurons, it is apparent that lamina IIa–stalked cells and islet cells have response properties of either nociceptive-specific or wide-dynamic-range neurons. The islet cells in lamina IIb responded principally to nonnoxious stimuli. Although there are similarities between the responses of the substantia gelatinosa neurons and those recorded in other laminae, there are some significant dissimilarities. Many substantia gelatinosa neurons show habituation to repeated stimulation whereas others that are spontaneously active are inhibited by peripheral stimulation. However, the key to the functional role of substantia gelatinosa neurons lies in the connections made by their dendritic trees.

Although there are interneurons throughout the dorsal horn, the interneurons of the substantia gelatinosa are the only ones that have been studied extensively. Interneurons are important in the mechanisms of the gate control hypothesis, and it is tempting to suggest that the interneurons of the substantia gelatinosa are involved in the synaptic gating mechanism proposed in the hypothesis. Indeed, some substantia gelatinosa neurons are inhibited by cutaneous stimulation, but many others are not. In addition, neurons in the substantia gelatinosa have responses similar to spinal gating transmission cells (T cells). Although the existence of certain response properties of neurons in the substantia gelatinosa might suggest a role in a spinal gating mechanism, that is not the sole function of substantia gelatinosa neurons.

ASCENDING NOCICEPTIVE TRACTS

Experimental evidence and clinical observations show that axons of dorsal horn nociceptive neurons cross the spinal cord and ascend in the ventrolateral (sometimes called anterolateral) quadrant. The role of this ascending tract in pain perception is demonstrated by the profound analgesia that results from transection of the tract. The analgesia is limited to the body area innervated caudal to the transection and is unilateral. These contralateral ascending systems have been classically designated as the major ascending pain pathway and are often sectioned (ventrolateral cordotomy) to reduce chronic pain. However, the ventrolateral quadrant contains several descending and ascending fiber tracts including the spinothalamic tract, spinoreticular tract, and spinotectal tract. Moreover, ventrolateral cordotomy is not always effective in blocking pain transmission. In a large percentage of individuals, pain sensitivity returns and so it is very likely that nociceptive information reaches higher brain center by other ascending tracts.

The spinothalamic tract has long been considered the major ascending tract conveying nociceptive information. The cells of origin of the tract are scattered over the entire gray matter of the spinal cord but are especially concentrated in laminae I and V. The cells of origin of the spinothalamic tract that terminates in the medial thalamus are situated in the deeper laminae, whereas those that project to the ventrobasal and posterior thalamus are located in the more superficial laminae (Fig. 2-8).

Neurons that project in the spinothalamic tract respond to different types of peripheral stimulation. The major proportions are nociceptive-specific and wide-dy-

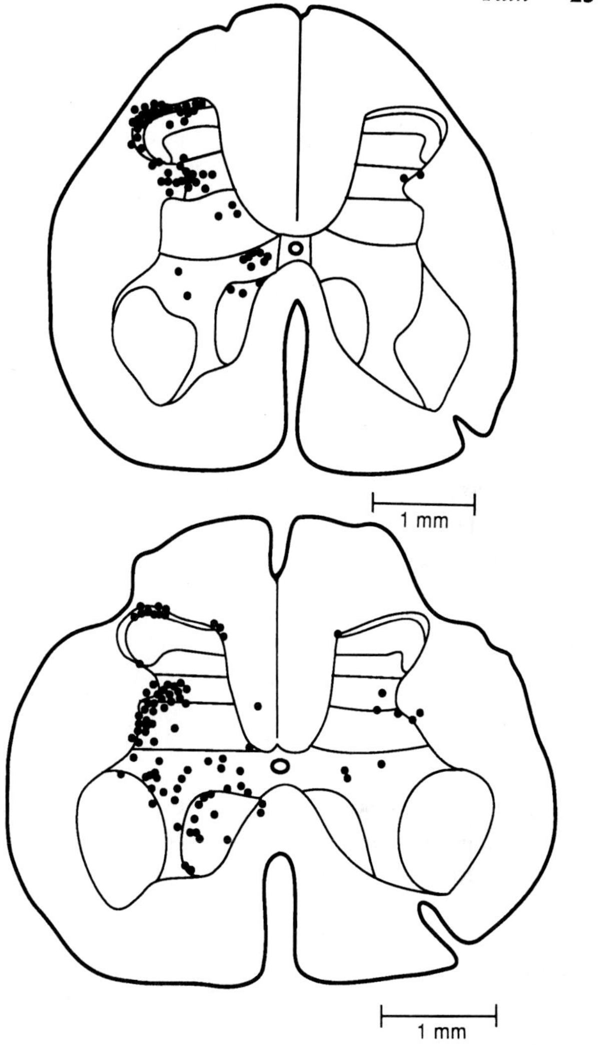

FIG. 2-8
Cross sections of the lumbosacral region of the spinal cord showing the location of the spinothalamic tract neurons (*dots*) that send their axons to **A**, the lateral and **B**, the medial thalamus. (From Willis WD, Kenshalo DR Jr, Leonard RB: *Journal of Comparative Neurology* 188:543-578, 1979. Reprinted by permission of Wiley-Liss, a division of John Wiley & Sons, Inc.)

namic-range neurons, but some are activated by nonnoxious and visceral stimulation. Spinothalamic tract neurons, located in deeper laminae of the spinal cord that project to the medial thalamus, also have nociceptive-specific or wide-dynamic-range response properties but respond to stimulation of large areas of the body.

Until recently the spinothalamic tract was thought to be confined to the ventrolateral quadrant of the spinal cord, but a second spinothalamic tract has been described in the dorsolateral spinal cord. The cells of origin of the dorsolateral spinothalamic tract are located in the contralateral lamina I of the dorsal horn. Because the cells of origin of this tract in lamina I respond exclusively to noxious peripheral stimulation it is thought to have a major role in pain transmission.

The reticular formation of the brain stem is known to be involved in nociception, and it is therefore assumed that nociceptive information travels in the spino-reticular tract. The spinoreticular tract originates from neurons with cell bodies in laminae V to VIII and ascends in the ventrolateral quadrant of the spinal cord with fibers of the spinothalamic tract. Fibers of the spinoreticular tract terminate in several nuclei in the reticular formation, some of which have no nociceptive function. The spinoreticular tract, therefore, transmits nociceptive and nonnociceptive information, and it is thought that the reticular formation nociceptive projection participates in the motivational-affective component of the pain response.

The spinomesencephalic tract, which also ascends in the ventrolateral quadrant of the spinal cord, may play an important role in pain transmission. The cells of origin in laminae I and V of the dorsal horn are often nociceptive-specific. The tract terminates bilaterally in several regions of the dorsal midbrain. These regions, important in nociceptive processing, include the parabrachial nucleus, the periaqueductal gray, and the intercollicular nucleus. Recordings from neurons in the parabrachial projection area of the spinomesencephalic tract have demonstrated that many of these neurons respond exclusively to noxious stimuli. This suggests that the spinomesencephalic tract is a major nociceptive projection pathway originating in lamina I.

The cells of origin of the spinocervical tract lie in laminae III, IV, and V of the dorsal horn, and their axons ascend in the dorsolateral quadrant of the spinal cord to terminate in the lateral cervical nucleus. Response characteristics indicate the existence of several types of spinocervical neurons including some nociceptive-specific neurons, and therefore indicate a role for this tract in pain transmission. However, although the tract has been identified in some mammals, it is much reduced or absent in primates, which shows that it is not significant in human pain perception. It is important to realize that other species differences exist in the pain projection pathways, and caution must be taken in interpreting results obtained in animals to pain mechanisms in humans.

It is apparent that there are multiple ascending projections of nociceptive neurons in the spinal cord. Therefore, surgical transection of only part of the spinal cord to treat chronic pain might product unpredictable results. The multiple projection pathways may serve different functions, thereby providing a physiologic basis for the multifaceted nature of the pain experience.

NOCICEPTIVE MECHANISMS IN THALAMUS AND CORTEX

Spinal and trigeminal nociceptive neurons have axons that terminate in the thalamus. Both the ventroposterolateral nuclei and the posterior group of nuclei receive projections from all major ascending pathways involved in nociception: the dorsal column, the spinocervical, and both ventral and lateral spinothalamic projections. The medial intralaminar complex receives projections from the spinoreticular and spinothalamic pathways. Nociceptive axons arising in the trigeminal system cross to the opposite side of the brain and ascend in the ventral trigeminothalamic tract to the ventral posteromedial nucleus of the thalamus. Despite the fact that all these pathways contain axons of nociceptive neurons, relatively few recordings have been obtained from thalamic neurons responding to nociceptive stimulation, and none of the thalamic nuclei respond exclusively to nociceptive stimulation. When neurons are encountered that respond to noxious cutaneous stimulation, they are subdivided into nociceptive-specific and wide-dynamic-range response types. The receptive fields of these neurons are restricted in size and located contralateral to the recording site. One of the reasons for the paucity of recordings from nociceptive neurons in the thalamus is that activity of thalamic neurons is depressed by anesthetics.

The primary (SI) and secondary (SII) somatosensory areas of the cortex receive input from the thalmus. In SI cortex, scattered among neurons responding to non-noxious cutaneous stimulation are a number of nociceptive neurons. These nociceptive neurons are either nociceptive-specific or wide-dynamic-range neurons with contralateral receptive fields that are small or with very large receptive fields that often include the entire body surface. Neurons of the secondary somatosensory cortex (SII) are generally excited by tactile and nonnociceptive cutaneous stimulation, although some neurons with large bilateral receptive fields and responding to intense mechanical stimulation have been described.

OTHER PROJECTIONS IMPORTANT IN NOCICEPTION

Using neural tract tracing techniques, investigators have found connections between the parabrachial area involved in nociception and the amygdala. In addition, pathways connecting dorsal horn neurons to the lateral hypothalamus and septal nuclei have been defined. These projections to the areas of the brain, believed to participate in emotional behaviors such as rage and aggression, could be involved in the emotional and motivational characteristics of the pain response, whereas the thalamocortical projection is responsible for the sensory-discriminative aspects of pain.

ENDOGENOUS PAIN CONTROL

One major proposition of the "gate control hypothesis" of pain mechanisms is descending control of the spinal gate (Box 2-3). Beginning in the early 1970s, the underlying neurobiology of this descending system began to emerge. Investigators interested in the mode of action of opiates (substances with morphine-like activity) demonstrated specific binding of opiate agonists and antagonists to synaptic membranes. It soon became apparent that neurons possess sites that bind opiates with all the properties of synaptic receptors. Investigators realized that opiate receptors had not evolved to respond to morphine, and, therefore, the body produces neurotransmitters called endogenous opiates (endorphins) that bind to the opiate receptors. Furthermore, from studies in which electrical stimulation of the periaqueductal gray area of the brain resulted in profound analgesia, it became evident that descending pathways exist that could inhibit pain transmission. Finally, because these analgesic effects could be inhibited by pretreatment with Naloxone (a specific morphine antagonist), it was inferred that the analgesia produced by electrical stimulation was caused by the release of endogenous opiates that could be antagonized by Naloxone. Therefore, the descending pain control system involves neural pathways that originate in the periaqueductal gray area which is mediated by newly discovered neurotransmitters. Details of the descending system have since been clarified, and there is a great deal of information on endogenous opiates including their role in functions other than nociception.

Endorphins

Three major classes of endorphins have been discovered: leucine and methionine enkephalins, β-endorphins and dynorphins. Each class is derived from a different precursor molecule and each has a distinctive anatomical distribution.

The enkephalins, which are small peptides, were the first endorphins to be discovered. The amino acid sequences are H-Try-Gly-Gly-Phe-Met-OH (methionine enkephalin) and H-Try-Gly-Gly-Phe-Leu-OH (leucine enkephalin). The enkephalins are produced by cleavage of a large precursor molecule called proenkephalin into six copies of metenkephalin and one copy of leuenkephalin (Fig. 2-9 and Table 2-1). Two of the metenkephalin sequences are extended as octapeptides and heptapeptides. The basic amino acid sequence of the enkephalins is important for opioid activity because all the endorphins contain this sequence in their protein chains (Table 2-1).

The second class of endorphins that was discovered—β-endorphin—is cleaved, together with ACTH (adrenocorticotrophic hormone) and three copies of a melanocyte-stimulating hormone from a common precursor molecule, proopiomelanocortin (Fig. 2-9 and Table 2-1). The site of production of proopiomelanocortin is localized in cells of the basal hypothalamus. Axons of these cells course caudally along the wall of the third ventricle toward the periaqueductal gray and locus coeruleus.

The precursor molecule for dynorphins and prodynorphins is cleaved into dynorphin and two other peptides containing a leuenkephalin sequence, α/β-neoendorphin, dynorphin-A, and dynorphin-B (Fig. 2-9 and Table 2-1). The distribution of dynorphins and enkephalins in the central nervous system is similar. They are found in a large number of locations but differ in concentration. For example, the substantia nigra contains much more dynorphin than enkephalin, whereas relative concentrations are reversed in the interpeduncular nucleus. Even when dynorphins and enkephalins are found in the same location, the distribution can vary as in the periaqueductal gray, where dynorphin-containing neurons are located more ventrally. Spinal and medullary dorsal horn neurons contain both enkephalins and dynorphins. Neurons containing enkephalins are found in laminae I, II and V, while dynorphin-containing neurons are localized in lamina I. The medulla is particularly rich in

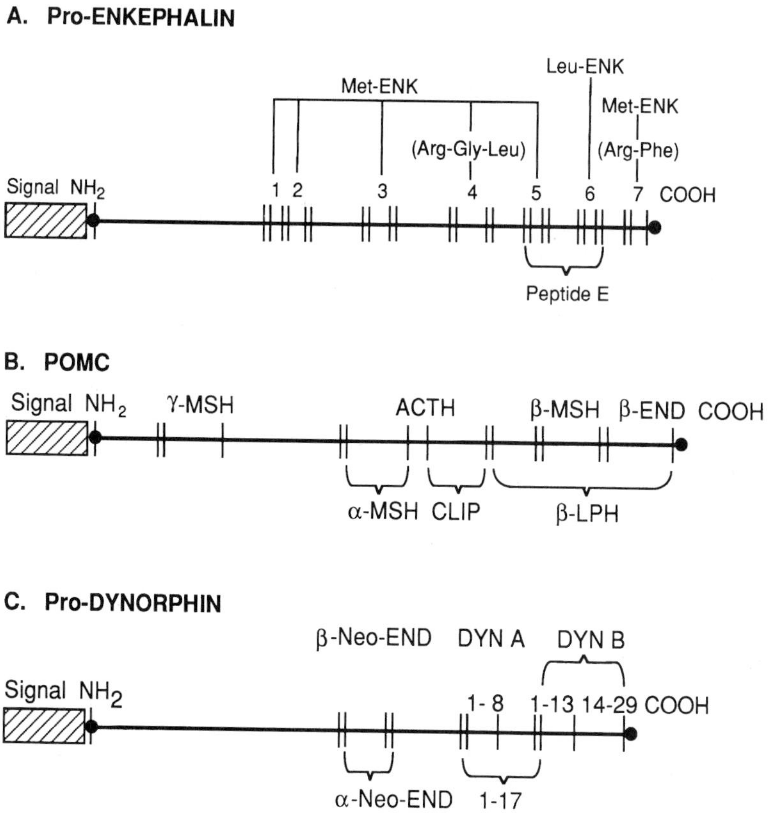

FIG. 2-9
The protein precursor structures of the three opioid peptide families. The double vertical lines represent dibasic amino acid cleavage site. From (Akil H and others: *Annual Review of Neuroscience* 7:223-255, 1984. Reprinted with permission from the *Annual Review of Neuroscience*, vol 7, © 1984 by Annual Reviews Inc.)

enkephalins and dynorphins, but, in general, there are more enkephalin- than dynorphin-containing neurons in the medulla.

One of the characteristics of the endorphins is their ability to bind strongly to opiate receptor sites in areas of the brain known to be involved in nociceptive transmission. Moreover, they have been shown to have profound analgesic effects when administered to experiment animals. This and other evidence strongly supports the role of the endorphins in pain mechanisms, but details are not yet clear. In addition, much recent research has focused on the role of the endorphins in other functions. Some of these functions such as stress and aggression, are related to pain, but other roles of the endorphins in eating, drinking, and cardiovascular control are less related to pain and illustrate the multiple biological functions of endorphins.

TABLE 2-1
Amino Acid Sequence of the Endogenous Opioids

Derived from Proenkephalin	
Leucine-enkephalin	Tyr-Gly-Gly-Phe-Leu
Methionine-enkephalin	Tyr-Gly-Gly-Phe-Met
Methionine-enkephalin-8	Tyr-Gly-Gly-Phe-Met-Arg-Gly-Leu
Methionine-enkephalin-Arg6-Phe7	Tyr-Gly-Gly-Phe-Met-Arg-Phe
Peptide E	Tyr-Gly-Gly-Phe-Met-Art-Arg-Val-Gly-Arg-Pro-Glu-Trp-Met-Asp-Tyr-Gln-Lys-Arg-Tyr-Gly-Gly-Phe-Leu
Derived from Proopiomelanocortin (POMC)	
β-Endorphin	*Tyr-Gly-Gly-Phe-Met*-Thr-Ser-Glu Lys-Ser-Gln-Thr-Pro-Leu-Val-Thr-Leu-Phe-Lys-Asn-Ala-Ile-Val-Lys Asn-Ala-His-Lys-Gly-Gln
Derived from Prodynorphin	
α-Neo-endorphin	*Tyr-Gly-Gly-Phe-Leu*-Arg-Lys-Tyr-Pro-Lys
β-Neo-endorphin	*Tyr-Gly-Gly-Phe-Leu*-Arg-Lys-Tyr-Pro
Dynorphin A-(1-8)	*Tyr-Gly-Gly-Phe-Leu*-Arg-Arg-Ile
Dynorphin A-(1-17)	*Tyr-Gly-Gly-Phe-Leu*-Arg-Arg-Ile-Arg-Pro-Lys-Leu-Lys-Tyr-Asp-Asn-Gln
Dynorphin B-(1-13)	*Tyr-Gly-Gly-Phe-Leu*-Arg-Arg-Gln-Phe-Lys-Val-Val-Thr

The amino acid sequence of leu and met enkephalin contained in larger peptides is italicized.

Opiate Receptors

The fact that more than one class of opiate receptor exists was suggested by experiments in which different classes of opiate drugs produced different behavioral effects. On the basis of these findings three opioid receptor types have been described—referred to as μ,δ, and κ. It is tempting to suggest that each receptor type is associated with one of the three types of endorphins, but no clear correlation emerges from comparisons between distributions of endorphins and opiate receptor types.

Opiate receptors are widely distributed throughout the brain with particularly dense binding in limbic structures, thalamic nuclei, and neural areas important in visceral functioning. The μ receptors are found in numerous locations including the neocortex, caudate-putamen, septum, thalamus, hippocampus, substantia nigra, inferior and superior colliculi, periaqueductal gray, locus coeruleus, and nucleus tractus solitarius. In contrast the distribution of δ receptors is more limited: they are found principally in forebrain structures such as neocortex, cudate-putamen, and amygdala. The widely distributed κ receptors are found in the preoptic area, hypothalamus, median eminence, caudate-putamen, amygdala, periaqueductal gray, and nucleus tractus solitarius. While there is some overlap in the distribution of the opiate receptor types, their exact distributions vary markedly. For example, all three receptor types are found in the caudate-putamen and nucleus accumbens, but the hippocampal area is particularly rich in μ receptors. More caudally in the mesencephalon and brain stem, μ and κ receptors predominate in regions such as the periaqueductal gray, superior and inferior colliculi, interpeduncular nucleus, raphe nuclei, locus coeruleus, parabrachial nuclei, nucleus tractus solitarius, and spinal trigeminal nucleus.

It is important to note, however, that marked species variation occurs in opiate receptor distribution in both relative concentrations and locations (Table 2-2). In general, the distribution of opiate receptor types is well conserved across species in brain stem and spinal cord areas and varies most in forebrain and midbrain structures.

All three opiate receptors have been shown to have a role in nociception, but the details of their differential involvement have not yet been elucidated. Supraspinal opioid analgesia is believed to be mediated by μ receptors, but δ receptors may be involved as well. In the spinal cord, μ, δ, and κ agonists have all been demonstratedto have analgesic actions. The κ agonists seem to block mechanical nociceptive responses, but μ and δ agonists mediate thermal nociceptive responses.

Descending Nociceptive Control System

The periaqueductal gray area plays a pivotal role in the descending pain control system. Electrical stimulation or injection of analgesic drugs into this area produces profound and lasting analgesia. Although it is usual in humans to stimulate more ros-

TABLE 2-2

Species differences in distribution of opiate receptors

Receptor	Brain Region	Rat	Monkey
μ	Central nucleus of amygdala	O	+++
	Caudate	++++	++
	Hypothalamus	+	++++
	Median eminence	O	+++
	Periventricular thalamus	O	++++
δ	Central nucleus of amygdala	O	++
	Hippocampus	+	++++
	Median eminence	O	+++
κ	Frontal cortex	+	+++
	Hippocampus	+	+++
	Caudate	+++	++
	Globus pallidus	+	++
	Medial mammillary nucleus	++	O
	Cerebellum	O	+++
	Median eminence	++++	+++

++++, very dense; +++, dense; ++, moderately dense; +, light; O, not detectable

tral brain areas for treatment of chronic pain syndromes, the analgesia is effected by connections to the periaqueductal gray. The fact that microinjections of opiates and electric stimulation inhibit firing of spinal and medullary dorsal horn nociceptive neurons indicates that opiate analgesia and stimulus-produced analgesia have common neural mechanisms. Moreover, the inhibition of the dorsal horn neurons is nociceptive-specific since the excitation of wide-dynamic-range neurons by nonnoxious stimuli is unaffected by periaqueductal gray area stimulation.

The periaqueductal gray area receives many inputs but those originating in hypothalamus, amygdala, and cortex are particularly relevant to analgesia. Descending tracts from the periaqueductal gray area connect to the rostral ventrolateral medulla, which includes the nucleus raphe magnus and adjacent reticular formation nuclei in the ventral medulla. All of these nuclei send axons to the spinal cord by way of the dorsolateral funiculus, and all produce analgesia when electrically stimulated (Fig. 2-10). Neurons in nucleus raphe magnus contain enkephalins, substance P, and other transmitters, each of which may play a different role in nociceptive transmission. This descending relay in the pain control system with connections to the medullary and spinal dorsal horns may therefore have different physiological roles, only one of which may be involved in nociception.

Within the rostral ventrolateral medulla, three classes of neurons alter their pattern of firing during noxious stimulation. One class, called "on-cells," shows a sudden increase in firing rate just before reflex responses to noxious stimulation. "Off-cells" are characterized by a sudden interruption in action potential generation just before reflex responses to noxious stimulation. The third class of neurons is unaffected by noxious stimulation and is called "neutral cells." Besides being involved in responses to noxious stimulation, on-cells and off-cells are excited by electrical stimulation of the periaqueductal gray area and are connected to the spinal cord and trigeminal sensory complex. Therefore, it is thought that these neurons in the rostral ventrolateral medulla are important in modulating nociceptive transmission.

The descending control or modulation of pain suggested in the "gate control hypothesis" now has a well defined neuroanatomic basis, using a discrete central nervous system pathway involving release of opioid peptides and other transmitters. Additional functions of this pathway indicate its relationship to other behaviors. If the behaviors controlled by this system can be defined, it will be possible to use it to alleviate pain and other nervous system disorders without the danger of addiction and other side effects of current therapies.

CLINICAL CONSIDERATIONS

Measuring Pain Responses in Humans

To determine the potency of a new analgesic drug or to diagnose objectively a patient in pain, methods of measuring a painful sensation are needed. The analgesic properties of a new drug are often tested by applying a painful stimulus to experi-

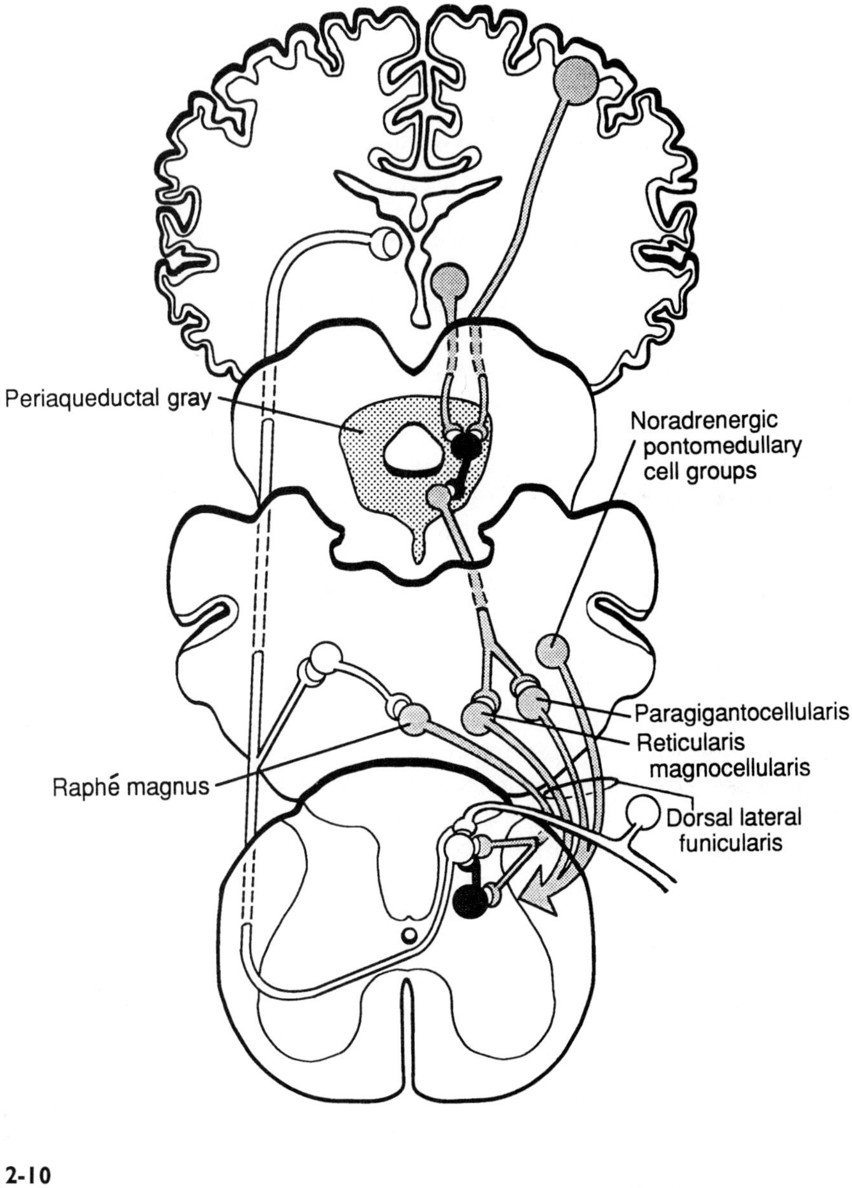

FIG. 2-10

Descending pain control pathways. The periaqueductal gray area receives input from higher centers and connects to the rostral ventrolateral medulla, which includes nucleus raphé magnus and adjacent reticular formation in the ventral medulla. All these nuclei send axons to the spinal cord through the dorsolateral funiculus. (from Fields HL, Basbaum AI: Endogenous pain control mechanisms. In Wall PD, Melzak R, editors: *Textbook of Pain*, New York, 1989, Churchill Livingstone, pp 206-217.)

mental subjects who are not in pain. This experimental measurement of pain sensation is quite different from clinical measurements made to aid in the diagnosis and treatment of individuals with pain. It is important, therefore, to understand the problems and techniques used to measure pain sensations and experiences so that objective evaluations of individuals with and without pain can be made.

Experimental Measurement of Pain Sensation

Although various types of stimuli, such as mechanical pressure, chemical, ischemia, cold, heat, and electric shock, have been used to initiate painful sensations in animals and humans, none of these stimuli is ideal. For example, electrical tooth pulp stimulation provides a controllable, repeatable sensation with minimal temporal effects, excites a relatively restricted group of primary afferent fibers, and exhibits a precise onset and offset. Therefore it is an ideal stimulus for many investigations. However, it is an inappropriate stimulus for studies that compare sensitivities between groups, since the range of intensities required to elicit pain sensation varies widely between individuals. Electrical tooth pulp stimulation also bypasses receptor mechanisms to produce a synchronous barrage of afferent activity and resultant unnatural sensation. Electrical stimulation of the skin produces unnatural sensations, but sensitivities are similar between individuals, permitting between-group comparisons. However, sensations evoked by electrical skin stimulation excite nonnociceptive fibers, therefore complicating sensory input. Radian heat stimulation produces similar sensations in different individuals, allowing comparison of pain sensitivity across groups; it excites a restricted group of primary afferent fibers; and its onset is rapid. Termination is slow, however, and therefore these methods are less appropriate for studies in which stimulation must be repeated quickly. Contact heat stimulation has a fast termination and can be used for such studies, although it excites mechanoreceptors and thermal receptors. Obviously no one method is ideal; the choice of stimulus is determined by the particular kind of experimental questions being posed.

Not only is it difficult to find an ideal pain stimulus, but it is also not an easy task to measure the response. The most commonly used method in humans is to elicit a verbal communication in a psychophysical test. In these procedures stimulus current is increased until subjects give a response to indicate when an electrical current becomes moderately painful. The current required for this response is the dependent variable used for analysis. Or a fixed set of stimuli such as electrical currents of increasing magnitude are given in a random sequence, and subjects indicate the painfulness by choosing numbers from 1 to 10. The numbers assigned to each electrical current strength are the dependent variable used for analysis. These numbers or descriptors, such as mild, moderate, and severe, constitute a categorical scale. However, such a scale assumes equal distances between numbers or descriptors, which may in fact not represent the true psychophysical function. Other scaling procedures have been developed to overcome this shortcoming such as the visual analog scale, in which subjects indicate their pain magnitude by marking on a 10 cm line labeled at the ends with "no pain" and "most intense pain imaginable" an appropriate place corresponding to their perceived painful sensation. Other methods include the magnitude estimation method in which subjects describe the magnitude of the sensation evoked by an initial stimulus with a number, and then they assign numbers to subsequent stimuli in proportion to this judgment. Another method is cross-modality matching in which subjects use any adjustable modality such as the length of a line, duration of a tone, or brightness of a light to indicate perceptual intensity. Both of these methods are also considered very effective to measure pain sensation.

Mistrust of verbal judgments has motivated the search for physiological and behavioral "objective measures" of pain magnitude. These are, of course, the only measures available for measurement of pain in experimental animals.

Behavioral measures such as grimaces, vocalization, licking, withdrawal, limping, and rubbing have been used because they often accompany painful stimuli. Both these naturally occurring reactions and trained operant behaviors (pressing a bar to escape a painful stimulus) have been used to assess pain magnitude. Pain magnitude has also been assessed with reaction time measures.

The search for physiological measures has a long and largely nonproductive history. Autonomic measures such as heart rate, skin conductance, and temperature have been correlated with painful stimuli. Although influenced by painful stimulation, these responses habituate quickly and respond nonspecifically to nonpainful stressing or novel stimulation. Measurements of cortical evoked potentials have been studied extensively and under certain conditions correlate with both stimulus intensity and verbal report. Cortical activity has also been assessed with use of nuclear magnetic resonance techniques.

Measuring Pain Sensation in Humans with Pain

Measurement of pain in the clinic takes place in a highly variable, emotional, and cognitive context and has to rely upon an indirect assessment of nociceptive input. Clinical measurement of pain is used to establish a diagnosis, to select the most appropriate treatment, and then to evaluate treatment efficacy, so that specific effects of therapies can be distinguished from the nonspecific or placebo effects. In addition, monitoring pain sensation over the course of treatment allows assessment of the degree and nature of the change that is brought about by treatment.

Methods used to evaluate pain in humans with pain are similar to those used in experimental analysis of pain. Rating scales and cross-modality matching have all been used successfully, but an important instrument is the questionnaire. One of the most universally used is the McGill pain questionnaire. With it patients describe their pain experience on a number of dimensions, using both "emotional" and "sensory" descriptors, thereby avoiding the use of unidimensional rating scales. Since its introduction the McGill pain questionnaire has become a frequently used tool in clinical evaluation and treatment trials. It permits evaluation of the sensory, affective, and evaluative dimensions of pain and yields a number of indices such as a pain rating index. The McGill pain questionnaire is useful in patient evaluation and permit comparisons between patients and with other investigations of pain mechanisms, such as clinical trials.

In conclusion, there are a number of methods in current use to evaluate pain. At present none of these methods is ideal to monitor and investigate pain mechanisms. Proponents of verbal scales have championed their scales, while behaviorists have discarded subjective experience in favor of direct measurements of behavior. Regardless of the methods used, it is important to avoid the unprofitable clinical question of the degree to which the "pain is real or in the mind." Such a dichotomous view of pain as real or imaginary bears little relation to what is known about the physiological basis of pain experience.

SUMMARY

Pain is a complex sensory experience often associated with tissue damage or as a warning that tissue damage may occur. For most individuals pain occurs relatively rarely, but for others it occurs frequently, often without any apparent cause. The mechanism of acute pain resulting from noxious cutaneous stimulation has been extensively studied. Two major groups of nociceptors have been described. The Aδ, high-threshold mechanoreceptors, are excited by intense mechanical stimulation, whereas the C polymodal nociceptors are activated by intense mechanical, thermal, and chemical stimuli. Other groups of nociceptors have been described in the skin, muscle, and joints.

Afferent fibers carrying nociceptive information synapse in the superficial laminae of the dorsal horn of the spinal cord and medulla. The nociceptive fibers synapse with two major types of second order neurons in the dorsal horn. Nociceptive specific neurons receive input only from nociceptive fibers, whereas wide-dynamic-range fibers receive projections from both nociceptive specific and nonnociceptive fibers. The substantia gelatinosa contains two morphologic types of interneuron: stalked cells and islet cells. Both of these cell types have responses that are either nociceptive-specific or wide-dynamic-range types.

Axons from dorsal horn nociceptive neurons cross the spinal cord and ascend in several fiber tracts to terminate in a number of brain areas. Nociceptive neurons in the thalamic pain relay are either of the nociceptive-specific or wide-dynamic-range type. Nociceptive neurons in these rostral brain areas differ in receptive field properties from nociceptive neurons in the spinal cord and medulla, because they often receive input from large areas of the body surface and viscera.

In recent years an endogenous pain control system has been delineated. This system involves defined pathways descending by way of the periaqueductal gray area to synapse and inhibit nociceptive neurons in the dorsal horn. Neurons in this descending system use endogenously produced opiates, or endorphins. The endorphins are of three types, called enkephalins, β-endorphins, and dynorphins. These endorphins bind to three types of opiate receptor. Besides being involved in analgesia, endogenous opiates have several other functions.

Investigators studying pain mechanisms and clinicians treating pain syndromes have used several techniques to evaluate pain experience. These include a number of stimulation techniques and methods to evaluate objectively pain responses. Although no one method is totally adequate, careful use of these techniques has led to remarkable advances in understanding the physiology of pain with improved methods of pain control treatments.

SELECTED READINGS

Beeson JM, Chaouch A: Peripheral and spinal mechanisms of nociception, *Physiological Reviews* 67: 67-186, 1987.

Brown, AG: The dorsal horn of the spinal cord, *Quarterly Journal of Experimental Physiology* 67: 193-212, 1982.

Dubner R, and Bennett GJ: Spinal and trigeminal mechanisms of nociception, *Annual Review of Neuroscience* 6: 381-418, 1983.

Fields HL, Heinricher MM, Mason P: Neurotransmitters in nociceptive modulatory circuits, *Annual Review of Neuroscience* 14: 219-245, 1991.

Fitzgerald M: Capsaicin and sensory neurones: a review, *Pain* 15: 109-130, 1983.

Light AR: *The initial processing of pain and its descending control: spinal and trigeminal systems*, Basel, 1992, Karger.

Mansour A and others: Anatomy of CNS opioid receptors, *Trends in Neuroscience* 11:308-314, 1988.

Melzak R and Wall D: *The challenge of pain*, ed 2, London, 1988, Penguin Books.

Perl ER: Characterization of nociceptors and their activation of neurons in the superficial dorsal horn: first steps in the sensation of pain. In Kruger L and Liebeskind JC, editors: *Advances in Pain Research and Therapy*, vol 6, New York, pp. 23-51, 1984, Raven.

Wall PD, Melzak R: *Textbook of pain*, ed 3, Edinburgh, 1994, Churchill Livingstone.

Wall PD, McMahon SB: Microneurography and its relation to perceived sensation: a critical review, *Pain*, 21:209-229, 1985.

Willis WD: *The pain system: the neural basis of nociceptive transmission in the mammalian nervous system*, Basel, 1985, Karger.

Willis WD Jr: Role of the forebrain in nociception, *Progress in brain research*, 87:1-12, 1991.

Yaksh TL, Hammond DL: Peripheral and central substrates involved in the rostrad transmission of nociceptive information, *Pain* 13:1-85, 1982.

3

Tooth Pulp Pain

- *Pulpal Nociceptors*
  - *Pulpal Innervation*
  - *Termination of Pulpal Fibers*
  - *Recordings from Pulpal Nociceptive Fibers*
  - *Transmission of Stimulus Across Dentin*
  - *Nonnociceptive Responses from Pulp*
- *Central Terminations of Pulpal Nociceptive Afferent Fibers*
- *Responses to Pulpal Stimulation in Thalamus and Cortex*
- *Plasticity of Pulpal Innervation*
  - *Regeneration*
  - *During Eruption and Shedding*
- *Summary*

LEARNING OBJECTIVES

At the end of this chapter you should be able to:

1. Define the characteristics of pulpal pain.
2. Identify the nerve supply to the dental pulp.
3. Define the termination of pulpal nerve fibers.
4. Describe the neurophysiologic responses of pulpal nerve fibers.
5. Identify the method by which painful stimuli are transmitted across dentin.
6. State the termination of pulpal nociceptive fibers in the trigeminal sensory nucleus.
7. Identify the ascending neural pathways transmitting pulpal nociceptive information.
8. Describe the regenerative properties of the pulpal innervation.
9. Define the changes in pulpal innervation during eruption of teeth.

Until the widespread use of fluoridated water supplies, dissolution of the protective enamel covering the tooth crown with exposure of the dentin was a prevalent condition and dental caries or tooth decay was a common occurrence. Dentin is also exposed as a result of gingival recession. When thermal or chemical stimuli, such as a draft of cold air or candy, contact exposed dentin, tooth pain or toothache occurs, first experienced as a twinge of sharp pain that develops into a severe, throbbing sensation. Individuals with toothache are dominated by this type of pain, which can be relieved only by dental treatment to remove diseased tooth structure and cover the exposed dentin with a protective filling material.

Investigators of pain mechanisms and dental clinicians have explored the pulpal pain mechanisms underlying this all-consuming tooth pain. In many investigations a tooth is electrically stimulated because it is considered a source of "pure" pain sensation. In other words, the hypothesis has been that stimulation of the pulpal innervation by any type of stimulus results only in a painful sensation. However, that assumption has been challenged in recent years by findings that nonnociceptive sensations can result from pulpal stimulation. The tooth does not always respond with pure pain sensations; it has nonnociceptive responses as well. However, because toothache is such a severe clinical problem, considerable scientific effort has been devoted to elucidate nociceptive mechanisms of the pulp, and, despite intense investigation, these mechanisms still remain unclear.

There are a number of factors hindering progress in understanding pulpal nociception. Histologic studies on the pulp are technically difficult to perform because the pulp is encased in dentin and enamel; a decalcification process is needed to prepare sections. Although recent technical advances have largely overcome the difficulties associated with recording electrophysiologic responses to stimulation of pulpal nociceptors, the process is still not easy, and exposure and dissection of small-diameter fibers that innervate the pulp is a challenging procedure. Many investigators continue to use electric stimulation of the tooth crown to stimulate pulpal nociceptors. Indeed this is also a common clinical procedure for testing pulpal health. Although it is convenient, what structures are stimulated by electrical pulp stimulation are not clear; investigators now tend to use more natural stimuli such as thermal, mechanical, and chemical. However, much of the information available on the central pathways of nociceptive transmission from the pulp are based on experiments using electrical stimulation, because this form of stimulation is easy to apply and control.

PULPAL NOCICEPTORS

The tooth pulp is innervated by neurons with cell bodies in the trigeminal ganglion and central terminations in the trigeminal principal and spinal nuclei. The axons of these nerves reach the teeth in the maxillary and mandibular branches of the trigeminal nerve. Morphologic studies of these nerves and their alveolar branches have revealed both myelinated and unmyelinated axons ranging in size from 0.2 to 15 μM. The largest myelinated axons probable do not innervate teeth, because electrical stimulation of teeth activates fibers with conduction velocities in the Aδ and C fiber ranges with a minimal contribution from large, faster conducting fibers. Therefore the tooth pulp is innervated by Aδ and C fibers which are involved in nociceptive transmission in other parts of the body (see Chapter 2). Analysis of pulpal innervation is complicated by the branching of afferent fibers so that a fiber may initially appear to be a C fiber in the pulp but may be instead a branch of a much larger-diameter parent axon.

Pulpal innervation

Fibers enter the tooth pulp at the root apex and the type, number, and diameter of the fibers at this location have been counted in various species (Table 3-1). Both myelinated and unmyelinated fibers are found at the apex with axonal diameters less than 7 μM, with most axons in the 2 to 4 μM range. Wide variability in the number of axons is often reported for particular teeth from one animal to another. This variability is in part caused by age differences: some counts were made in young animals that have fewer pulpal axons, but, because many axons branch in the first 1 to 2 mm of the root pulp, some of this variability could be accounted for by the exact site of sampling.

Once inside the pulp, branching becomes extensive in the coronal pulp. Between the root apex and the midcrown region, the ratio of branching is 1:3, but more extensive branching occurs toward the crown tip. Therefore, input from large number of dentinal nerve endings converges on a single afferent pulpal fiber, indicating that integration of sensory information takes place within the pulp.

TABLE 3-1

Number and Type of Axons Entering the Dental Pulp at the Root Apex*

Species	Myelinated	Unmyelinated
Human		
Incisor	359 ± 46†	1591 ± 728†
Canines	361 ± 82†	2240 ± 966†
Cat		
Incisor	126 ± 31†	432 ± 63†
Canine	193 – 529‡	375 – 1376‡
Dog§		
Canine	536	1553

*Only studies using electron microscopic analysis have been included. Table partly from data in Byers MR: Dental sensory receptors, *International Review of Neurobiology* 25: 39-94, 1984.

†. Data are given as mean ± standard deviation.

‡. Data are given as a range of values.

§. Data are means taken from Hirvonen TJ: *Acta Anatomica* 128: 134-139, 1987.

Dental pulp axons can be grouped into afferent sensory fibers and autonomic efferent fibers. Immunocytochemical staining has revealed subdivisions of these two groups: the first subdivision comprises large-diameter and small-diameter afferent fibers that are cholinergic; the second is small-diameter substance P–containing afferent fibers; and the third consists of sympathetic unmyelinated axons containing norepinephrine or vasoactive intestinal peptide, or both. Sensory fibers of the dental pulp also contain calcitonin gene–related peptide, a neuroactive substance that is expressed in many small-diameter nerve fibers. The pulpal calcitonin gene–related peptide fibers course through the pulp and enter the dentinal tubules.

Termination of Pulpal Fibers

The controversy that once raged over the question of whether dentin is innervated has now been settled with modern anatomical techniques. Electron microscopic examination in the 1970s demonstrated nerve-like processes in dentinal tubules that degenerated after transection of the inferior alveolar nerve. When neural tracing techniques (Chapter 2, Box 2) are applied to pulpal innervation, the trans-

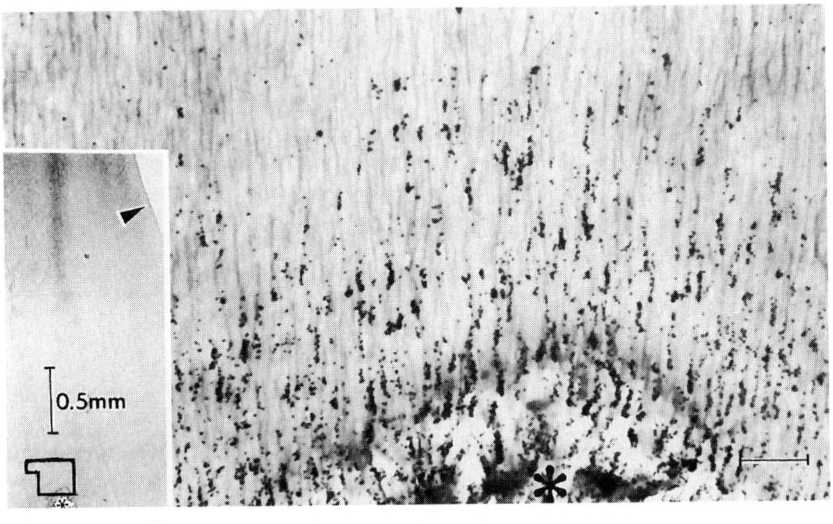

FIG. 3-1
Autoradiography of radioactive proline transported from the trigeminal ganglion to the dentinal tubules in a canine tooth. Inset, low-magnification orientation micrograph of the cusp of this tooth, showing most of the crown tip and the large span of of dentin present between the apex of the pulp (*) and the dentinoenamel junction (*arrowhead*). Outline, position of the high-magnification photomicrograph of the dentin pulp junction at the pulp apex. Scale bar is 0.5 mm In the high magnification photomicrograph numerous silver grains are seen, indicating the location of the transported proline in the dentinal tubules adjacent to the tip of the pulpal apex (*). Scale bar is 20 μm. (From Byers ME, Dong WK: *Anatomical Record*, 205:441-454, 1983. Reprinted by permission of Wiley-Liss, a division of John Wiley & Sons, Inc. Copyright © 1983.)

ported label is found in nerve terminals extending only a short distance (0.1 to 0.2 mm) into the dentinal tubules, and fibers have never been described that penetrate the whole length of the dentinal tubule (Fig. 3-1). The terminal arbors of pulpal afferent fibers have been traced and single pulpal afferent fibers have been shown to branch repeatedly so that up to 100 dentinal endings are connected to a single afferent fiber. Once the fibers enter the dentin they run parallel to the axis of the dentinal tubules. The innervation density of dentin is not uniform, it is greatest near the tip of the pulp, reduced along the sides of the crown, and least along the roots (Fig. 3-2). The density of dentin innervation does not correlate with dentinal pain sensitivity. For example, areas of the dentin with a relatively low density of innervation, such as the junction of the crown with the root (cervical dentin), are very sensitive and contribute to the clinical problem of hypersensitive dentin.

Inside the dentinal tubule the nerve fibers run alongside the odontoblast process, sometimes in a groove. The nerve fiber endings are relatively unspecialized and consist of thin regions with successive dilations. The whole ending, including both

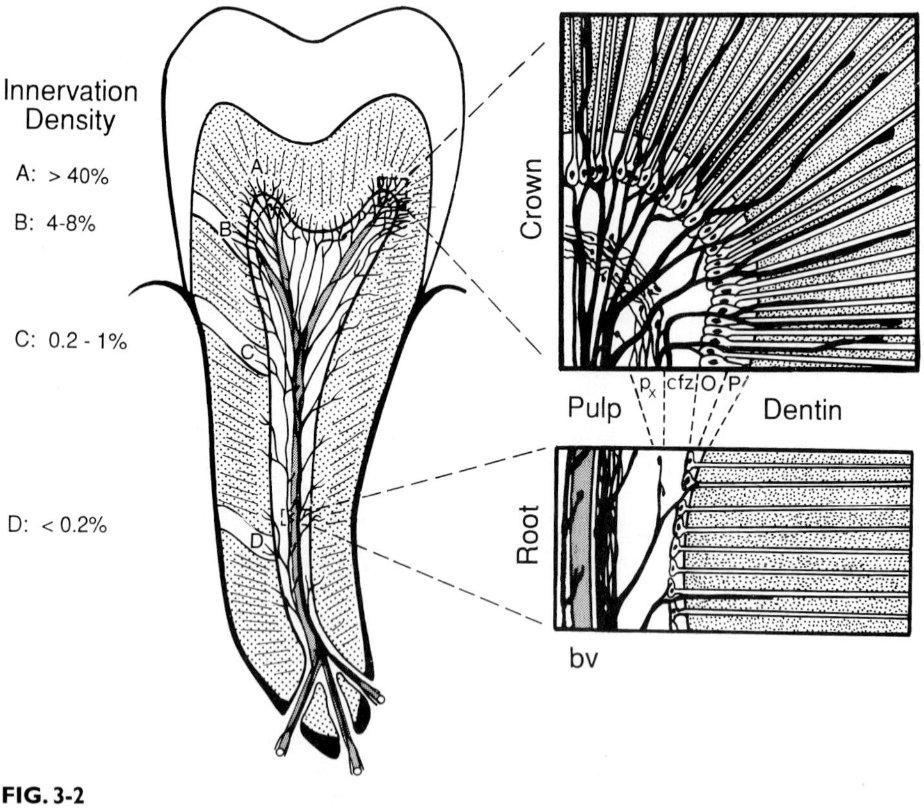

FIG. 3-2
Innervation of the pulp and dentin, with an indication of the innervation density at different areas of the tooth. P_x is the neural plexus bordering the cell free zone (*cfz*). *O*, Odontoblast layer; *P*, predentin; *bv*, blood vessels. (From Byers MR: *International Review of Neurobiology* 25:39-94, 1984.)

thin regions and dilations, contains microtubules and microfilaments, whereas the dilations contain additional organelles such as mitochondria and various kinds of vesicles. No classical synapses, tight junctions, or gap junctions connect the dentinal nerve terminals to the odontoblasts. However, most investigators have described a close apposition between the nerve terminals and the odontoblasts. Whether this apposition has any functional significance is not clear, but it at least suggests that the odontoblast may be coupled to the pulpal nerve terminal.

Recordings from Pulpal Nociceptive Fibers

Investigators examining pulpal nociceptive mechanisms have recorded from single afferent fibers either by dissecting alveolar nerves or by using extracellular recordings from the cell bodies of the afferent fibers located in the trigeminal ganglion. A further technique used to record neural activity from the pulp involves applying an elec-

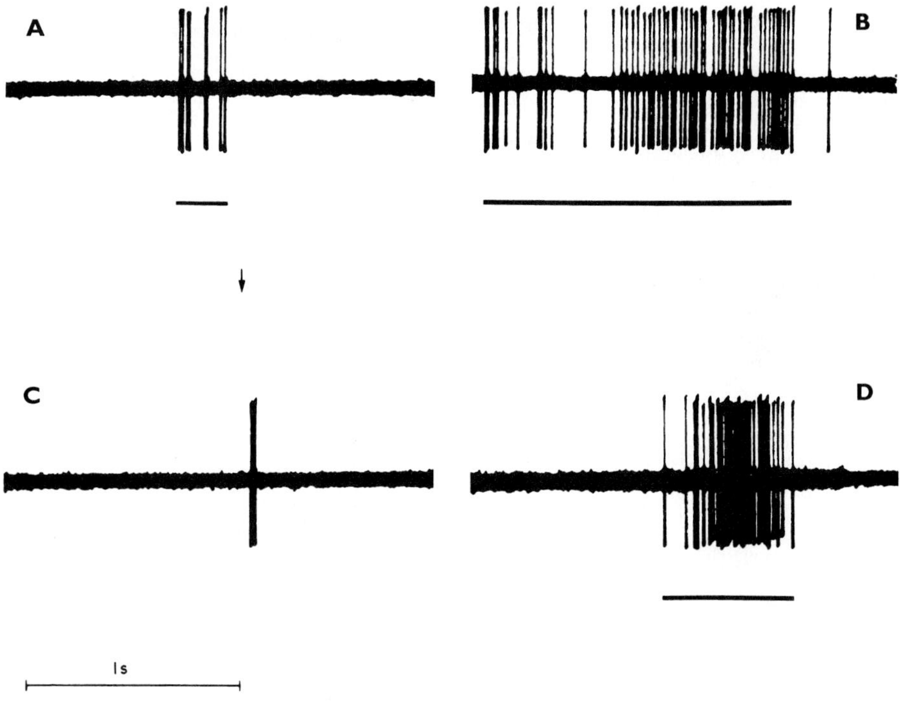

FIG. 3-3
Responses of pulpal nerve fibers to stimulation by superficial dentin by **A**, scraping with a probe; **B**, an air blast; **C**, 4.9M $CaCl_2$ solution, and **D**, drilling with a bur. Time of application indicated by a horizontal bar, except for chemical stimulation, indicated by a small arrow. (Reprinted from Närhi MVO, Hirvonen TJ, Hakumäki MOK: Activation of intradental nerves in the dog to some stimuli applied to the dentine, *Archives of Oral Biology* 27, 1053-1058, Copyright 1982, with permission from Pergamon Press Ltd, Headington Hill Hall, Oxford, UK.

trode to dentin at the base of a tooth cavity. This latter technique is useful because it permits recordings to be made from human teeth, a unique opportunity because the other recording methods cannot be used in humans. All three recording techniques have been used in animals to obtained responses to stimulation of dentin with thermal, mechanical, and chemical stimuli. These stimuli, when applied to exposed dentin in unanesthetized human teeth, produced only a painful sensation. Therefore the recordings obtained in animals are considered to be from pulpal nociceptors.

Based on measurements of conduction velocity the pulpal recordings were obtained from both Aδ and C fibers. Afferent pulpal nerve fibers are not spontaneously active and respond after a short latency to stimuli applied to the enamel sur-

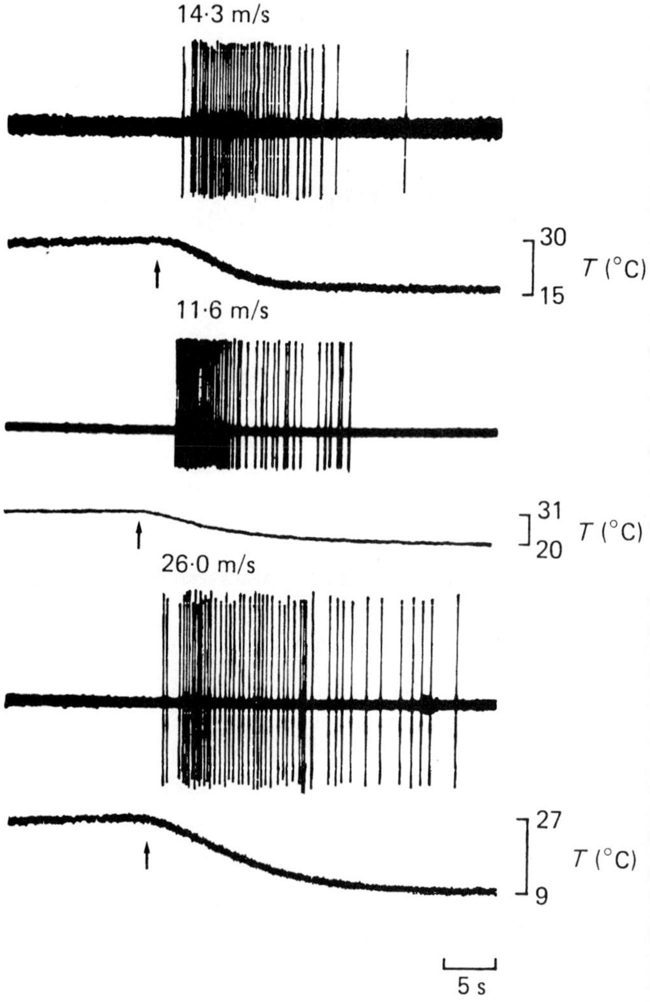

FIG. 3-4
Response of three Aδ pulpal nerve fibers to cold stimulation of crown tip of cat canines. Tooth was maintained at a steady temperature and then, as indicated by the arrow, cooled to a lower temperature. Cooling step is different for each fiber. Conduction velocity for each fiber in meters/second (*m/s*) is indicated above each response. Note absence of spontaneous neural activity and the short latency between start of cooling step and initiation of neural discharges. (From Jyväsjärvi E, Kniffki KD: *Journal of Physiology* [Lond] 391:193-207, 1987.)

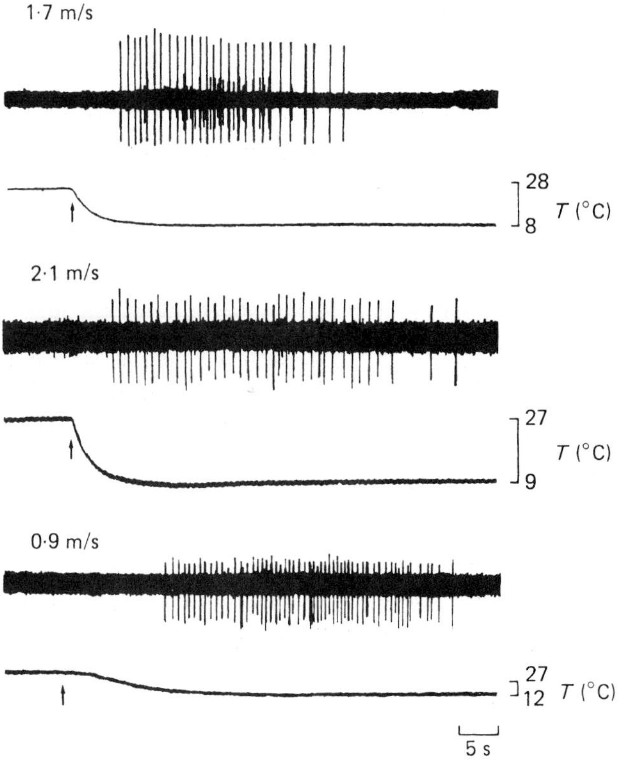

FIG. 3-5
Responses of three pulpal C fibers to cold stimulation of crown tip of canines. Tooth was maintained at a steady temperature and then, as indicated by the arrow, cooled to a lower temperature. Cooling step is different for each fiber. Conduction velocity for each fiber in meters/second (*m/s*) is indicated above each response. Note the absence of spontaneous neural activity and the long latency (compare with Fig. 3-4) between start of cooling step and initiation of neural discharges. (From Jyväsjärvi E, Kniffki KD: *Journal of Physiology* [Lond] 391:193-207, 1987.)

face or exposed dentin. Some Aδ pulpal fibers respond to mechanical stimulation of dentin such as drilling, air blasts, and probing (Fig. 3-3); others respond to thermal stimuli (Fig. 3-4). Pulpal C fibers also respond to thermal stimuli (Fig. 3-5). While some pulpal fibers seem to respond to only one type of stimulus, others respond to more than one. The pulp therefore contains two types of nociceptor, one of which responds to a single type of stimulus and another that responds to several different types of stimuli.

Most of the information on pulpal nociceptive mechanisms has been obtained from healthy, noninflamed dental pulps. However, toothache usually occurs in diseased pulps that are inflamed. To examine the nociceptive responses of diseased pulps investigators have induced inflammation experimentally. Inflammatory changes in the dental pulp can markedly affect responses of pulpal afferent fibers.

Fibers become spontaneously active and responses to dentinal stimulation are enhanced. These functional changes probably contribute to the clinical phenomenon of hypersensitive dentin in diseased teeth or in dentin that has been exposed to the oral environment for several days.

Transmission of Stimulus Across Dentin

It is clear from the neuroanatomical studies outlined previously that pulpal nerve-fiber endings do not penetrate through the dentin to the junction between the enamel and dentin. Despite this lack of nerve endings, the area is acutely sensitive to stimulation with thermal, mechanical, and chemical stimuli when the enamel is removed to expose the dentin. Therefore an area without nerve endings initiates a painful response when stimulated. Also, the distribution of intradentinal nerve terminals is not uniform (see Fig. 3-2), and areas of the dentin containing relatively few dentinal fibers are often highly sensitive to stimulation. For example, a comparison of dentinal innervation density shows that relatively few nerve fibers enter root dentin, yet exposed radicular dentin of human teeth is extremely sensitive to mechanical and chemical stimuli. If all dentinal nerve endings are similarly sensitive, the overall sensitivity of a particular area of the dentin is not correlated with innervation density. Therefore, the sensory responses recorded from pulpal nerve fibers are not induced by direct activation of nerve endings, and the response that is induced is not correlated with the innervation density of the dentin.

Most investigators of dentinal sensitivity now believe that the stimulus applied to dentin is transmitted and amplified by flow in the dentinal tubules. The application of thermal, mechanical, and heat stimuli to dentin causes fluid to flow in dentinal tubules; this flow, if rapid, causes distortion of the pulp tissue at the pulp dentin border where the nerve endings are located. Not only does this fluid flow transmit the stimulus across the dentin to the nerve endings in the dentinal tubules, but, because of the geometry of the dentinal tubules, it also is capable of concentrating the stimulus at the pulpal side of the tubules. This proposed mechanism of stimulus-induced fluid flow is therefore capable of explaining both the transmission of a stimulus across the dentin to pulpal nerve endings and amplification of the stimulus. Much experimental evidence has been gathered that supports this theory (often referred to as the *hydrodynamic hypothesis of dentinal sensitivity*).

Electrophysiologic recordings from pulpal nerve fibers indicate that any type of stimulus that causes fluid flow in the dentinal tubules results in activation of pulpal afferent fibers, presumably by mechanical distortion of the nerve endings. This explains why stimuli as diverse as chemical and thermal initiate a similar painful sensation. Moreover, the condition of the dentin surface has been shown to influence the dentinal response, which, if blocked effectively, reduces sensitivity to applied stimuli. The hydrodynamic mechanism implies that the actual stimulus applied to the nerve ending is mechanical in the form of pressure.

The exposed pulp is also extremely sensitive to stimuli, which cause an intense toothache. Once the pulp is opened, the pulpal innervation is directly exposed to external stimuli. It is possible that stimulation of the pulp activates both Aδ and C fibers directly, bypassing any receptor system at the nerve endings in the dentin. This is similar to the exposed base of a skin blister, which is also extremely sensitive to various stimuli.

Nonnociceptive Responses from Pulp

Although investigators formerly thought that only painful responses could result from stimulation of tooth pulp and dentin, there have been a number of reports in both humans and animals that responses that are not painful can be evoked from the pulp. Moreover, nerve fibers in the Aβ range have been reported in the pulp that may be responsible for transmitting nonnociceptive responses. The pulp is thought to contain low-threshold mechanoreceptors innervated by Aβ fibers that respond to mechanical stimulation in the nonnoxious range. These intradental mechanoreceptors may be responsible for prepain sensations sometimes reported when teeth are electrically stimulated; they may also play an important role in the control of mastication by transmitting information on mechanical forces applied to the teeth during chewing. Also, the tooth is not a "pure source" of pain sensation, because nonnociceptive sensations can be evoked by tooth stimulation.

CENTRAL TERMINATIONS OF PULPAL NOCICEPTIVE AFFERENT FIBERS

Electrical stimulation and central tracing experiments have demonstrated that pulpal nociceptive-afferent fibers from the tooth terminate in the medullary dorsal horn. This termination is not surprising because this is a major relay in the trigeminal nociceptive pathway. However, more rostral terminations in the principal and subnucleus oralis have been described. The function of substantial projections in rostral trigeminal nuclei is difficult to explain because the tooth pulp is innervated primarily by afferent fibers involved in nociception and because these rostral areas are not usually associated with pain transmission. However, the electrophysiologic evidence for the tooth pulp afferent fiber projections to the brain stem is based on evoked responses to electric stimulation of the tooth so that although there is little doubt that these projections exist, there is no direct evidence implicating them in nociceptive mechanisms, because electrical stimulation could initiate impulses in pulpal Aβ, Aδ, and C fibers directly. Only neurons in the medullary dorsal horn respond when noxious thermal stimuli are applied to teeth, and the medullary dorsal horn neurons activated by noxious pulpal thermal stimulation are nociceptive-specific and wide-dynamic-range types, both of which are involved in nociceptive transmission. Therefore, nociceptive transmission from the dental pulp is apparently relayed primarily through neurons in the medullary dorsal horn. However, because section of the descending trigeminal tract in humans does not eliminate nociceptive and aversive responses to noxious facial and pulpal stimulation, the more rostral projections from the tooth pulp must play some role in pain transmission. One possibility is that the rostral projections are involved in dental prepain sensations that accompany low-intensity electric stimulation of the pulp. A further possibility is that the more rostral projections are involved in spatiotemporal discriminative aspects of dental pulp pain.

RESPONSES TO PULPAL STIMULATION IN THALAMUS AND CORTEX

Electric stimulation of the tooth pulp activates neurons in the ventromedial and ventrobasal complex of the thalamus. These projections are assumed to transmit nociceptive information but were determined by using electrical stimulation of the pulp. Thalamic projections have not been analyzed by the use of natural stimulation applied to the dentin or tooth pulp. Also a projection to the intralaminar complex has been reported, and is thought to be associated with cortical arousal and direction of attention.

Recordings of evoked and single-unit activity indicate that the tooth pulp projects to the oral area of the primary somatosensory cortex (SI). Most of the neurons activated by electric stimulation of the tooth pulp are also activated by nonnoxious peripheral stimulation. Convergence at the cortical level is therefore indicated. Cortical neurons activated by tooth pulp stimulation have different response latencies. Some respond after a latency of less than 20 msec, while others have response latencies longer than 20 msec. The short latency neurons also contain a group that demonstrates a profound burst of impulses as the stimulus is removed.

From the discussion of the response characteristics of neurons that relay nociceptive information from the tooth pulp at each ascending level of the neural pathway, it should be apparent that significant differences are found at each level. Considerable processing occurs, consisting of alteration in the response patterns recorded in the primary afferent fibers, and convergence of other sensory systems. The result is a decrease in specificity of the neurons responding to tooth pulp stimulation. This neural processing probably underlies the complex behaviors induced by toothache.

PLASTICITY OF PULPAL INNERVATION

Regeneration

After section or crush of the inferior alveolar nerve, regeneration occurs and nerve fibers reenter the dental pulp. The regenerating fibers ascend the pulp chamber and enter the dentinal tubules to the same depth as in normal teeth. The studies that show this also confirm the importance of dentinal nerve fibers in tooth sensitivity, because the point in time when nerve fibers enter into the dentin correlates with the recovery of sensitivity to electric stimulation. Dental nerves also reinnervate teeth that have been extracted and reimplanted. Regeneration of reimplanted teeth does not seem to be as complete as teeth denervated in situ and varies between 7% and 75% of the number of axons counted in unoperated teeth.

During Eruption and Shedding

When root resorption of the deciduous dentition begins before tooth shedding, the nerve supply in the deciduous dental pulp degenerates and myelinated fibers begin to appear in the permanent tooth pulp. Examination of the deciduous and permanent canines in cats indicates that, for a brief time during eruption and shedding, both teeth are supplied by branches of the same axon. Therefore, during development the permanent teeth are supplied by nerves that originally supplied the deciduous predecessor.

SUMMARY

Toothache is a severe pain resulting from stimulation of tooth dentin exposed because of a carious lesion or gingival recession. Various stimuli applied to exposed dentin elicit toothache. Besides pain other nonnoxious sensations can be initiated by dentinal stimulation. Although the dental pulp is highly innervated, dentin is not. Nerve fibers only penetrate dentin for a short distance and do not reach the enamel-dentin junction. Also, the dentinal innervation is not uniform, the major innervation being at the tooth crown. Within the dentin the nerve fibers travel in the dentinal tubules along a groove in the odontoblast process.

Electrophysiologic recordings from dentinal nerve fibers have revealed both Aδ and C fibers that respond to stimulation of the dentin. Some of these fibers respond only to one stimulus modality whereas others respond to more than one. Effective stimuli are thermal, mechanical, and chemical. These same stimuli applied to exposed human dentin induce toothache. The transmission of the stimulus across the dentin is mediated by movement of fluid through the odontoblast tubules that stimulates nerve endings in the dentin and at the border between dentin and pulp.

The cell bodies of dentinal-fibers are in the trigeminal ganglion. The fibers terminate in the medullary dorsal horn and synapse with second order nociceptive specific and wide-dynamic-range neurons. In addition to this caudal termination there is also a more rostral termination in the trigeminal sensory nucleus. The caudal termination together with termination of other orofacial afferent nociceptive fibers forms the first relay in the trigeminal pain pathway. The function of the rostral pulpal nociceptive projection is not known but may be important in spatiotemporal discrimination related to pulpal sensation.

From the trigeminal nucleus, pulpal nociceptive information first connects in the thalamus and then projects to the somatosensory cortex. Cortical neurons responding to dentinal stimulation often receive nonnoxious convergent input as well, so that these neurons have characteristics of wide-dynamic-range neurons.

Pulpal innervation is capable of regenerating and reinnervating dentinal tubules.

Some reinnervation even takes place when teeth are reimplanted. During transition between deciduous and permanent dentitions a single nerve supply transiently supplies both a deciduous tooth and its permanent successor.

SELECTED READINGS

Brännström M: *Dentin and Pulp in Restorative Dentistry*, Nacka, Sweden, 1981.

Byers MR: Dental sensory receptors, *International Review of Neurobiology* 25:39-94, 1984.

Light AR: *The Initial Processing of Pain and Its Descending Control: Spinal and Trigeminal Systems*, Basel, 1992, Karger.

Närhi MVO: Dentin sensitivity: a review, *Journale Biologie Buccale* 13:75-96, 1985.

4 Mechanoreceptors

LEARNING OBJECTIVES

At the end of this chapter you should be able to:

1. Name the four kinds of mechanoreceptors.
2. Identify the structure of four kinds of mechanoreceptors.
3. Give a classification of mechanoreceptors based on response characteristics.
4. Define the receptive field characteristics of mechanoreceptors.
5. Describe the response properties of facial mechanoreceptors.
6. Give the morphology of periodontal mechanoreceptors.
7. Identify the response properties of periodontal mechanoreceptors.
8. Define the directional sensitivity of periodontal mechanoreceptors.
9. Name the location of two types of periodontal mechanoreceptors in the periodontal ligament.
10. Identify the response characteristics of human periodontal mechanoreceptors.
11. Describe the regenerative properties of periodontal mechanoreceptors.
12. Name the central terminations of periodontal mechanoreceptive fibers.
13. State the functional properties of mechanoreceptive neurons in the trigeminal sensory nucleus and thalamus.

Mechanoreceptors, as their name implies, are receptors designed to respond to mechanical stimuli. There are many kinds of morphologically distinct mechanoreceptor endings, each designed to respond to a particular kind of mechanical stimulus. Some are found in just one species of animals while others occur in most vertebrates. Certain of these receptors are associated with hairs whereas others are found in large numbers in nonhairy or glabrous skin. For example, the glabrous skin of the human hand has an estimated 17,000 mechanoreceptors.

In the orofacial area mechanoreceptors serve two major functions. First, they are responsible for transmitting textural information, an important component of the flavor of foods. Foods provide tactile oral stimulation, and the sensations of texture such as crunchy, crisp, smooth, and chewy, all originate from mechanoreceptors situated in the oral mucosa.

Second, mechanoreceptors provide sensory feedback essential in the control of orofacial motor functions. During mastication, mechanoreceptors provide information on the position of food in the mouth, and, during speech, monitor tongue position. They are therefore important in guiding manipulation and formation of the food bolus during chewing and prevent biting of the tongue and cheek. This is often apparent after all or part of the mouth has been anesthetized for a dental procedure, when speech is impaired and accidental tongue biting sometimes occurs. Also, the inhibition of swallowing after application of topical anesthesia to the oral mucosa demonstrates the necessity of sensory feedback from mechanoreceptors for swallowing.

The periodontal ligament that supports and attaches the teeth in their sockets is also supplied with mechanoreceptors, which are stimulated when pressure is applied to the teeth. This occurs when the teeth come into contact, when food is bitten during mastication, and when the tongue touches the teeth during speech production. Therefore periodontal mechanoreceptors also serve an important function in sensory feedback control of orofacial motor functions.

MECHANORECEPTORS

The structure and function of mechanoreceptors of the skin have been investigated extensively. They are innervated by large-diameter, fast-conducting, myelinated Aα fibers. The adequate stimulus for these mechanoreceptors is mechanical deformation of their receptive fields. Two major classes of mechanoreceptors have been defined by their neurophysiologic response to a controlled stimulus. The definitions are based on receptor responses during a phase of application and removal of the stimulus, called the dynamic phase of the stimulus; and during a phase of steady application of the stimulus, called the static phase. Mechanoreceptors that only generate action potentials during the dynamic phase of stimulus application are called rapidly adapting receptors (RA). Mechanoreceptors that fire action potentials during the dynamic and static phases of stimulus application are called slowly adapting receptors (SA).

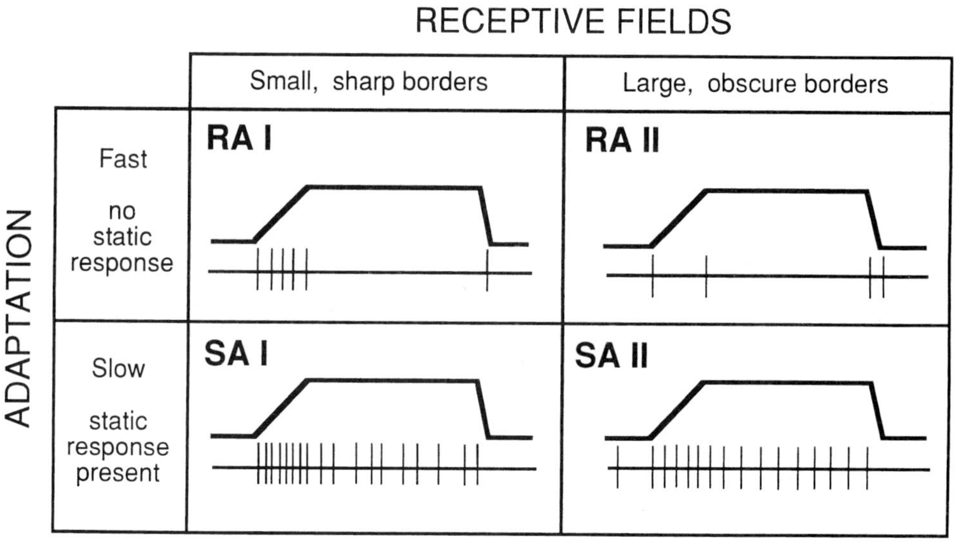

FIG. 4-1
Classification of cutaneous mechanoreceptors based on response adaptation pattern and receptive field properties. (From Johansson RS, Vallbo ÅB: *Trends in Neuroscience* 6:27-32, 1983.)

Within these two major classes of mechanoreceptors several other subclasses can be distinguished through other response characteristics of the receptor. For example, the mechanoreceptors of the glabrous skin of the human hand have been studied extensively and because of their receptive field properties have been divided into two types of rapidly adapting and two types of slowly adapting receptors. Rapidly adapting type I (RA I) and slowly adapting type I (SA I) have small, circumscribed, receptive fields, whereas rapidly adapting type II (RA II) and slowly adapting type II (SA II) have large receptive fields with ill-defined borders (Fig. 4-1).

Structure

Because of correlations between function and structure in animals the RA1 mechanoreceptors are Meissner's corpuscles, located in the papillary ridges of the dermis. These receptors consist of a series of cross lamination interleaved with nerve endings to form a column. Several nerve fibers enter the receptor and form small-diameter terminals. Collagen fibers between the laminae connect the corpuscle to the basement membrane of the epithelium (Fig. 4-2). The SA I mechanoreceptors are Merkel cell neurite complexes, consisting of a modified epithelial cell associated with a plate or disk-like expansion of nerve fiber terminals. Desmosomes connect the modified epithelial cell with the surrounding epithelium (Fig. 4-3). The SA II response originates in Ruffini endings, that are long spindle-shaped

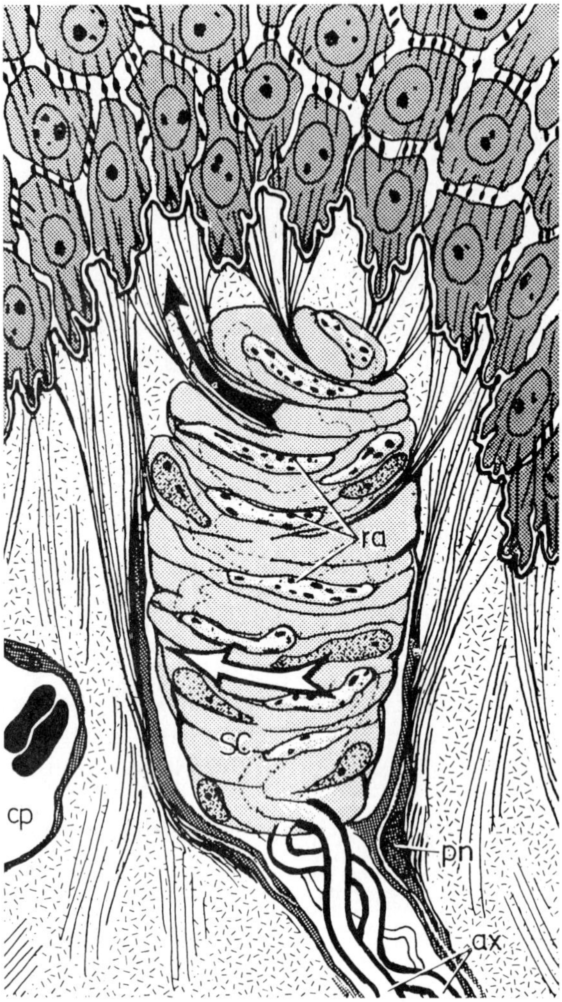

FIG. 4-2
Meissner corpuscle. *ax*, Axon; *ra*, coiled receptor axon; *SC* Schwann cell; *pn*, cup-shaped perineural sheath; *cp*, capillary. (From Andres KH, Von Düring M: Morphology of cutaneous receptors. In Iggo A, editor: *Handbook of Sensory Physiology*, vol 2, *Somatosensory Systems*. Berlin, 1973, Springer Verlag, p. 16.)

structures made up of several nerve fibers that branch inside the receptor capsule and are surrounded by connective tissue elements and fluid-filled spaces. Collagen fibers in contact with the ends of the nerve fibers are also attached to the surrounding connective tissue so that tension can be directly transferred from the subepithelial tissue to the receptor terminals (Fig. 4-4). The RA II receptors are

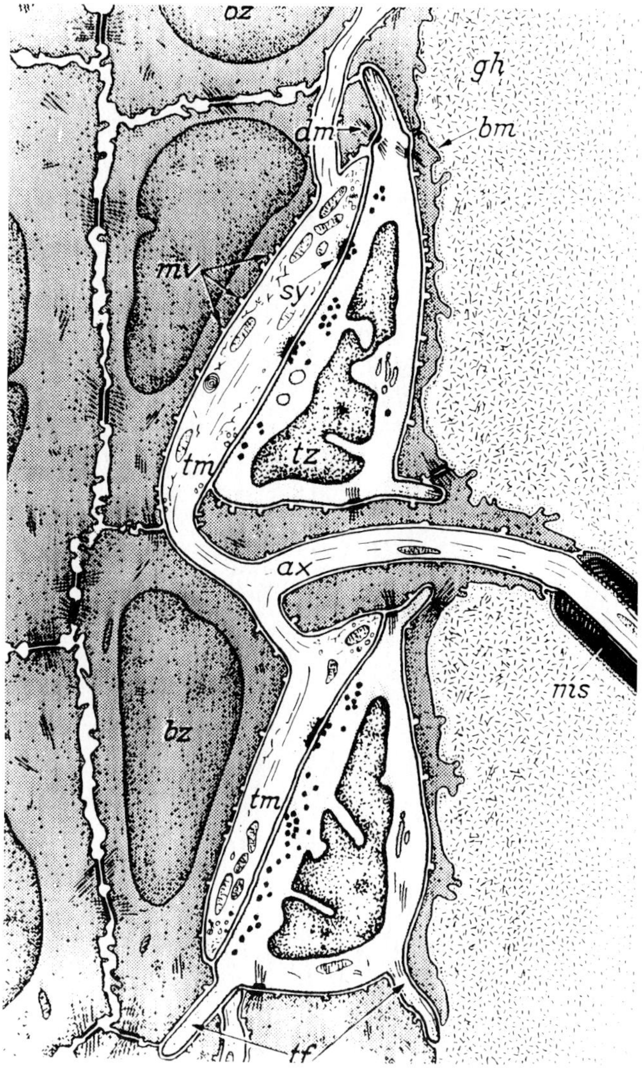

FIG. 4-3
Merkel cell–neurite complex. *ax*, Axon; *bm*, basement membrane; *bz*, basal cell; *dm*, desmosome; *gh*, glassy membrane; *tf*, fingerlike process of touch cell; *tz*, touch cell; *tm*, touch meniscus; *sy*, contact zone to the Merkel cell; *ms*, myelin sheath. (From Andres KH, Von Düring M: Morphology of cutaneous receptors. In Iggo A, editor: *Handbook of Sensory Physiology*, vol 2, *Somatosensory Systems*. Berlin, 1973, Springer Verlag, p. 16.)

FIG. 4-4
Ruffini corpuscle. Branched terminals lie between the interlaced collagenous fibers of inner core. *AX*, Axon; *IC*, inner core; *C*, capsule; *CS*, capsule space; *EC*, endoneural cell; *IC*, inner core; *KF*, collagenous fibers; *NF*, myelinated axon with perineural sheath; *SC*, Schwann cell; *TB*, branched terminals. (From Chambers MR et al: *Quarterly Journal of Experimental Physiology* 57:417-445, 1972.)

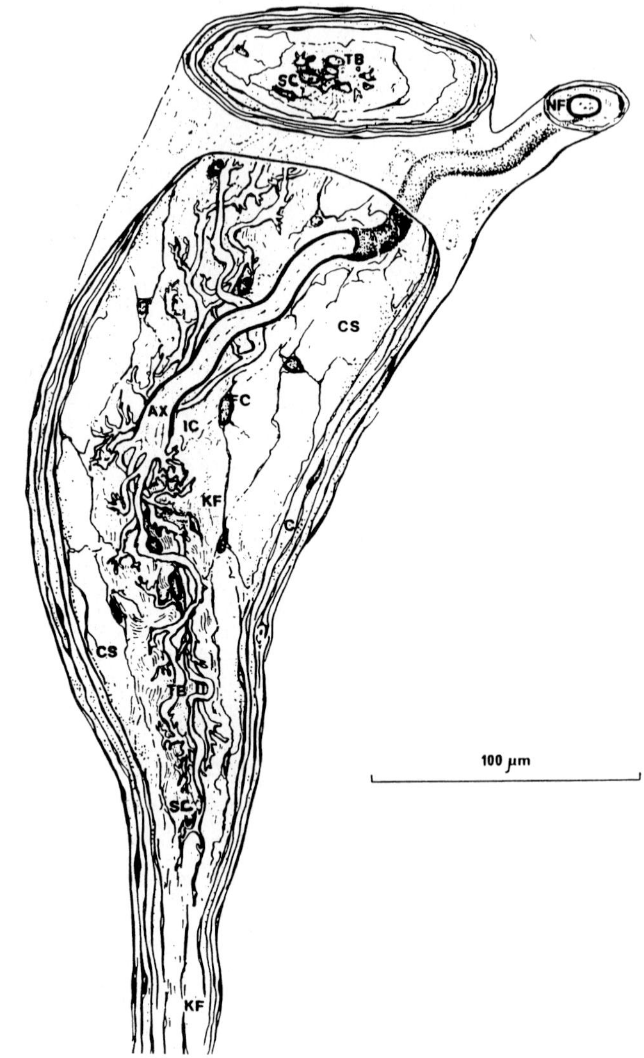

Pacinian corpuscles, which are constructed of concentric layers of Schwann's cell lamellae surrounding a central-receptor axon terminal (Fig. 4-5).

Response Characteristics of Cutaneous Mechanoreceptors

The receptive field of the RA I and SA I mechanoreceptors is small (3 to 5 mm in diameter) and circular or oval (Fig. 4-6). The sensitivity is high and relatively uniform across the center of these receptive fields, and declines rapidly at

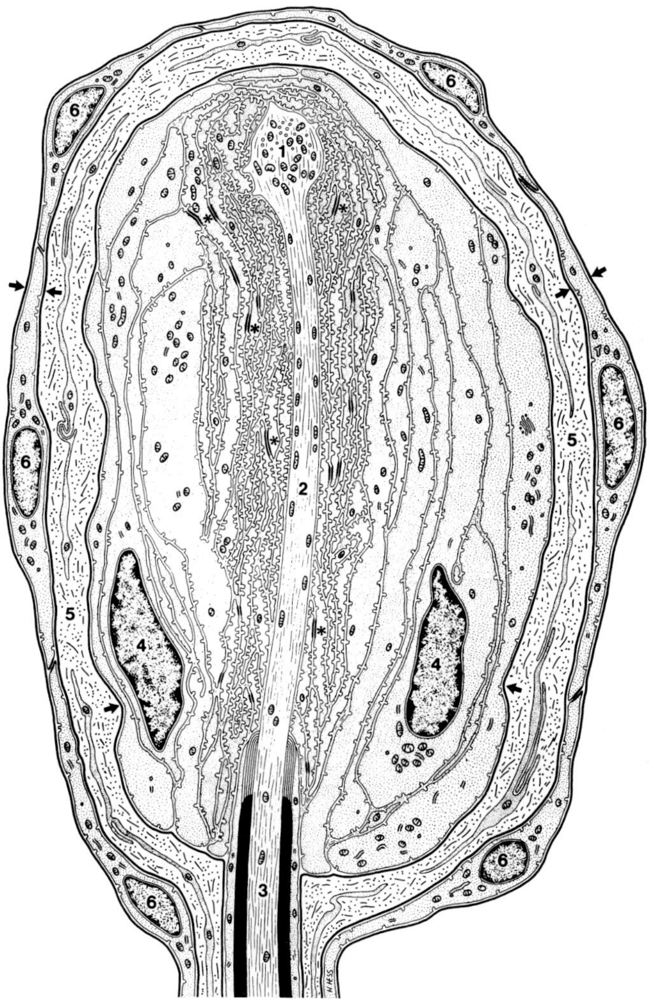

FIG. 4-5
Pacinian corpuscle. *1*, Bead-like expansion of axon; *2*, middle portion of axon running inside middle core; *3*, myelinated afferent fiber; *4*, inner core made up of Schwann cell lamellae; *, lamellae linked by desmosomes; *5*, subcapsular space containing fibrocytes and collagen fibers; *6*, capsule covered by a basal lamina (↑). (From Halata Z: *Advances in Anatomy and Cell Biology* 50:31, 1975.)

the edges. Several small zones of maximal sensitivity are located within the area of high sensitivity. An important characteristic of RA I and SA I mechanoreceptors is their ability to show a pronounced response when stimulated across the edge of their receptive fields. They are therefore ideally suited to transmit information on the contour and texture of mechanical stimuli. Moreover, because these receptors are found in the highest density on the finger tips, they are probably important in spatial discrimination of objects held in the fingers. The RA I mechanoreceptors are particularly responsive to low-frequency (5 to 40 Hz) vibratory stimuli and are therefore responsible for the sensation of "flutter" transmitted from the skin.

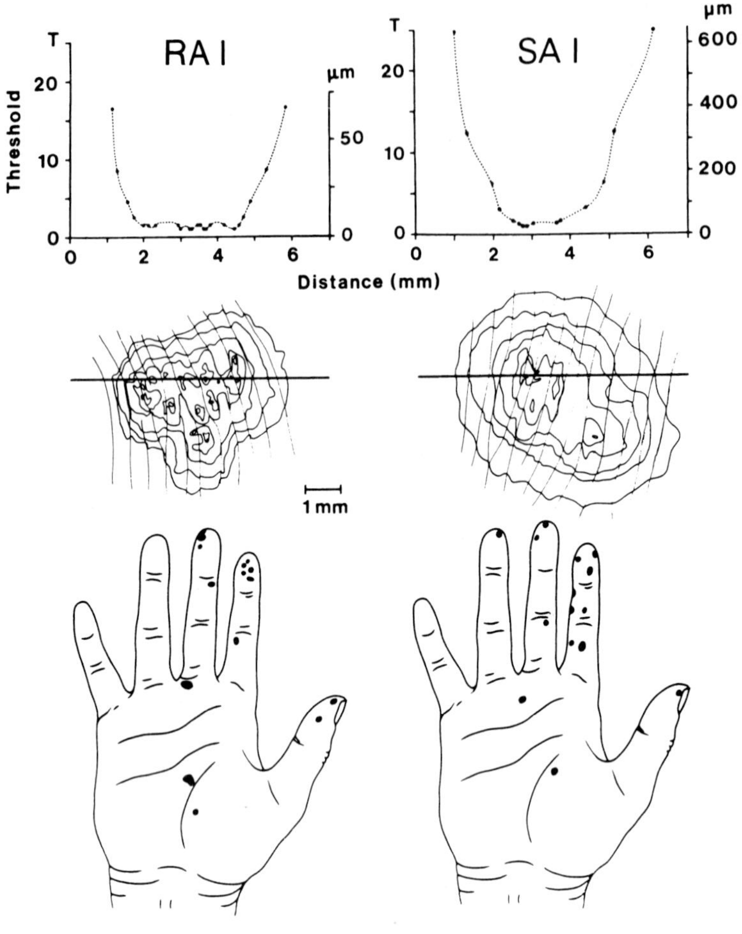

FIG. 4-6
Receptive fields of rapidly adapting (*RA I*) and slowly adapting (*SA I*) type I mechanoreceptors based on microneurographic recordings from human radial nerves. *Bottom*, Locations of small, punctate receptive fields on the hand. *Middle*, Equal sensitivity contours for receptive fields; faint lines represent the fingerprint lines. *Top*, Threshold sensitivity and indentation depth across center of receptive field (thick line in middle receptive field diagrams). (From Johansson RS, Vallbo ÅB: *Trends in Neuroscience* 6:27-32, 1983.)

In contrast the receptive field of RA II and SA II mechanoreceptors is large, with a central zone of maximal sensitivity that slowly declines with increasing distance from the center (Fig. 4-7). The receptive field of RA II mechanoreceptors covers a wide area such as a whole finger or a major part of the palm. They are sensitive to remote mechanical transients, particularly vibratory stimuli that range between 100 and 300 Hz. Vibratory stimuli with an amplitude of only 1 µm are often sufficient to

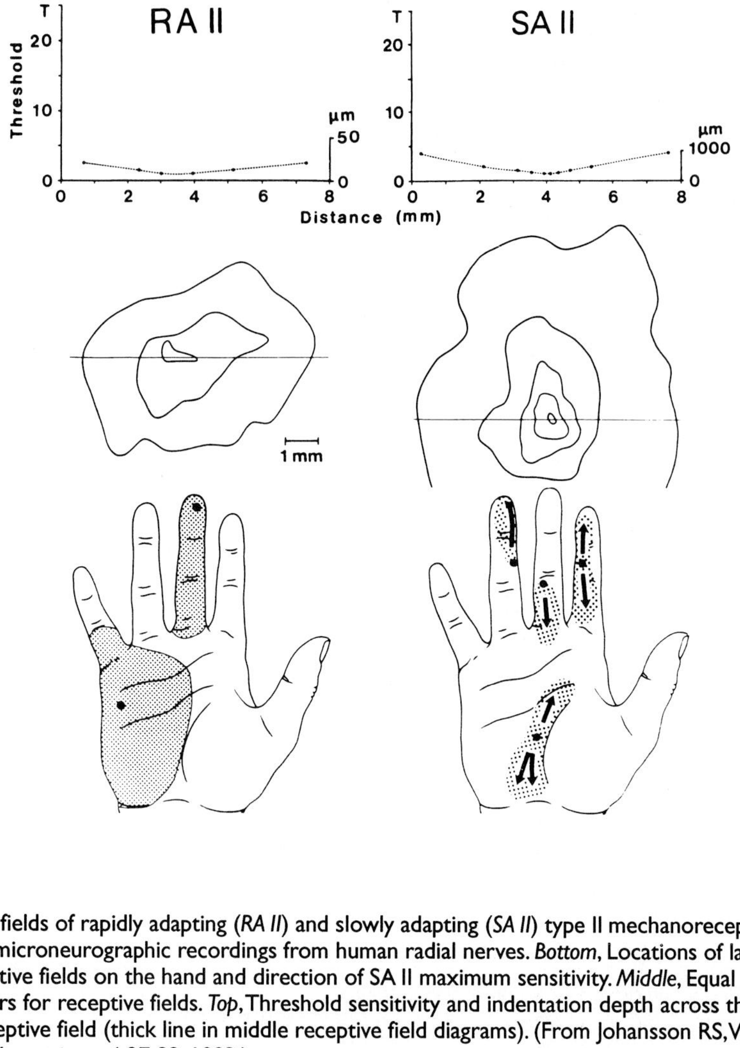

FIG. 4-7
Receptive fields of rapidly adapting (*RA II*) and slowly adapting (*SA II*) type II mechanoreceptors based on microneurographic recordings from human radial nerves. *Bottom*, Locations of large, diffuse receptive fields on the hand and direction of SA II maximum sensitivity. *Middle*, Equal sensitivity contours for receptive fields. *Top*, Threshold sensitivity and indentation depth across the center of the receptive field (thick line in middle receptive field diagrams). (From Johansson RS, Vallbo ÅB: *Trends in Neuroscience* 6:27-32, 1983.)

elicit a nerve impulse from these mechanoreceptors. The sense of vibration for frequencies above 40 Hz is derived from RA II mechanoreceptors. A characteristic of SA II mechanoreceptors is spontaneous generation of action potentials in the apparent absence of any stimulus. These mechanoreceptors have large receptive fields and respond maximally to stretches that occur in a particular direction. They transmit information on the direction and magnitude of lateral tension in the skin. SA II mechanoreceptors in the hand play an important role in the control of grip.

Response Characteristics of Facial Mechanoreceptors

Recordings have been made from mechanoreceptive fibers in the human infraorbital nerve with receptive fields on the facial skin. Most of the mechanoreceptive responses derive from slowly adapting receptors with small, well defined receptive fields although rapidly adapting responses are also recorded. Response characteristics of RA mechanoreceptors located in facial skin are similar to the RA I in glabrous skin

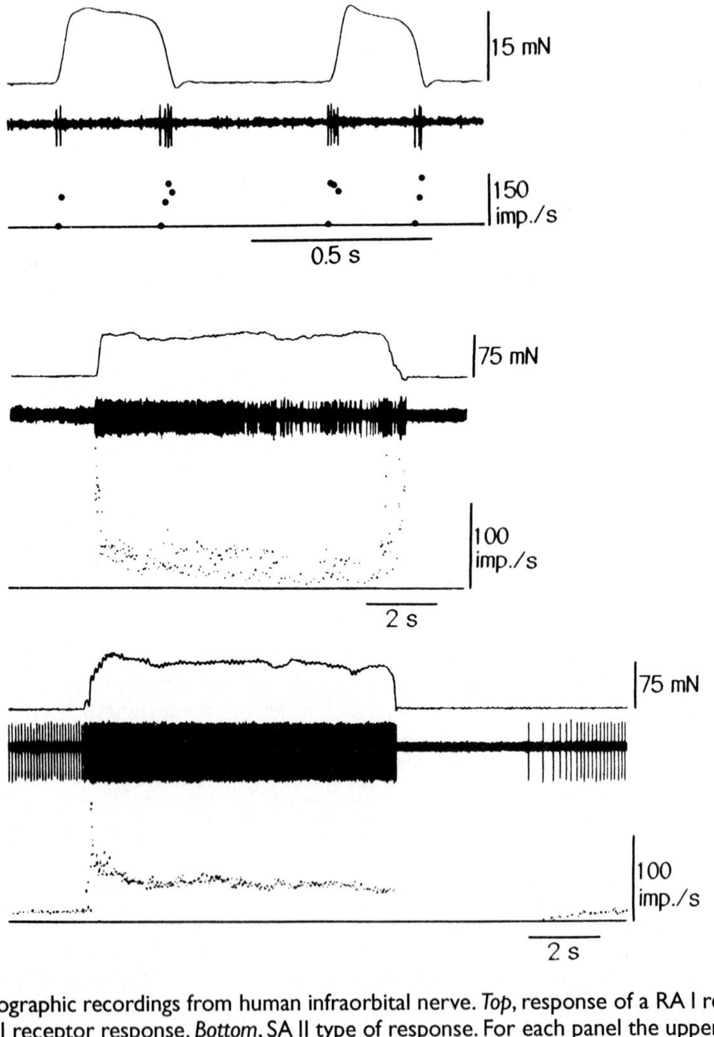

FIG. 4-8
Microneurographic recordings from human infraorbital nerve. *Top*, response of a RA I receptor. *Middle*, SA I receptor response. *Bottom*, SA II type of response. For each panel the upper tracing is the force applied in milli-Newtons, the middle trace is the response of the fiber, and the lower trace is the instantaneous frequency response in impulses per second. (From Johansson RS, Trulsson M, Olsson KÅ, Westberg K-G: *Experimental Brain Research* 72: 204-208, 1988.)

of the hand (Fig. 4-8). Responses from RA II units typical of Pacinian corpuscles are not found in the skin of the human face. Both subclasses of SA responses (SA I and SA II) are found in the infraorbital nerve although differences between facial and glabrous skin mechanoreceptors are apparent (Fig. 4-8). For example, facial SA I mechanoreceptors respond with burst of discharges when the stimulus is removed ("off response"), and this is rarely encountered in glabrous mechanoreceptor responses (Fig. 4-8).

PERIODONTAL MECHANORECEPTORS

Mechanoreceptors in the periodontal ligament are Ruffini-type endings supplied by large-diameter (1 to 15 μm) myelinated fibers. The Ruffini endings are unencapsulated and vary in complexity from large-branched endings with finger-like extensions in contact with collagen ligaments to small endings that lack neural fingers (Fig. 4-9). Therefore, although the only type of mechanoreceptor in the periodontal ligament is Ruffini endings, there is considerable variability in their morphology.

Periodontal mechanoreceptors are innervated by afferent fibers with cell bodies in either the trigeminal ganglion (TG) or the trigeminal mesencephalic nucleus (MS) (see Fig. 4-17). Both TG and MS periodontal mechanoreceptors are distributed

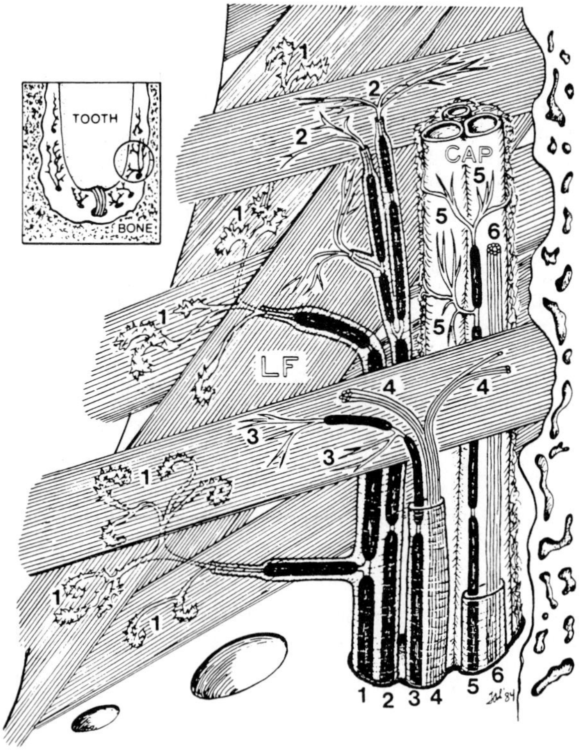

FIG. 4-9
Sensory endings in rat periodontal ligament. Receptors among ligament fibers (*LF*): *1*, complex Ruffini-like endings, ensheathed preterminal axon; *2*, simple Ruffini-like endings, ensheathed preterminal axons can form paired branches; *3*, simple Ruffini-like endings branching from free, small, myelinated axons; *4*, bundles of free unmyelinated axons. Receptors in loose connective tissue around capillaries (*CAP*): *5*, simple Ruffini-like endings branching from from free, small, myelinated axons; *6*, bundles of free unmyelinated axons. The tooth inset indicates the location of the schematic diagram in the periodontal ligament. (From Byers MR: *Journal of Comparative Neurology* 231:500-518, 1985. Copyright © 1985. Reprinted by permission of Wiley-Liss, a division of John Wiley & Sons, Inc.)

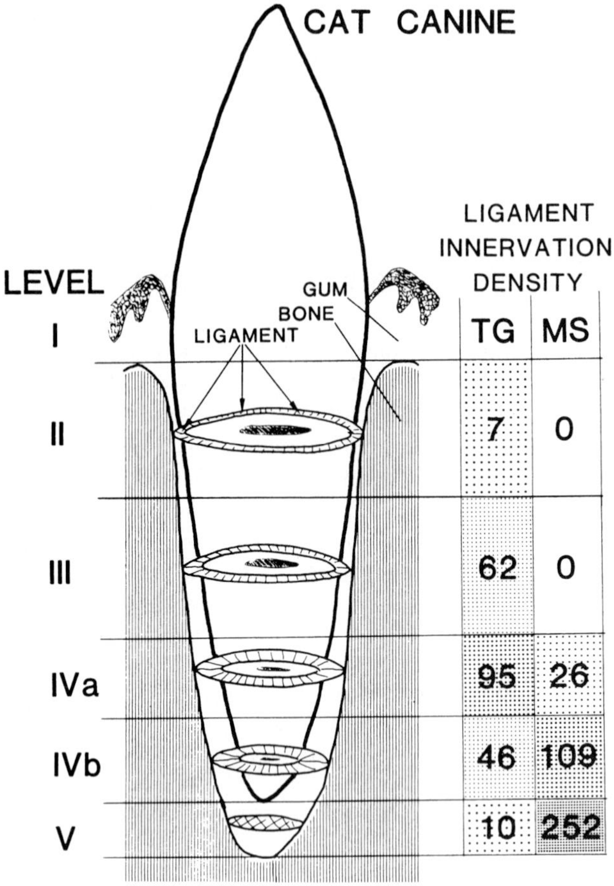

FIG. 4-10
Site of termination of afferent fibers with cell bodies in the trigeminal ganglion (*TG*) and trigeminal mesencephalic nucleus (*MS*) in the periodontal ligament of a cat canine tooth. *Right,* Relative densities of the innervation. (From Byers MR, Dong WK: *Journal of Comparative Neurology* 279:117-127, 1989. Copyright © 1989. Reprinted by permission of Wiley-Liss, a division of John Wiley & Sons, Inc.)

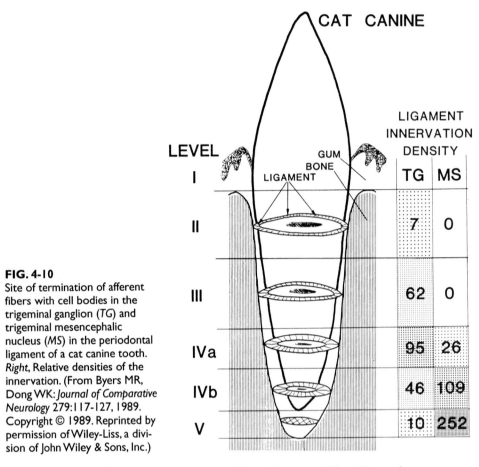

throughout different areas of the periodontal ligament. The MS mechanoreceptors are concentrated near the root apex while the TG mechanoreceptors are found around the middle of the root (Fig. 4-10).

Recordings from Periodontal Afferent Mechanoreceptive Fibers

Mechanical forces applied to a tooth move the tooth in its socket, and, as a result, secondarily generate tension in the periodontal ligament, causing activation of periodontal mechanoreceptors. Therefore the degree of stimulation and subsequently the response of a mechanoreceptor depend not only on the intrinsic properties of the mechanoreceptor but also on the amount of force required to move the tooth in its socket sufficient to activate the receptor. In addition, the location of the mechanoreceptor in the ligament influences response characteristics, because the tooth rotates about a fulcrum situated near the junction of the crown and the root. The same force applied to the crown of a tooth would stimulate receptors situated near the fulcrum less than it would near the root apex. The coupling between a periodontal receptor and the applied stimulus is therefore complex and is an important factor in determining response characteristics.

Single-fiber recordings from afferent fibers innervating the periodontal ligament have revealed both RA and SA mechanoreceptor classes. Rapidly adapting periodontal mechanoreceptors respond to tooth movement with just a few action potentials (Fig. 4-11, A). These receptors respond only during the application of the stimulus to the tooth, and the number of impulses produced depends on the rate of application of the stimulus. If the stimulus is applied slowly a single action potential is generated (Fig. 4-11, A). At faster applications more neural impulses are produced. The number of impulses produced is also related to the magnitude of the applied load. Therefore, these receptors are sensitive to both the rate of application and the magnitude of the applied tooth displacement, but only respond when the displacement is being applied. Also, as the rate of stimulus application is increased, the time to produce a response decreases; that is, the response latency is shortened (Fig. 4-11, B).

Slowly adapting periodontal mechanoreceptors have lower response thresholds than the rapidly adapting class. The magnitude of the SA dynamic phase responses is determined by the rate of stimulus application. The frequency of the static phase responses is related to the intensity of the applied stimulus (Fig. 4-12). When lower forces are applied some SA units stop responding before the force is removed from the tooth. Therefore when low stimulus forces are applied to some SA units, they begin to resemble RA units suggesting that RA and SA responses might originate in the same type of mechanoreceptor. However, if a ratio is calculated by using the number of action potentials that occur during the static phase divided by the number of impulses that occur during the dynamic phase (the dynamic index), RA units have a very low dynamic index that is clearly different from the index of SA units (Fig. 4-13). Therefore, even if RA and SA responses derive from the same receptor type, there is strong evidence to support two distinct response types.

Both RA and SA periodontal mechanoreceptors respond to the direction of the applied tooth displacement (Fig. 4-14). Most investigations on directional sensitivity of periodontal mechanoreceptors have used canine teeth, and the direction of maximal sensitivity is not evenly distributed around these teeth. Although the mechanoreceptors are maximally sensitive in one direction, they will respond to other directional forces as well. For example, mechanoreceptors in the cat canine respond to forces directed over a 300 degree arc (Fig. 4-14). The direction of maximal sensitivity for the majority of periodontal mechanoreceptors lies in a 120 degree arc toward the distolingual direction. The arc of sensitivity is directly dependent on the applied forces and is smaller with lower applied forces. Directional sensitivity is not considered a property of the mechanoreceptive ending itself but rather reflects its location in the periodontal ligament and its relationship to the periodontal fibers. Some periodontal mechanoreceptors have bidirectional sensitivity that is presumably related to the complex collagen arrangement of the periodontal ligament.

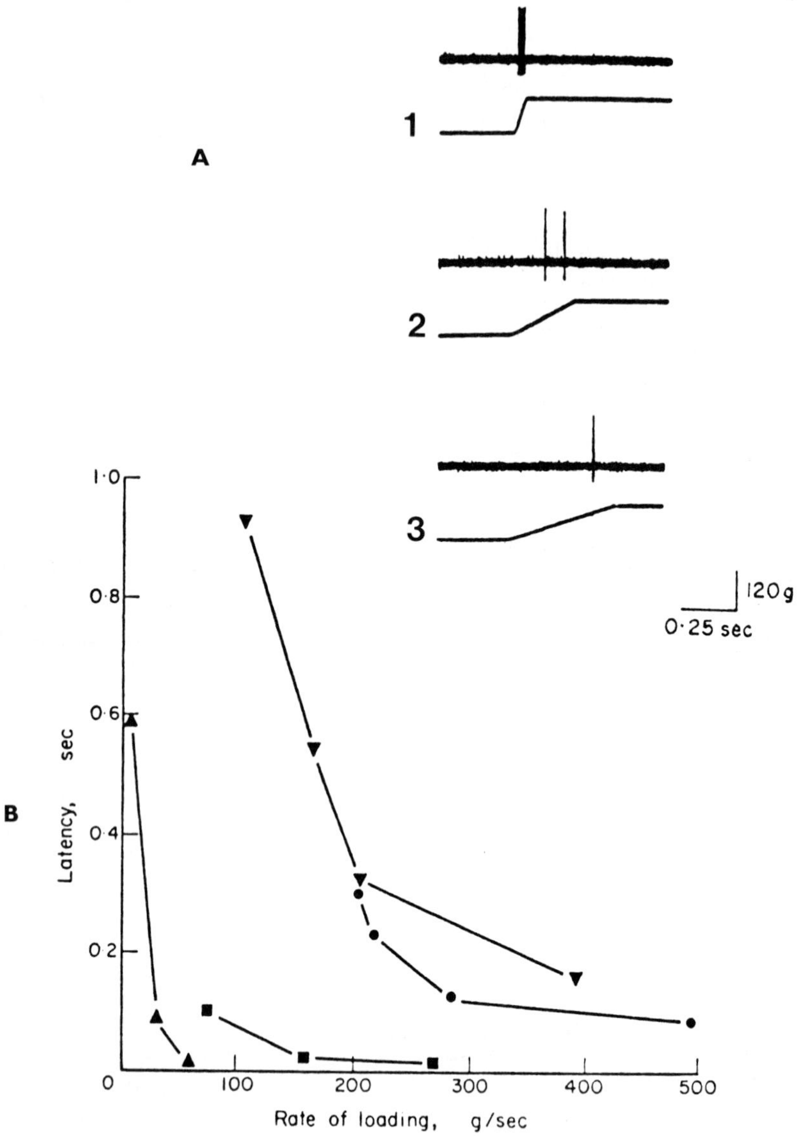

FIG. 4-11
A, Action potentials recorded from a rapidly adapting periodontal ligament receptor to ramp forces applied to a canine tooth, Note that at low rates of stimulus application (*3*) only a single action potential is generated. At higher rates of stimulus application (*1* and *2*), increasing numbers of action potentials are generated. **B**, Latency of response in four rapidly adapting periodontal mechanoreceptors as a function of rate of application of a load to a tooth. (Reprinted from Hannam AG: The response of periodontal mechanoreceptors in the dog to controlled loading of the teeth, *Archives of Oral Biology*, 14: 781-791, copyright © 1969, with permission from Pergamon Press Ltd, Headington Hill Hall, Oxford, UK.)

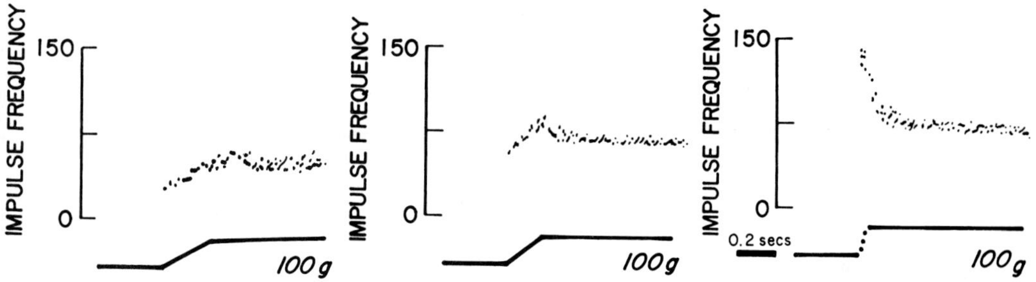

FIG. 4-12
Instantaneous response frequency of a slowly adapting periodontal mechanoreceptor to the same load applied at three different rates. (Reprinted from Hannam, AG: The response of periodontal mechanoreceptors in the dog to controlled loading of the teeth, *Archives of Oral Biology,* 14: 781-791, copyright © 1969, with permission from Pergamon Press Ltd, Headington Hill Hall, Oxford, UK.)

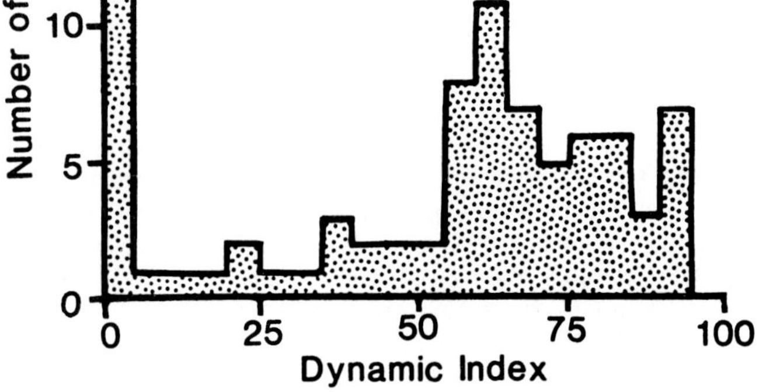

FIG. 4-13
Histogram of dynamic index of 91 periodontal mechanoreceptive afferent fibers. Rapidly adapting (*RA*) receptors with a low dynamic index form a separate peak from slowly adapting (*SA*) units with a high dynamic index. (From Loescher AR, Robinson PP: *Journal of Neurophysiology* 62:971-978, 1989.)

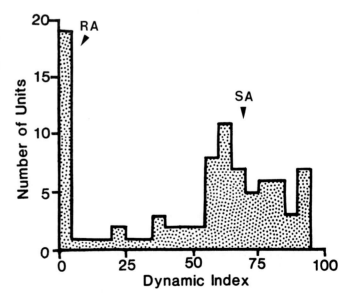

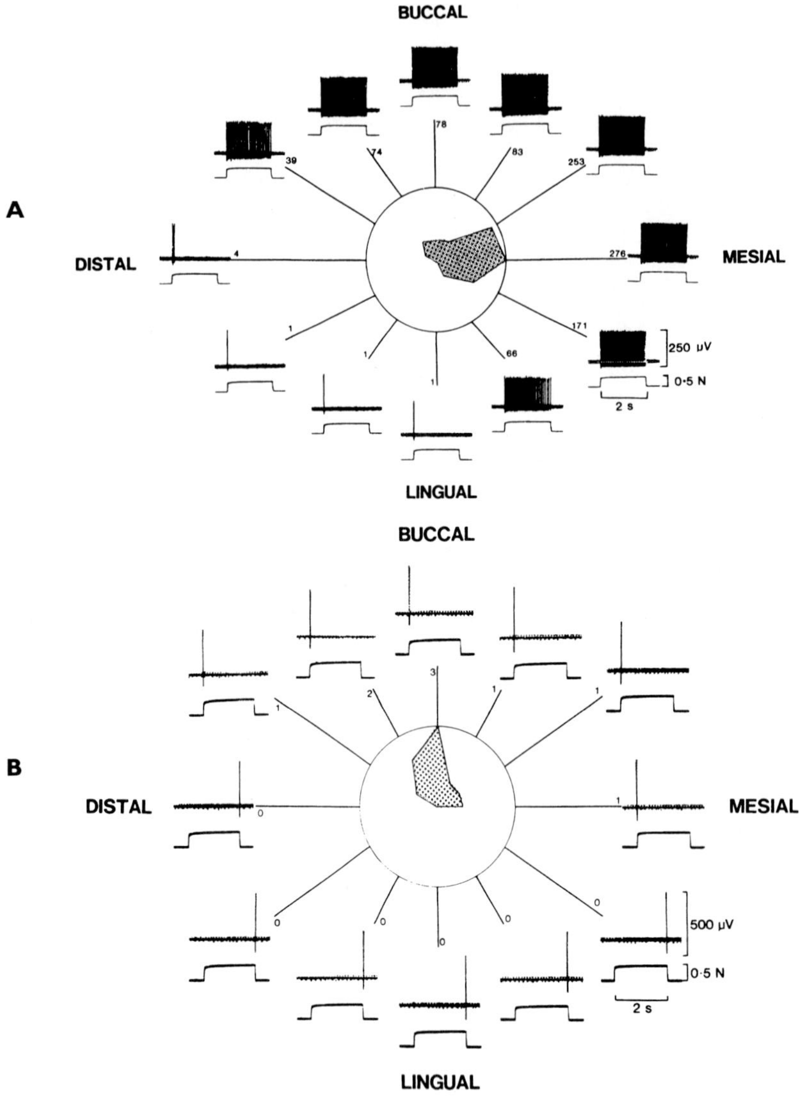

FIG. 4-14
Response of **A**, slowly adapting and **B**, rapidly adapting periodontal mechanoreceptive afferent fibers to the same force applied at 30-degree intervals around the crown of a cat's canine tooth. For each direction of the applied force, the neural response is shown together with the stimulus. The arc of maximum sensitivity is represented by the shaded area in the central circle. The number of action potentials initiated at each angle of stimulation is given at the end of each of the radial lines, (From Loescher AR, Robinson PP: *Journal of Neurophysiology* 62:971-978, 1989.)

Anatomic and electrophysiologic experiments indicate that periodontal mechanoreceptors are located primarily below the tooth fulcrum and concentrated in the apical one third of the tooth (Fig. 4-15). Moreover, RA mechanoreceptors seem to be concentrated near the fulcrum of the tooth, with SA mechanoreceptors occurring more frequently toward the root apex.

The response properties of the SA periodontal mechanoreceptors are similar to SA II Ruffini endings in glabrous skin. In fact, Ruffini endings are the principal mechanoreceptive ending in the periodontal ligament. It is therefore reasonable to assume that SA responses recorded from the periodontal ligament originate in the Ruffini endings. This then raises the question of the identity of the receptor responsible for the RA response.

One suggestion advanced proposes that only one type of periodontal mechanoreceptor may exist, and the location of this receptor in the periodontal ligament is

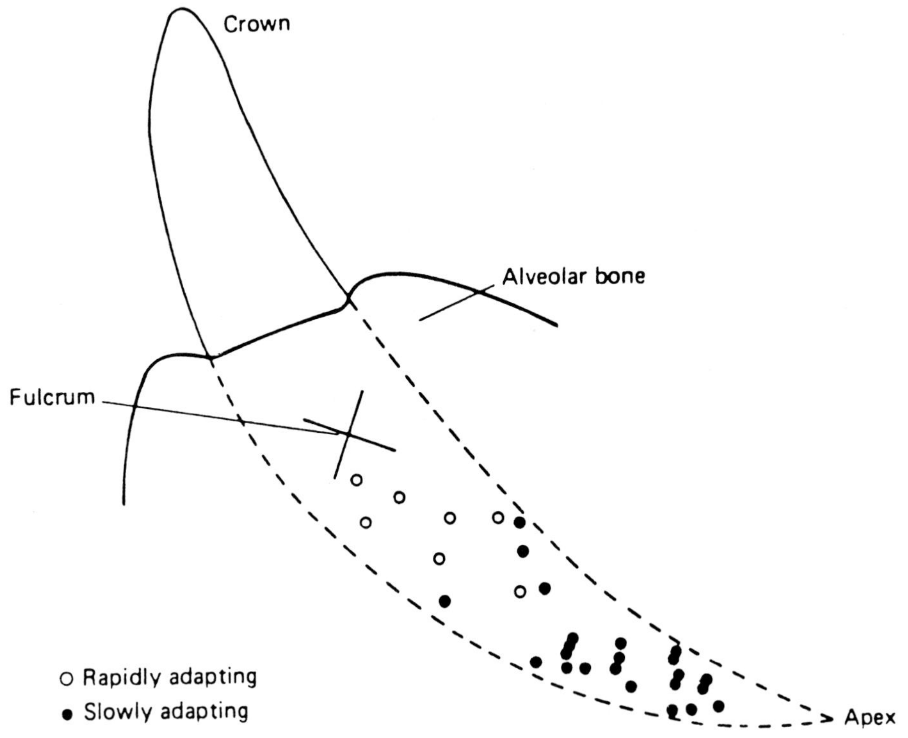

FIG. 4-15
Distribution of rapidly and slowly adapting receptors on the labial surface of the cat canine. (From Cash RM, Linden RWA: *Journal of Physiology* [Lond] 330:439-447, 1982.)

responsible for its adaptation pattern and threshold. If this were the case, receptors situated close to the tooth fulcrum would receive a smaller stimulus for a given applied force to the crown than a similar mechanoreceptor situated at the root apex. The receptor at the fulcrum would appear to have a higher threshold and adapt more rapidly than the root apex receptor. Experimental evidence supporting this proposition is that RA mechanoreceptors are located close to the fulcrum of the tooth (see Fig. 4-15). Furthermore, the observation that RA responses can be elicited from receptors located at the apex by applying a reduced force to the crown supports this hypothesis of only one type of mechanoreceptor, in the periodontal ligament. An alternative explanation is that the different response types relate to the variation in morphology of the Ruffini ending, the more complex morphological type giving rise to one response while the other type of response originates in the simpler receptor ending.

Responses from Human Periodontal Mechanoreceptors

The investigations on periodontal mechanoreceptors have been conducted mostly with animals; however, recordings using the technique of microneurography have been used to record from human periodontal ligament mechanoreceptors (see Box 2-1). Recordings have been made from single afferent fibers located in the alveolar nerve when forces were applied in the lingual, labial, mesial, and distal horizontal plane and in an axial (up and down) direction. Periodontal mechanoreceptors in the human appear to be composed entirely of the SA type, responding with increasing action potential frequencies to increasing magnitudes of stimulation. Also, they are directionally sensitive to forces that are applied in two, three, or four horizontal directions and are responsive to forces applied in an axial direction as well (Fig. 4-16). More than 50% of the human periodontal mechanoreceptive-afferent fibers are spontaneously active and produce action potentials in the absence of any applied load. Some of the afferent fibers respond to stimulation of more than one tooth, possibly because of mechanical coupling between the teeth rather than branching of the single fiber to innervate the periodontal ligament of adjacent teeth. These results of human experiments are similar to those obtained in animals, and indicate that periodontal mechanoreceptors have a similar role in most vertebrates.

Responses of Reinnervated Periodontal Mechanoreceptors

Periodontal mechanoreceptors regenerate after their innervation is interrupted by nerve section or damage (nerve crush or freezing), and mechanoreceptive responses return as early as 6 weeks after injury. However, response characteristics of the regenerated receptors show differences such as reduced arc of sensitivity, reduced maximum response frequencies, and decreased dynamic indices. These response characteristics approximate control recordings as regeneration time increases, but even after a long recovery, the response characteristics do not return

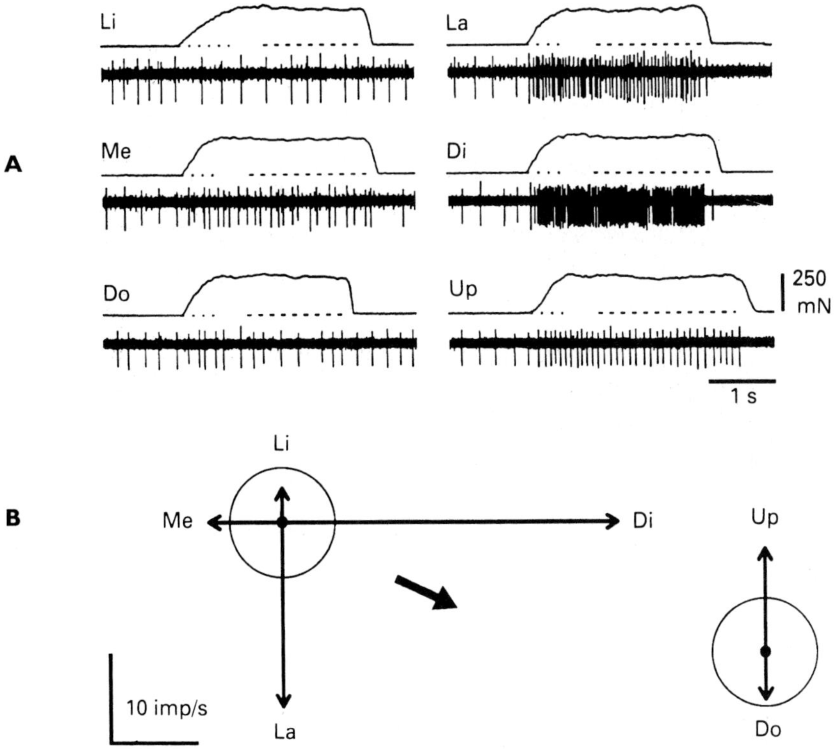

FIG. 4-16
A, Single fiber recordings from human inferior alveolar nerve innervating premolar periodontal mechanoreceptors, showing directional sensitivity to forces applied in the labial (*La*), lingual (*Li*), distal (*Di*), mesial (*Me*), downward (*Do*), and upward (*Up*) directions. **B**, Vectorial representation of the steady state response to stimulation in the horizontal (*left*) and axial (*right*) directions. The length of each vector is proportional to the mean impulse frequency of the response in each direction. (From Trulsson M, Johansson RS, Olsson KÅ: *Journal of Physiology* [Lond] 447:372-389, 1992.)

to normal values. Therefore, even though periodontal receptors regenerate, there is a permanent alteration in their function. This alteration may be caused by either changes in the receptor or changes in the regenerating nerve fibers.

Recordings from Trigeminal Sensory and Mesencephalic Nucleus Neurons

TG periodontal-mechanoreceptive afferent fibers connect with second-order neurons located in the principal and spinal divisions of the trigeminal sensory nucleus. Mesencephalic nucleus periodontal mechanoreceptors (MS) have cell bodies located within the mesencephalic nucleus. This is an exception to the general rule in which cell bodies of afferent fibers are located in a peripheral ganglion (Fig. 4-17). So responses that are recorded from the mesencephalic nucleus periodontal neurons are derived from primary afferent fibers. Those recorded from neurons that receive input from TG periodontal mechanoreceptors have passed through a synapse.

Neurons that synapse with TG periodontal mechanoreceptors are found in the principal sensory nucleus and the subnucleus oralis, interpolaris, and medullary dorsal horn of the spinal trigeminal nucleus (Fig. 4-17). Recordings made form second-order periodontal mechanoreceptive units in the principal and subnucleus oralis during stimulation of the teeth reveal that these neurons are directionally sensitive SA neurons that have receptive fields of single teeth. They, therefore, have similar response properties to primary afferent fibers. In contrast, second-order neurons in the subnucleus interpolaris and the medullary dorsal horn respond to stimulation of more than one tooth indicating convergence of peripheral input to these neurons. Because recordings made from the mesencephalic nucleus are recordings from the cell bodies of primary afferent fibers their responses should be similar to peripheral single-fiber recordings. In fact, recordings made in the mesencephalic nucleus closely resemble peripheral fiber recordings in that they are generally SA responses from single teeth. However, during prolonged application of force to a tooth, mesencephalic periodontal mechanoreceptive neurons are not capable of firing beyond 10 seconds, which has not been reported for peripheral fibers. This may indicate some inhibitory synaptic activity within the trigeminal mesencephalic nucleus.

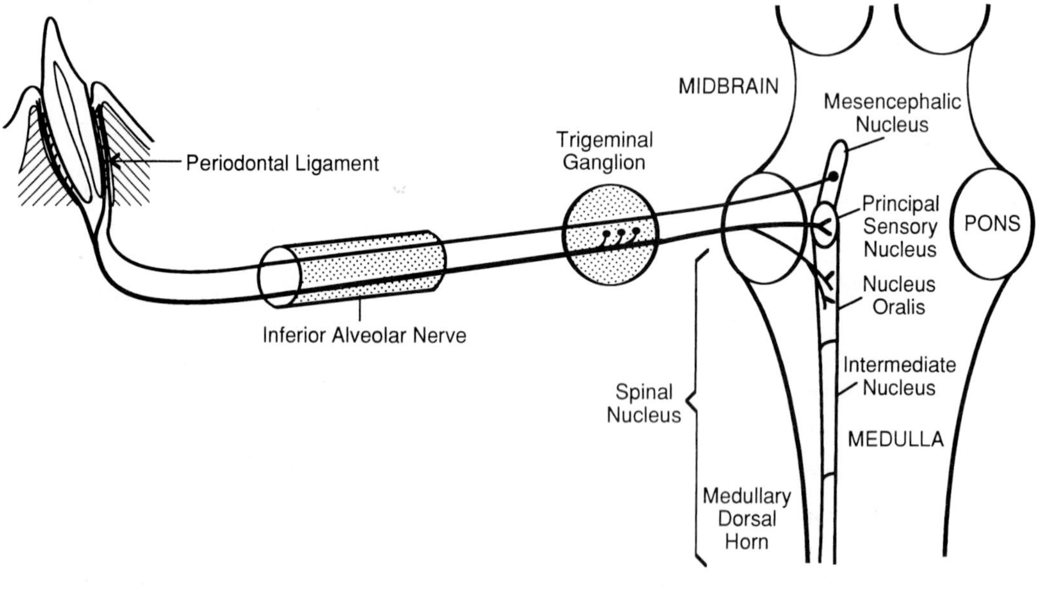

FIG. 4-17
Termination of periodontal primary afferent fibers in the trigeminal sensory nucleus.

Recordings from Thalamus

Responses at the thalamic level to periodontal stimulation are recorded in the ventral posteromedial nucleus. Both RA and SA units are present and responsive to single teeth. Other units that respond to stimulation of two, three, and four quadrants of the dentition are also present. Although some thalamic periodontal neurons are directionally sensitive, others respond to stimulation of the tooth from all directions. As a result, there is considerable difference in response characteristics among peripheral, trigeminal, and thalamic periodontal units, suggesting a convergence of many fibers at the thalamic level.

SUMMARY

Rapidly acting (RA) and slowly adapting (SA) mechanoreceptors can be separated into different groups on the basis of their response to skin indentation and receptive field characteristics. Mechanoreceptors respond to sustained skin indentation either during the application of the stimulus only (rapidly adapting) or during both the application and steady deformation of the receptive field (slowly adapting). RA I and SA I receptors have small, receptive fields with well defined borders, whereas SA II receptors have large, receptive fields with ill defined edges. The different types of receptors correspond with different receptor morphologies that probably subserve different functions in the glabrous skin. Similar types of receptors are found in the skin of the face although RA II receptors are absent.

Mechanoreceptors in the periodontal ligament are all varieties of Ruffini endings. Both RA and SA response types are found by use of electrophysiological recordings. RA receptors are located near the fulcrum of the tooth; SA receptors closer to the apex. Periodontal receptors are directionally sensitive, responding to an arc with a size that depends on the type of tooth and the magnitude of the applied force. A hypothesis suggests that only one type of periodontal mechanoreceptor exists and that the difference in responses is caused by the receptor location in the Periodontal ligament. Receptors that are situated closer to the fulcrum will be less stimulated than those at the tooth apex, when the same force is applied to each group of receptors.

Fibers innervating periodontal ligament mechanoreceptors have their cell bodies either in the trigeminal ganglion or in the mesencephalic nucleus. Mechanoreceptors with cell bodies in the mesencephalic nucleus are concentrated near the tooth apex in comparison with trigeminal ganglion mechanoreceptors that are most numerous near the middle of the root. Recordings from the projection areas of the mesencephalic and trigeminal ganglion periodontal mechanoreceptors reveal differences in response properties.

Periodontal mechanoreceptors regenerate after an interruption of innervation. However, significant differences exist between responses of normal and regenerated periodontal mechanoreceptors.

SELECTED READINGS

Johannsson RS, Vallbo ÅB: Tactile sensory coding in the glabrous skin of the human hand, *Trends in Neuroscience* 6: 27-32, 1983.

Linden RWA: Periodontal mechanoreceptors and their function. In Taylor A, editor: *Neurophysiology of the jaws and teeth*, Basingstoke, 1990, Macmillan.

Loescher AR, Robinson PP: Receptor characteristics of periodontal mechanosensitive units supplying the cat's lower canine, *Journal of Neurophysiology* 62: 971-978, 1989.

5

Kinesthesia

LEARNING OBJECTIVES

At the end of this chapter you should be able to:

1. Name the types of receptors responsible for the senses of movement and position.
2. Describe the morphology of a muscle spindle.
3. Give the functional properties of a muscle spindle.
4. Define the morphology of a Golgi tendon organ.
5. List the functional properties of a Golgi tendon organ.
6. Describe the structure and function of joint receptors.
7. Describe the structure and function of muscle receptors in the muscles controlling the jaws and face.
8. Name the structure and function of temporomandibular joint receptors.

Kinesthesia is the sense of movement and position of limbs and other body parts. In dentistry this is important in sensing jaw movements and position. A number of receptors are responsible for generating the information important in kinesthesia including muscle receptors, joint receptors, and mechanoreceptors in the skin and mucosa (see Chapter 4 for a discussion of mechanoreceptors). Because these receptors respond to stimuli produced from within the body, receptors responsible for kinesthesis are called *proprioceptors* to distinguish them from receptors responding to external stimuli, termed *exteroceptors*.

Until recently it was thought that joint receptors provided the major contribution to kinesthesia. Afferent activity derived from muscle receptors was not considered to reach conscious levels. However, even though joint receptors would seem to be an obvious candidate to signal joint position, electrophysiologic experiments in animals have conclusively demonstrated that most joint receptors respond only to the extremes of the joint angle, and, therefore, joint receptors are probably not the primary kinesthetic detectors. Moreover, when it became possible to replace diseased joints (and thereby remove the joint receptors) in humans, there was no loss in kinesthetic sense. Also, investigators found that vibratory stimuli, when applied to muscle tendons in animals, excited muscle spindle receptors and that this same kind of vibration, applied over human muscle tendons, produced a striking illusion of movement. The conclusion was that not only can impulses from muscle receptors reach conscious levels, but they can also elicit kinesthetic sensations. It is now concluded that muscle receptors do contribute to kinesthesia, whereas joint receptors seem hardly involved at all.

RECEPTORS INVOLVED IN KINESTHESIA

Muscle Spindles

Muscle spindles not only contribute to kinesthesia, but are also important as a sensory feedback system in the control of muscle movements and reflex load compensation. Moreover, the same information provided by muscle spindles may be utilized in diverse ways by various muscle groups and within different species. For example, the function of limb muscle spindles is primarily load compensation; however, extraocular eye muscles contain numerous muscle spindles which are involved mostly in movement control.

Structure

A muscle spindle, as its name implies, is a fusiform structure contained in a capsule that is attached at the poles to either the muscle fibers (extrafusal fibers) or filaments of tendons (Fig. 5-1). Muscle spindles are complex sensory receptors containing a number of structures such as modified muscle fibers with an independent neuromuscular innervation and two types of sensory endings. The spindles have a dual innervation consisting of fibers that carry information from the central nervous sys-

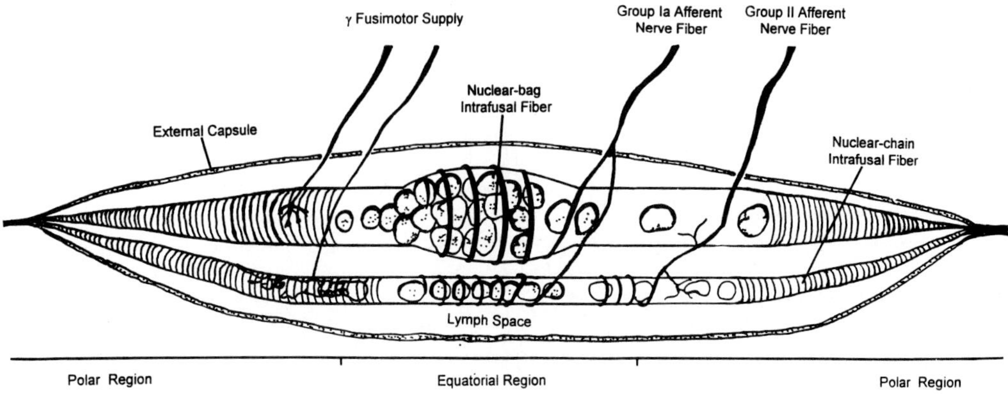

FIG. 5-1
Basic components of mammalian muscle spindle.

tem to the spindle (efferent supply), and a sensory innervation that transmits information from the muscle spindle to the central nervous system (afferent supply). The specialized muscle fibers, or intrafusal fibers, are striated toward the poles of the spindle, but at the equatorial region there is a clear area known as the lymph space. The intrafusal fibers are capable of contracting. The contraction is not initiated by the α motor fibers that produce contraction in extrafusal fibers of the main muscle, but by an independent motor innervation called the γ fusimotor efferent innervation. The sensory terminals provide afferent information to the central nervous system on the length of the muscle spindle.

Intrafusal Fibers

Based on fiber diameter, histochemical staining, and the arrangement of nuclei within the fibers, two major types of intrafusal fibers have been described: nuclear-bag fibers and nuclear-chain fibers (see Fig. 5-1). The nuclei of nuclear bag fibers are concentrated at the equatorial region of the fibers, whereas the nuclei of nuclear chain fibers are distributed along the length of the fibers. The nuclear bag fibers have been subdivided into two types of fibers called bag_1 and bag_2 fibers. A muscle spindle contains 2 to 3 nuclear bag type intrafusal fibers and 4 to 6 nuclear chain intrafusal fibers.

γ Fusimotor Innervation

Three types of motor fibers that innervate the intrafusal fibers have been identified, one terminating in a plate-like arrangement innervated by γ1 fusimotor fibers, one ending in a fine network called trail endings supplied by γ2 fusimotor fibers, and in about one third of the spindles dynamic β axons have been identified (Fig. 5-2). These different types of motor endings can be found innervating both nuclear-bag and nuclear-chain intrafusal fibers. A muscle spindles contains 10 or more γ fusimotor fibers.

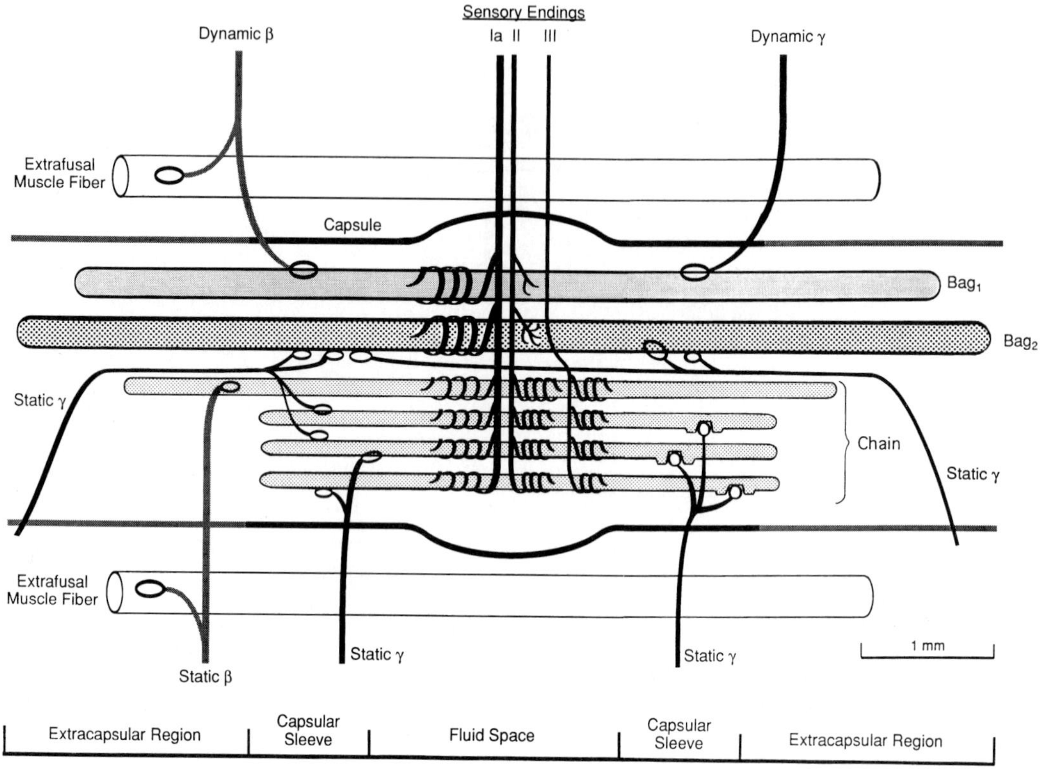

FIG. 5-2
Structure and innervation of a muscle spindle, showing different intrafusal fibers, afferent sensory innervation, and efferent fusimotor innervation. (From Boyd LA: Muscle spindle and stretch reflexes. In Swash M, Kennard C, editors: *Scientific Basis of Clinical Neurology* Edinburgh, 1985, Churchill Livingstone, pp. 74-97.)

Sensory Innervation

Nuclear-bag and nuclear-chain fibers have sensory terminals (annulospiral endings) that spiral around the equatorial region of the intrafusal fibers that are supplied by large-diameter group Ia afferent axons (Fig. 5-2). A second, smaller-diameter afferent (group II) ending found primarily on the nuclear-chain intrafusal fibers terminates laterally to the annulospiral endings. These two sensory terminals are called the primary and secondary endings respectively.

Response Characteristics of Muscle Spindle Sensory Endings. When a muscle spindle is stretched, the primary and secondary afferent sensory endings respond with increasing frequencies of neural discharges. However, the patterns of response recorded from primary and secondary endings differ. In response to a stimulus in which the spindle is stretched and then held at a new length for a time

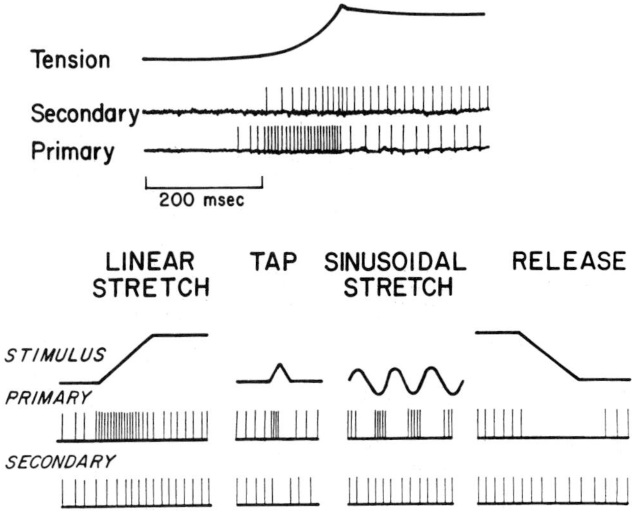

FIG. 5-3
A, Contrasting response of primary and secondary afferent endings of mammalian muscle spindles on application of a rapid stretch. **B**, Comparison of typical responses of primary and secondary endings of mammalian muscle spindles to various kinds of stimuli. (**A** from Matthews PBC: *Mammalian Muscle Receptors and Their Central Actions,* London, 1972, Arnold.) (**B** from Matthews PBC: *Physiology Review* 44:219-288, 1964.)

before being allowed to return to its initial length, the primary endings respond with a marked increase in action-potential frequency that is much greater than the secondary endings during the dynamic stretching phase. Both types of sensory endings usually produce action potentials at a similar rate during the static phase of the stimulus (Fig. 5-3, *A*). It is possible that the difference in relative sensitivity of these two endings to static and dynamic stimuli enables the central nervous system, by comparing discharge patterns, to monitor several conditions of a muscle. For example, muscle spindles provide information on the length of a muscle, whether it is moving or still, and the velocity and direction of any movement. Furthermore, primary endings are more sensitive than secondary endings to release of stretch, sinusoidal stretching, and brief tapping (Fig. 5-3, *B*). Therefore, muscle-spindle afferent endings provide a wealth of information essential to coordination of muscle contraction and provide a fundamental input required for kinesthesia.

Effect of γ Fusimotor Stimulation on Muscle Spindles. When the γ fusimotor supply to a muscle spindle is stimulated, the intrafusal fibers contract. Because the contractile, striated portion of the intrafusal fibers is situated near the poles of the spindle, the contraction stretches the equatorial region containing the sensory endings. Therefore, activation of the γ fusimotor supply increases the discharge fre-

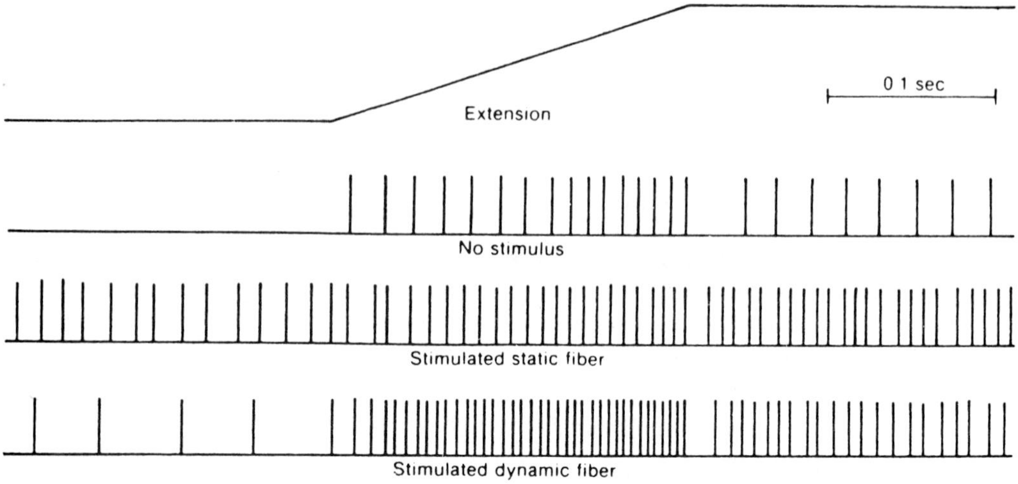

FIG. 5-4
Effects of stimulation of static and dynamic fusimotor supply on the response of spindle primary afferent fibers during muscle spindle stretching. (From Crowe A, Matthews PBC: *Journal of Physiology [Lond]* 174:109-131, 1964.)

quency of the primary and secondary sensory endings. On the basis of the effect of stimulation of the γ efferent innervation during the application of stretch to the spindle, investigators have divided the γ efferent supply into static and dynamic fusimotor supplies. Stimulation of the *static* γ fusimotor supply *reduces* the sensitivity of the primary ending during the dynamic phase of stretching the spindle, whereas stimulation of the *dynamic* γ fusimotor supply *enhances* the sensitivity of the primary ending during the dynamic phase of stretching the spindle (Fig. 5-4).

There are some differences in the patterns of innervation of the static and dynamic γ fusimotor fibers (see Fig. 5-2). Dynamic γ fusimotor fibers innervate bag_1 fibers at one or both poles of the muscle spindle. The dynamic β axon also innervates about one third of the bag_1 fibers and innervates a subset of the extrafusal fibers. Both dynamic β and γ axons have the same action on the muscle spindle, and in combination they have been called the dynamic fusimotor system. Static fusimotor axons innervate both bag_2 and nuclear-chain fibers. Although dynamic and static γ fusimotor fibers are distinguished by their effect on the action potential discharge pattern of the afferent sensory endings (see Fig 5-3), the differences are not an intrinsic property of the fusimotor endings but are apparently caused by the mechanical properties of the intrafusal fiber that they innervate.

Possible Role of γ Fusimotor Supply to Muscle Spindles on Muscle Function. The γ fusimotor supply to a spindle can change both the length of the spindle and the response characteristics of the sensory innervation of the spindle. Therefore, the γ fusimotor innervation is capable of complex control of the muscle spindle and several possible roles have been suggested for this independent motor control.

It has been proposed that fusimotor activity provides a way of maintaining the sensitivity of the spindle during contraction of the surrounding muscle. This can be best understood by considering the output of the spindle sensory endings without γ fusimotor control of the intrafusal fibers. According to this proposition, contraction of the surrounding muscle shortens the spindle. Because this removes tension on the sensory endings, they become silent during contraction. Consequently the central nervous system is deprived of any information on muscle length necessary for control of muscle movement. Synchronized γ fusimotor activity during main muscle contraction therefore maintains tension on the spindle sensory endings and provides sensory output during contraction of the surrounding muscle. The γ fusimotor supply therefore contributes peripheral adjustments for maintaining the constancy of output of the spindle sensory endings. These endings are important in the reflex control of muscle contraction under a wide range of differing conditions.

A second role for the γ fusimotor system was suggested after the discovery of the static and dynamic fusimotor innervation of muscle spindles. It was hypothesized that the major function of the γ fusimotor system was to regulate the responsiveness of the spindle sensory endings to suit the requirements of very different types of muscle activity. Therefore, with the capability to vary its calibration the spindle becomes a much more versatile sensory receptor. This is sometimes called parameter control, because fusimotor activity changes the response parameters of the ending.

Finally, it has been suggested that the sensory output of muscle spindles comprises the input to a servomotor system, which reflexively initiates contraction of the main muscle by way of the stretch reflex. So after γ fusimotor–initiated contraction of the intrafusal fibers, the frequency of discharge of the spindle sensory endings increases. This output, when it reaches the central nervous system, reflexively activates the α motor supply to the main muscle and causes muscle contraction. This mechanism by which the γ fusimotor system results in contraction of extrafusal fibers during the stretch reflex is often called the γ loop.

Recordings from Human Muscle Spindles. Most of the neurophysiologic experiments defining the properties of muscle spindles were conducted in animals either in vivo or in an isolated muscle spindle preparation. Based on the technique of microneurography (see Box 2-1), recordings have been made from human muscle spindles. However, in these experiments the origin of the response must rely on a set of criteria rather than a direct visualization of the receptor. Human muscle spindles have response characteristics similar to those of animals. They respond to stretch and are silenced during muscle shortening. In response to a ramp stretch, human muscle spindles contain both primary and secondary endings (Fig. 5-5).

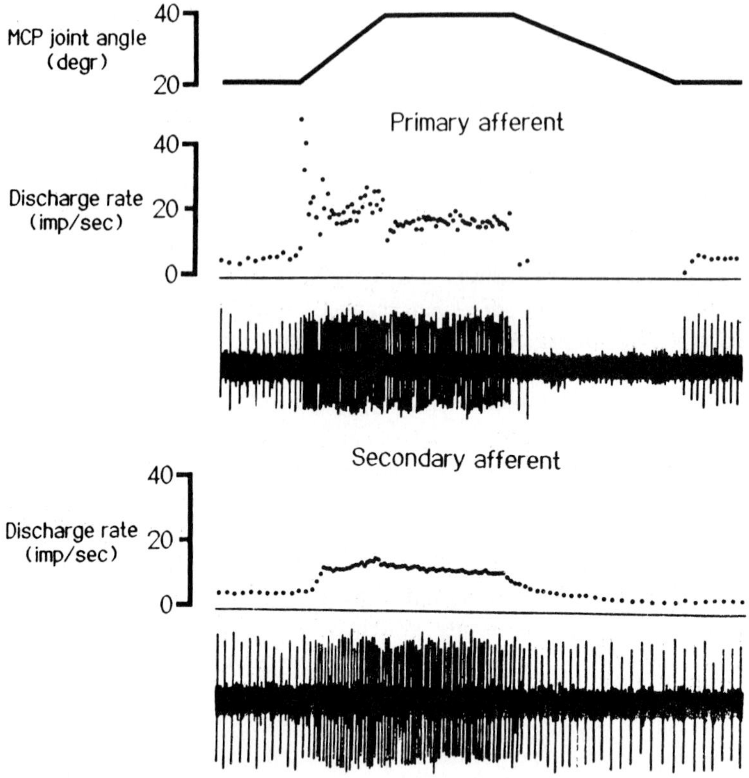

FIG. 5-5
Responses of primary and secondary afferent fibers of human muscle spindles (From Edin BB, Vallbo ÅB: *Journal of Neurophysiology* 63:1297-1306, 1990.)

Golgi Tendon Organs

The Golgi tendon organ consists of a thinly encapsulated bundle of small tendon fascicles with a fusiform (spindle-like) shape, innervated by a single large-diameter group Ib afferent nerve fiber. Fifty or more tendon organs are situated at the junction between a muscle and its tendon in series with a small group of extrafusal muscle fibers (Fig. 5-6). This special anatomical arrangement of a tendon organ at the aponeurotic junction underlies the functional characteristics of these receptors. Because of this arrangement, only a limited number of muscle motor units (the number of muscle fibers innervated by a single α motor neuron) activate a given tendon organ. For example, the cat soleus muscle contains more than 100 motor units, but each tendon organ is activated by only 4 to 15 of these. The extrafusal fibers of the few motor units that activate Golgi tendon organs are directly in series with the receptors.

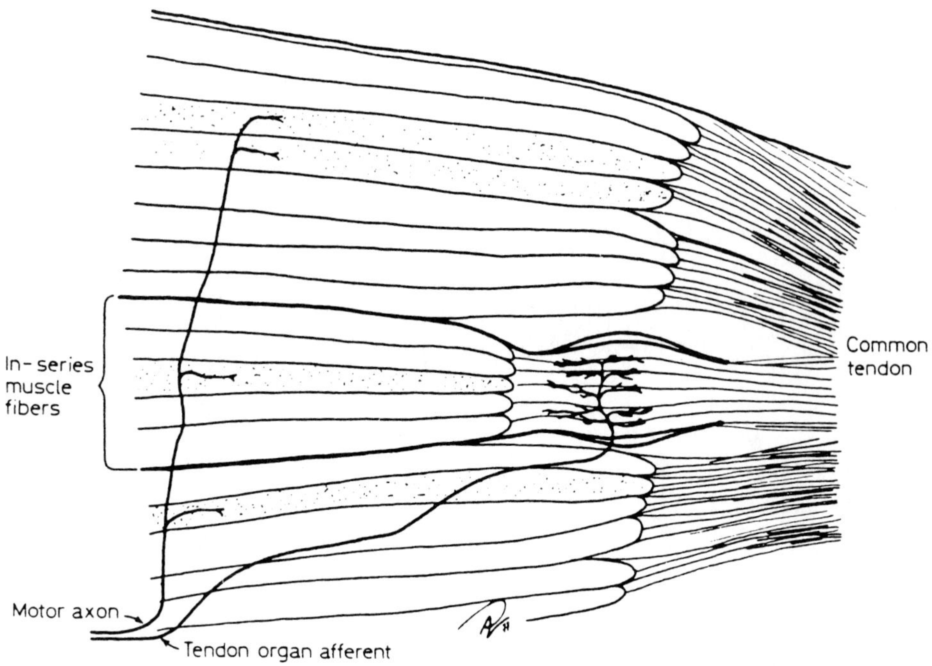

FIG. 5-6
Anatomical relationships between muscle fibers, a motor unit (stippled), and a tendon organ. (From Houk, JC, Crago PE, Rymer WZ: Functional properties of the Golgi tendon organs. In Desmedt JE, editor: *Spinal and Supraspinal Mechanisms of Voluntary Motor Control and Locomotion*, Basel, 1980, Karger, pp 33-43.)

Tendon organs are very sensitive receptors responding to a force of only 30 mg. Tendon organs respond with a steady frequency of action potentials when a single muscle motor unit connected to the tendon organ is activated. Some motor units have only one muscle fiber in series with the tendon organ receptor. If the entire muscle is stretched passively, tendon organs respond weakly. Therefore, the most effective stimulus for tendon organs is the active contraction of a small group of in-series muscle fibers. Because the number of muscle fibers connected in series with a tendon organ represents less than 0.1% of the fibers in a muscle, the response of an individual tendon organ provides limited information on total muscle force.

Recordings made from isolated tendon organs have confirmed their high sensitivity. When tension is applied to the tendon organ, the size of the generator potential (the depolarization of the receptor ending resulting from stimulation) and the frequency of action potential discharge are proportional to the rate of application and to the magnitude of the steady state-applied force (Fig. 5-7). The slope of the relationship between the applied tension and impulse discharge is directly related to the mechanical characteristics or stiffness of the tendon organ, which varies among

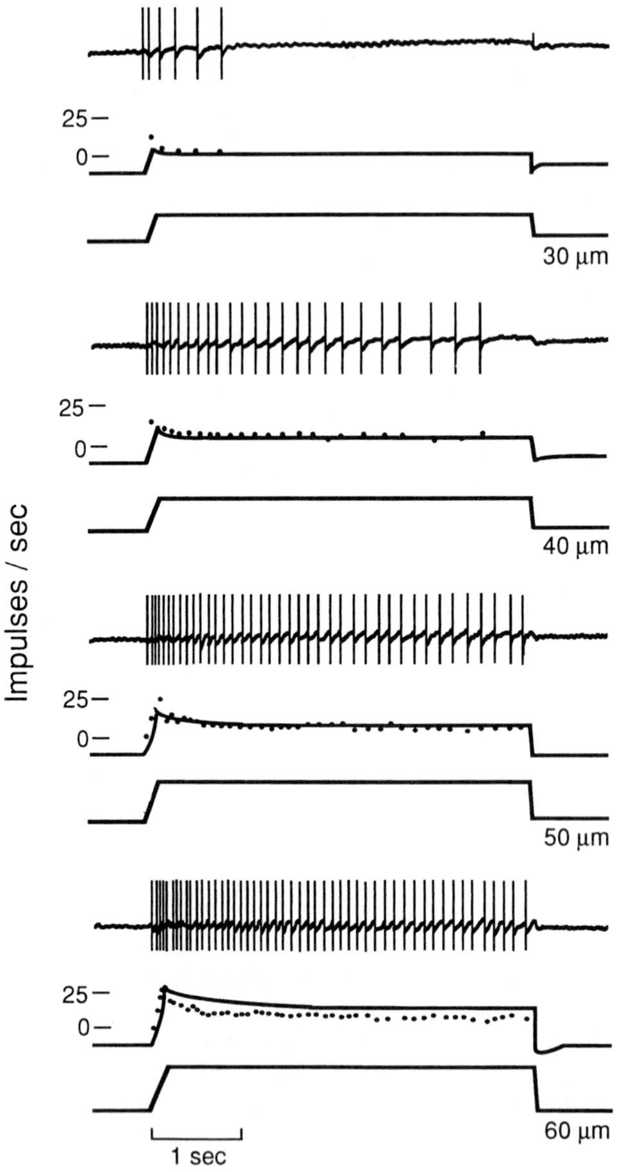

FIG. 5-7
Responses of an isolated tendon organ to different magnitudes of stretch. (From Fukami Y, Wilkinson RS: *Journal of Physiology [London]* 265:673-689, 1977.)

the isolated tendon organs. A tendon organ with low stiffness responds with greater sensitivity to increases in tension than tendon organs with higher stiffness values. This variability of stiffness provides a range of response for the entire population of tendon organ receptors so that during a graded muscle contraction, the afferent discharge from tendon organs increases progressively as more motor units are activated or recruited.

Joint Receptors

The ligaments and capsules of joints contain numerous slowly adapting mechanoreceptors that respond to the stretching of ligaments and the stretching or bending of capsules. In the ligaments, slowly adapting responses arise mainly from Golgi tendon organ-type endings formed by profuse branching of the nerve terminals. In the capsule, slowly adapting response originate from Ruffini-type endings. As previously mentioned, joint receptors mainly respond at extremes of joint rotation and therefore have a minor role in kinesthesia. Only a few responses are encountered at the midposition of the joint, and these responses probably originate in muscle receptors behind the joint—not in the joint itself. However, although joint receptors do not contribute to kinesthesia, they may have other roles. Careful examination of the response of the Ruffini endings of joints suggests that they respond to torque rather than joint angle. Moreover, because joint receptors respond to extremes in joint rotation, they play a protective role, providing a fast mechanism to prevent hyperextension of the joint such as when a person tries to kick a ball and misses.

MUSCLE AND JOINT RECEPTORS IN THE OROFACIAL AREA

Muscle Spindles and Golgi Tendon Organs

Muscle spindles are present in the masseter, temporalis, and medial pterygoid muscles and are therefore found in jaw-elevator, but not depressor, muscles. The spindles are not evenly distributed in the muscles and are concentrated in the deep and anterior parts of the muscles. Jaw muscle spindles are similar to limb muscle spindles, having both primary and secondary endings, a γ-efferent supply, and intrafusal fibers of chain, bag_1, and bag_2 types. Muscle spindles are absent from the tongue in most species but have been reported in primates.

Small numbers of Golgi tendon organs are situated deep in the masseter and temporalis muscles at the point of insertion into the mandible.

Temporomandibular Joint Receptors

The temporomandibular joint is different from other joints in that the condyle not only rotates but also translates jaw movements. Furthermore, because the human mandible is a singular bone, the temporomandibular joints of both sides move together simultaneously but not symmetrically. All the receptor endings found in other joints have been described in the temporomandibular joint of various species. In some animals, such as the mouse, only free nerve endings are found in the joint, other types of sensory ending being absent. There are, therefore, significant species differences in the innervation of the temporomandibular joint.

Central Connections of Orofacial Muscle and Joint Receptors

The cell bodies of the afferent innervation of muscle spindles in the jaw muscles are located in the trigeminal mesencephalic nucleus. Neurons innervating the muscle spindles are multipolar, with a complex dendritic tree. If the spindles are stimulated by stretching the jaw muscles, both rapidly adapting and slowly adapting responses are recorded in the mesencephalic nucleus. Because these are recordings from primary afferent fibers these response patterns either originate in the sensory endings of the jaw muscle spindles, or result from reflex synaptic modulation of the spindle input within the mesencephalic nucleus.

The cell bodies of the afferent innervation of the temporomandibular joint are in the posterolateral part of the trigeminal ganglion. The central processes of these neurons are distributed to all parts of the sensory trigeminal nucleus with the greatest density in the main sensory nucleus. Electrophysiologic recordings from either the trigeminal ganglion or the auriculotemporal nerve have shown responses to the rotation of the temporomandibular joint. Both slowly adapting and rapidly adapting responses have been reported.

SUMMARY

The sense of movement, or kinesthesia, is derived from muscle spindles, Golgi tendon organs, and cutaneous mechanoreceptors. Joint receptors are not a significant factor in kinesthesia.

Muscle spindles are complex sensory organs containing specialized muscle fibers, sensory endings, and a specialized motor innervation. Afferent sensory information derived from muscle spindles reaches conscious levels and is important in the control of muscle length. Golgi tendon organs are found at the junction of a muscle and its tendon, and are associated with relatively few motor units within a muscle. Golgi tendon organs are important in the control of muscle tension. Joint receptors are found in the ligament and capsule of the joint, respond to extremes of joint rotation, and may be important in preventing overflexion of the joint.

In the orofacial area, muscle spindles are found only in jaw elevator muscles, not in jaw depressor muscles. Only a few Golgi tendon organs have been described in jaw muscles. Joint receptors are associated with the temporomandibular joint.

SELECTED READINGS

Appenteng K: Jaw muscle spindles and their central connections. In Taylor A, editor: *Neurophysiology of the jaws and teeth*, Basingstoke, 1990, Macmillan.

Boyd IA: Muscle spindle and stretch reflexes. In Swash M and Kennard C, editors: *Scientific basis of clinical neurology*, Edinburgh, 1985, Churchill Livingstone.

Boyd IA and Gladden MH, editors: *The muscle spindle*, New York, 1985, Stockton Press.

Clark, FJ and Horch KW: Kinesthesia. In Boff KR and other, editors: *Handbook of perception and human performance, vol 1 Sensory Processes and Perception*, New York, 1986, John Wiley.

Houk JC, Crago PE and Rymer WZ: Functional properties of the Golgi tendon organs. In Desmedt JE, editor: *Spinal and supraspinal mechanisms of voluntary motor control and locomotion*, Basel, 1980, Karger.

Prochazka A and Hulliger M: Muscle function and its significance for motor control mechanisms during voluntary movements in cat, monkey, and man. In Desmedt JE, editor: *Motor control mechanisms in health and disease*, New York, 1983, Raven Press.

Proske U: The Golgi tendon organ, *Trends in Neuroscience* 2: 7-8, 1979.

6 Taste

LEARNING OBJECTIVES

At the end of this chapter you should be able to:

1. List the distribution of taste buds in the oropharynx and larynx.
2. List the characteristic features of a taste bud.
3. Describe the turnover of taste buds.
4. Describe the regenerative properties of taste buds.
5. Define the dependence of taste buds on their nerve supply.
6. Identify the various stages of transduction in taste receptors.
7. Name the four taste qualities.
8. State how taste bud cells respond to the four taste qualities.
9. Describe the response properties of afferent taste fibers.
10. Name the processes involved in neural coding in taste.

11. List the receptive field properties of afferent taste fibers.
12. Name the central terminations of afferent chemosensory fibers in the central nervous system.
13. Describe the structure and function of the nucleus tractus solitarius.
14. Describe the structure and function of the pontine taste relay nucleus.
15. Define the ascending neural pathways that transmit taste information to thalamus and cortex.
16. Name the ascending neural pathways that transmit taste information to other forebrain areas.
17. Identify the changes that take place in the taste system during development and aging.
18. Define the role of saliva in taste function.
19. List the etiology of disorders of the chemosenses.

All animals possess receptors that respond to environmental chemicals that signal the presence of food, a mate, or hazardous conditions. Single-cell animals such as bacteria have surface chemoreceptors sensitive to a variety of chemicals. Invertebrate chemosensitivity is based on discrete chemosensory organs contained in special appendages. For example, chemoreceptors in the leg hairs of many insects detect chemicals in the surface on which they are standing.

In most air-breathing vertebrates, chemosensitivity is divided into a contact chemical sense called taste and a distance chemical sense called smell. In taste, chemicals in solution are brought into contact with the chemoreceptors; in olfaction, the chemicals are carried to the chemoreceptors as a vapor in the inspired air. Although taste and smell are chemosenses, they have surprisingly little else in common. Receptor structure and function and central processing are entirely different for the two senses. The mammalian taste system consists of taste buds situated in the oropharynx and larynx that have afferent fibers projecting to relay nuclei in the medulla, pons, and thalamus. In contrast, the olfactory receptors are situated in the nasal cavity and have connections to a specialized structure called the olfactory bulb, with projections to the telencephalon referred to as the primary olfactory cortex.

TASTE RECEPTORS

Mammalian taste buds are widely distributed throughout the oral cavity pharynx and larynx (Table 6-1). Most lingual taste buds are confined to the dorsal and lateral borders of the tongue and are associated with specialized structures called papillae. There are four main types of tongue papillae: the filiform, fungiform, circumvallate, and foliate (Fig. 6-1). The most numerous are the filiform, located over the anterior and posterior tongue dorsum, which do not contain taste buds and therefore have no gustatory function. The fungiform papillae contain one or more taste buds on their upper surface and are confined to the anterior two thirds of the tongue. There are large numbers of fungiform papillae, about 200 in the human, for example.

TABLE 6-1
Quantitative Distribution of Taste Buds in Various Mammals

Species	Number	Percentage	Species	Number	Percentage
Rat[a]			**Cat**[c]		
Fungiform	185	12	Fungiform	2735	100
Foliate	460	30	**Monkey**[d]		
Circumvallate	467	30	Fungiform	1296	16
Nasoincisor ducts	67	4	Foliate	4296	50
Soft palate	54	10	Circumvallate	2896	35
Buccal wall	46	3	**Cow**[e]		
Sublingual organ	34	2	Fungiform	1707	9
Epiglottis	42	9	Circumvallate	16519	91
Hamster[b]			**Sheep**[f]		
Fungiform	130	18	Fungiform	2635	50
Foliate	230	32	Epiglottis	3000	50
Circumvallate	168	23	**Human**[g]		
Nasoincisor ducts	12	2	Fungiform	2635	50
Soft palate	88	12	Foliate	1279	16
Buccal wall	10	1	Circumvallate	2440	31
Sublingual organ	5	1	Nasoincisor ducts	0	0
Epiglottis	80	11	Soft palate	419	5
			Epiglottis	2164	27

a. Miller IJ: Gustatory receptors of the palate. In Katsuki Y and others: *Food intake and the chemical senses*, Tokyo, 1977, University of Tokyo Press.

Iida M, Yoshioka I, and Muto H: Taste bud papillae on the retromolar mucosa of the rat, mouse and golden hamster, *Acta Anat.* 117: 374-381, 1983.

Travers SP and Nicklas K: Taste bud distribution in the rat pharanx and larynx, *Anat. Rec.* 227: 373-379, 1990.

b. Miller IJ and Smith DV: Quantitative taste bud distribution in the hamster, *Physiol. Behav.* 32: 275-285, 1984.

c. Robinson PP and Winkles PA: Quantitative study of fungiform papillae and taste buds on the cats tongue, *Anat. Rec.* 225: 108-111, 1990.

d. Bradley RM, Stedman HM and Mistretta CM: Age does not affect taste buds and papillae in adult rhesus monkeys, *Anat. Rec.* 212: 246-249, 1985.

e. Davies RO, Kare MR, and Kagan RH: Distribution of taste buds on fungiform and circumvallate papillae of bovine tongue, *Anat. Rec.* 195: 443-446, 1976.

f. Bradley RM, Cheal ML, and Kim YH: Quantitative analysis of developing epiglottal taste buds in sheep, *J. Anat.* 130: 25-32, 1980.

Mistretta CM, Gurkan S, and Bradley RM: Morphology of chorda tympani fiber receptive fields and proposed neural rearrangements during development, *J. Neuroscience* 8: 73-78, 1988.

g. Human data from a table in Travers SP and Nicklas K: Taste bud distribution in the rat pharynx and larynx, *Anat. Rec.* 227: 373-379, 1990, and is based on estimates form several sources in the literature.

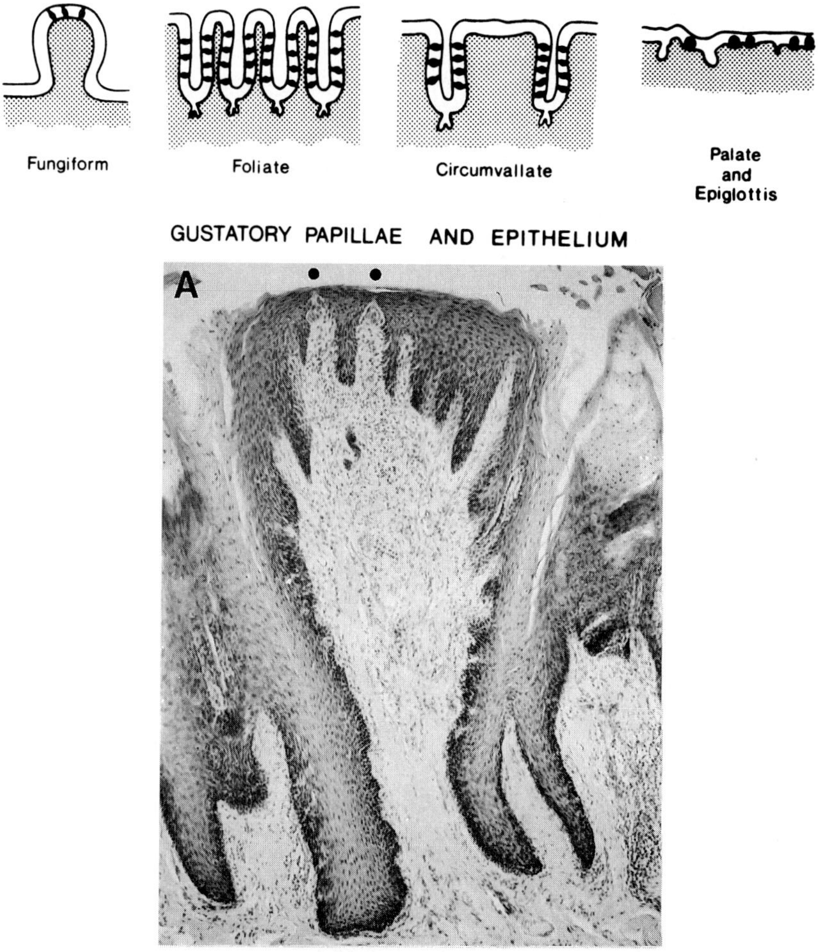

FIG. 6-1
Top, Location of taste buds in the fungiform, foliate, and circumvallate papillae as well as in the epithelium of the soft palate and epiglottis. Light micrographs of fungiform, circumvallate, and foliate papillae from rhesus monkey tongue to illustrate distribution of taste buds. **A**, Sagittal section through a fungiform papilla with two taste buds on its dorsum (×63). *Overleaf*, **B**, Circumvallate papilla sectioned parallel to the surface of the tongue, illustrating numerous taste buds in the papilla wall (×40). **C**, Cross section through clefts of a foliate papilla, illustrating numerous taste buds in the epithelium of the cleft wall (×40). (From Bradley RM, Stedman HM, Mistretta CM: A quantitative study of lingual taste buds and papillae in the aging rhesus monkey tongue. In Davis RT, Leathers CW, editors: *Behavior and Pathology of Aging Rhesus Monkeys*. New York, 1985, Alan Liss. pp. 197-199, Copyright © 1985, Reprinted by permission of Wiley-Liss, a division of John Wiley & Sons, Inc.)

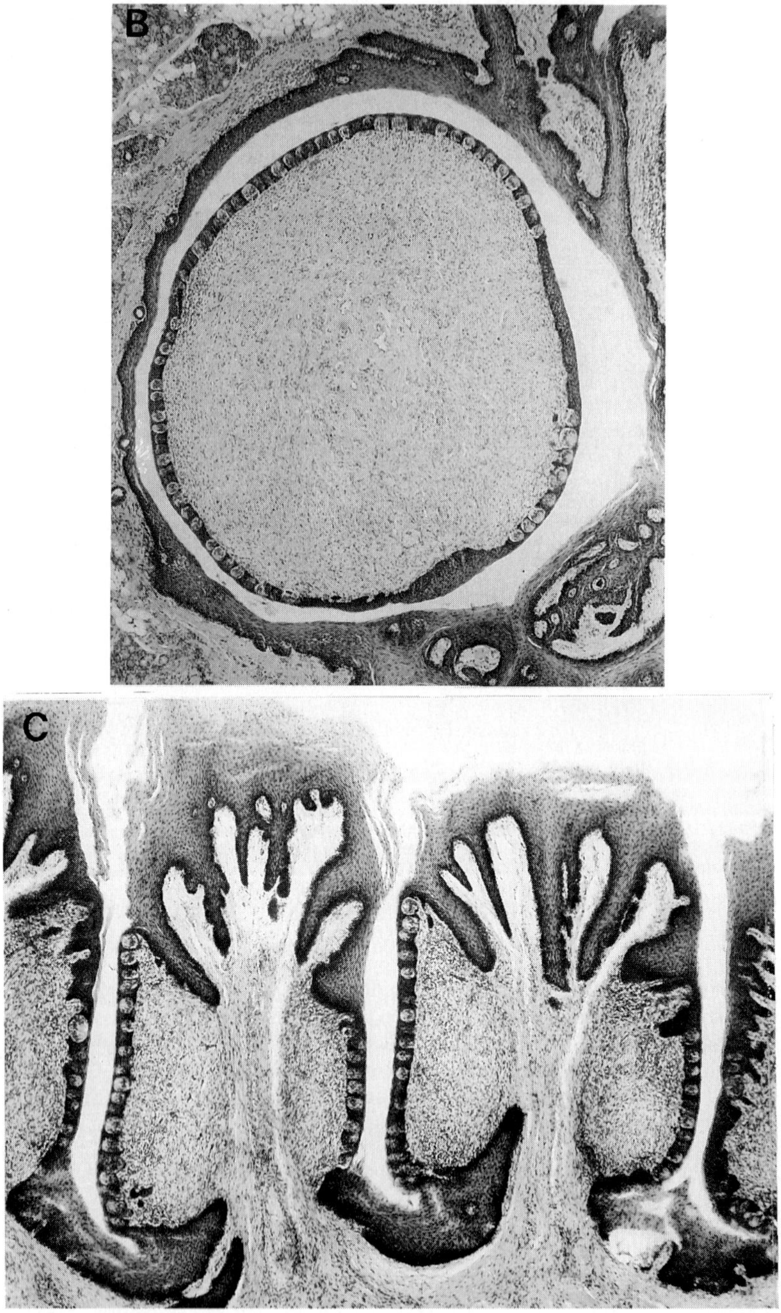
B
C

The circumvallate papillae are found at the junction of the oral and pharyngeal parts of the tongue. Taste buds are located on the sides of the papillae and sometimes in the wall surrounding the papillae. Species differ in the number of these papillae, the rat having a single, centrally placed papilla whereas other animals can have 30 or more. Humans have 8 to 12 circumvallate papillae arranged in a chevron.

The foliate papillae, found on the posterior, lateral border of the tongue, consist of a series of folds forming clefts in the tongue surface. Taste buds are found in the epithelium of the cleft walls. Some mammals, such as sheep, have no foliate papillae but have more circumvallate papillae.

Not all taste buds are confined to the tongue. Significant numbers of them are found on the palate and larynx. In these locations the taste buds are not contained on specialized papillae but are distributed in the surface epithelium.

Counts of taste buds have revealed wide variation in the total numbers present in different species (see Table 6-1). This may be because species differences in surface area of the oropharynx and larynx impose different limits on the packing density of taste buds. Fungiform taste buds have been extensively studied because it is relatively easy to stimulate the anterior tongue and record from the chorda tympani branch of the facial nerve. However, the major gustatory input from the tongue, originating in taste buds contained in papillae innervated by the glossopharyngeal nerve, has been the least studied. Only recently have investigators begun to study the response properties of extralingual taste buds.

Structure

Taste buds are goblet-shaped structures spanning the depth of the epithelium in which they are situated. Each bud consists of about 50 spindle-shaped, modified, epithelial cells that extend from the basement membrane to the epithelial surface. At the epithelial surface the tapered apical ends of the taste buds are in contact with the fluid environment of the oropharynx and larynx through a narrow channel called the taste pore. Terminal branches of gustatory nerve fibers enter the taste bud at its base and distribute among the taste cells (Fig. 6-2). Synaptic transmission occurs between the taste bud cells and gustatory nerve terminals.

Ultrastructural examination of taste buds has revealed that they contain a number of different cell types based on morphological features. Not all cells can be unequivocally categorized, possibly because the different cell shapes observed in a fixed specimen represent various stages in the life cycle of a single cell type.

There is a consistency in the classification of cell types, despite this limitation on interpretation of taste bud cell morphology, variations in histological techniques, and the use of taste buds in different papillae and species. The most frequently encountered taste bud cells, Type I cells, are long and narrow, extending from the base of the taste bud to the taste pore; they compose approximately 60% of the total cell population. These electron-dense cells (sometimes called dark cells) are characterized by large, dense-cored vesicles in the apical cytoplasm as well as deeply-

A

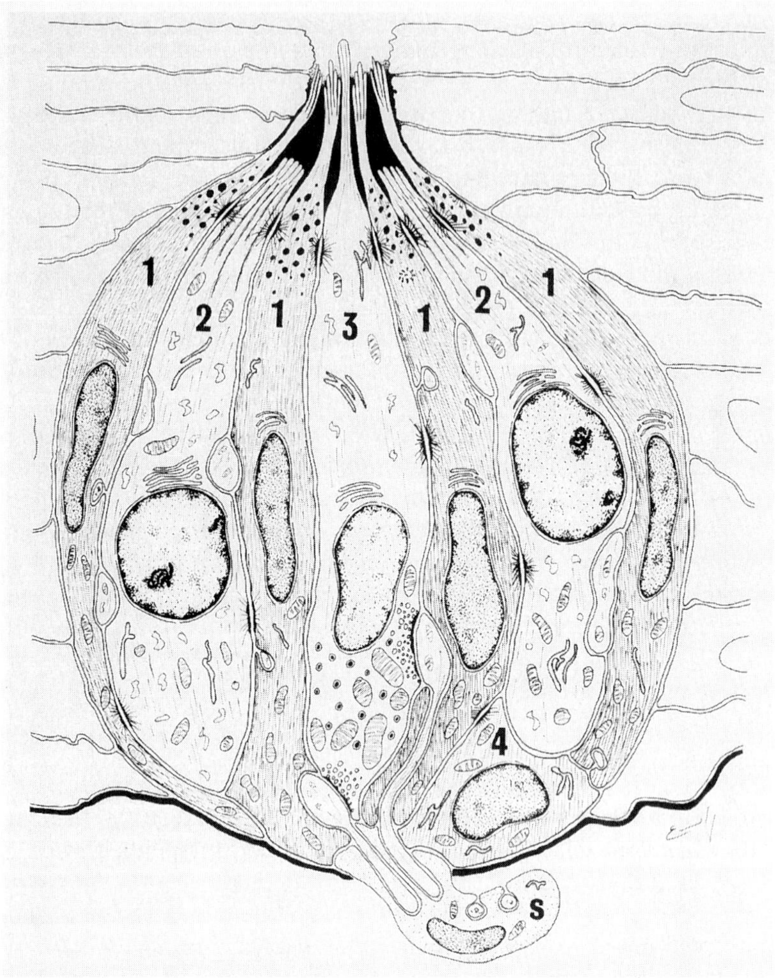

FIG. 6-2
A, Sagittal section of a taste bud from a rabbit foliate papilla, showing the taste pore with apical specialization of taste bud cells. Different cell types are indicated by numbers. A nerve bundle covered in a Schwann cell enters the taste bud at the basal end. Nerve fibers within the taste bud pass between the taste bud cells, making synapses. (From Murray RG: *Journal of Ultrastructure and Molecular Structure Research* 95:175-188, 1986.)

indented, irregularly shaped nuclei. Type II cells (often referred to as light cells) also extend from the basement membrane to the taste pore, but they are characterized by electron-lucent cytoplasm and large, round or oval nuclei. These cells are less numerous than Type I cells, composing about 30% of the population. Type III cells also have apical specializations that extend into the taste pore and are similar in morphology to Type II cells. However, these cells are infrequently encountered in the taste bud and contain numerous dense-cored vesicles concentrated in the basal portion of the cell. The Type IV cell contacts the basement membrane, but, unlike

B

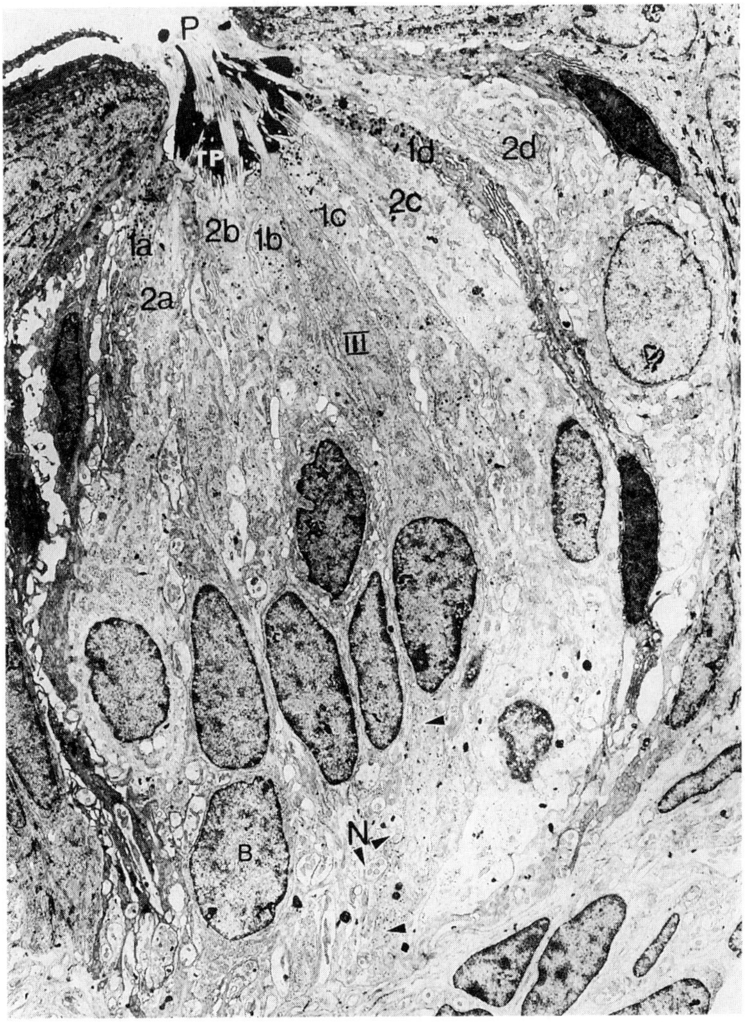

FIG. 6-2–CONT'D
B, Electron micrograph of a cross section through a rabbit foliate pappila taste bud. Type *I* cells (*Ia*, *Ib*, *Ic*, and *Id*) are identified by the dark granules in their apical ends. Type II cells (*2a*, *2b*, *2c* and *2d*) have lighter staining cytoplasm and no dark apical granules. A Type III cell (III) is shown in the center of the bud. Apical ends of Type I, II, and III cells have specialized structural ending in the taste pore (*P*). Cross sections of several nerve fibers (N) can be seen at the basal end of bud as well as a basal (*B*) or Type IV cell (×5000).

the other cells in the taste bud, does not extend to the taste pore; it is most often called a basal cell.

The initial contact between the taste stimuli and taste receptors takes place in the taste pore. Tight junctions join the apices of the taste bud cells at the base of the pore, effectively separating the external environment of the oral cavity and the internal environment below the tight junctions of the taste bud. Each of the three types of taste bud cells that extend into the taste pore has a different apical structure. Type I cells have long, finger-like microvilli that arise from a short neck. Type II cells have shorter microvilli, and Type III cells end in a blunt, club-shaped structure (Fig. 6-2, *B*).

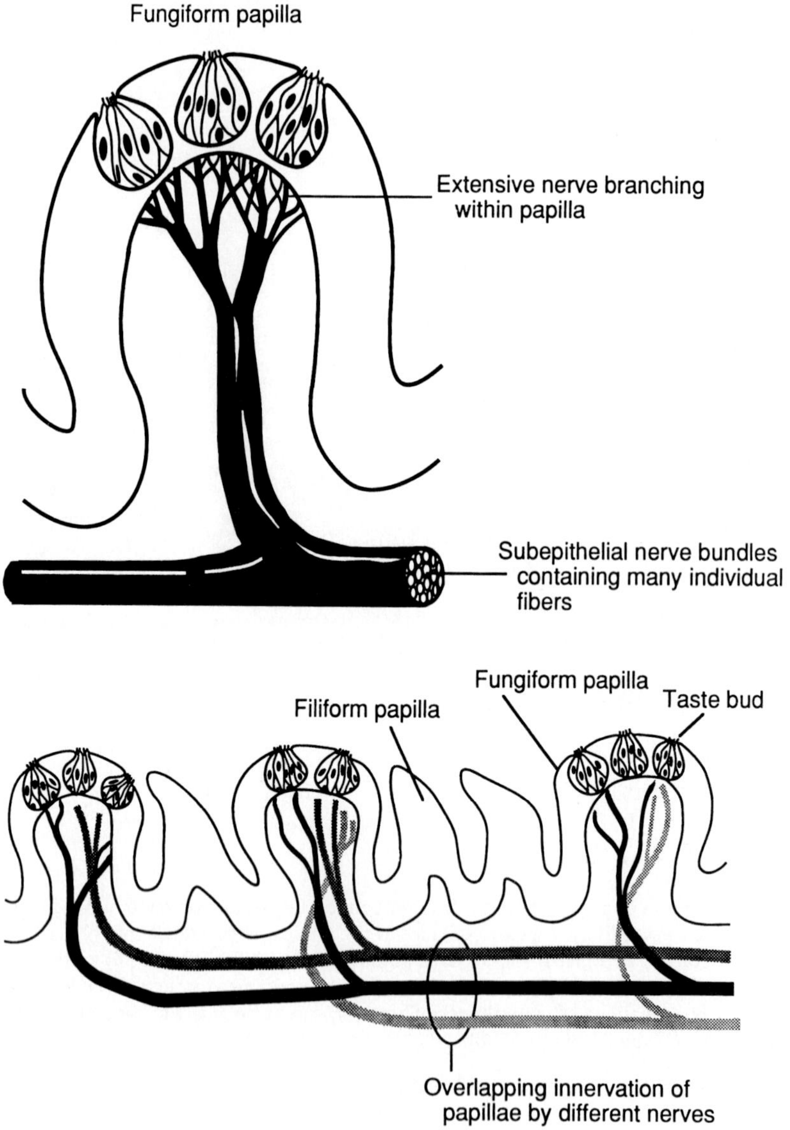

FIG. 6-3
Top, Innervation of a fungiform papilla. Multiple branching of fibers in the core of the papilla. *Bottom*, Distribution of three single fibers to fungiform papillae with overlap of receptive fields.

Nerve fibers enter the taste bud by penetrating the basal lamina. Within the taste bud the nerve processes branch, widen, then narrow again, and are often in contact with other nerve processes. In counts made of nerve fiber profiles in taste bud cross sections, about 50 fibers enter the taste bud, and increase to more than 200 fibers within the bud, indicating extensive branching (Fig. 6-3). These nerve fibers make ill-defined contacts with the taste bud cells, and relatively few typical synapses have been reported. The primitive nature of the contact between taste cell nerve terminals is possibly because of the short life span of taste cells, requiring a very transient form of synaptic contact. The scarcity of classical synapses may also indicate that taste cells communicate with afferent taste fibers by transmembrane transport of amino acid transmitters instead of release of synaptic vesicles. Synapses have been observed on Types I, II, and III cells in the taste bud; this observation suggests that any or all three types could act as the chemoreceptor transduction cell.

Dynamic properties of taste buds

Taste bud cells, like surrounding epithelial cells, are rapidly replaced. When the turnover of taste buds is studied with autoradiographic techniques, the basal cells of

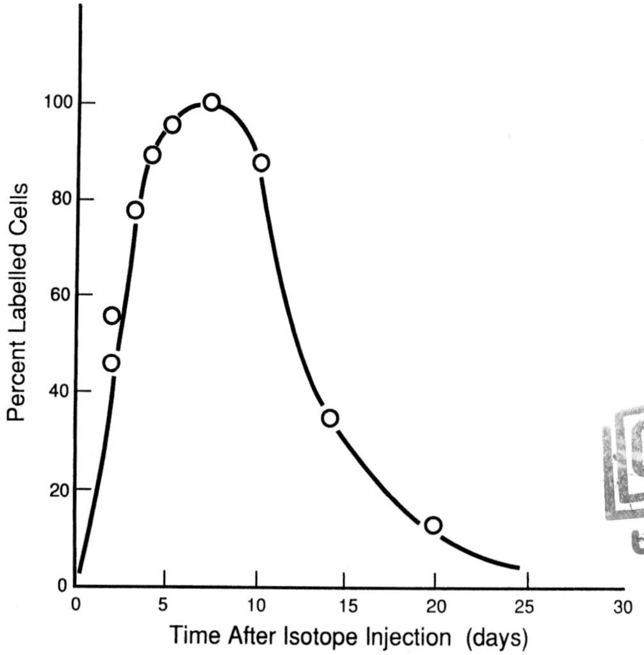

FIG. 6-4
Number of labeled cells in a taste bud after an injection of tritiated thymidine at time 0. Number of labeled cells increases to a maximum at approximately 7 days and then declines. (Data from Conger AD, Wells MA: *Radiation Research* 37:31-49, 1969.)

the taste bud are first labeled, followed by the Type I cells and then by Types III and II cells, suggesting that these cell types are transitional forms of a single cell line. The half-life of a taste bud cell is approximately 10 days (Fig. 6-4). Studies of taste bud turnover also reveal that during turnover taste cells migrate, or move from the periphery to the center of the bud.

This dynamic property of taste receptors poses questions about the relationship of the innervating nerve terminals to the taste bud cells, because the cells migrate from the periphery to the center of the taste bud during their life cycle. One possibility is that taste bud cells are passed along from one set of nerve endings to another during migration. However, it is just as conceivable that a fiber, once it connects with a taste cell at the periphery of the taste bud, will remain with that cell for the life of the taste cell and then retract to connect with another newly formed taste cell at the periphery of the taste bud.

The relationship of a nerve fiber to a migrating taste cell could have significant implications for the response stability of an afferent taste fiber, because the response properties of a taste cell could alter during its life. If fibers connect and reconnect during migration, the response of the afferent fibers would remain stable. On the other hand, if the nerve fibers remain attached with a taste bud cell for its life, the response of a single afferent fiber could potentially change with time. Until techniques to examine the response properties of afferent taste fibers over time are available, the peripheral mechanism responsible for stability of the response of taste receptors will remain unknown.

Another dynamic property of taste buds is their ability to regenerate. Transection of a gustatory nerve results in disappearance of the taste buds innervated by that nerve. Taste buds reappear once the nerve regenerates and reaches the epithelium. Only gustatory nerves promote regeneration of taste buds. When the proximal stumps of cut taste nerves are sutured to the central cut ends of nongustatory nerves, taste buds do not reform. By cross-union it is possible to cause the glossopharyngeal nerve, which normally innervates posterior tongue taste buds, to innervate and promote regeneration of anterior tongue taste buds normally supplied by the chorda tympani nerve. The opposite is also true. It is even possible for the branch of the glossopharyngeal nerve that innervates the carotid body (a chemoreceptor sensitive to blood gas levels) to support reinnervation of taste buds. These and many other experiments support the hypothesis that sensory axons innervating chemoreceptors secrete a substance, called a trophic substance, that causes epithelial basal cells to differentiate into taste bud cells rather than into stratified squamous epithelial cells.

Regardless of the source of reinnervation, regenerated taste buds are functional and exhibit neural responses to chemical stimulation of their receptive fields. Moreover, after cross-nerve regeneration, response characteristics of the receptive field are identical to those recorded from the normal neural innervation; so the response properties of a particular taste nerve are determined by the receptors that it innervates, and are not inherent characteristics of the sensory innervation.

Receptor mechanisms

In the early 1960s, intracellular recording techniques were used to study receptor mechanisms in taste buds (Box 6-1). Because mammalian taste buds are surrounded by a tough, keratinized epithelium, penetration of the taste cells with glass microelectrodes was made through the taste pore. Because it is not easy to see taste pores in live tongues, the number of successful penetrations was limited in these early studies. Furthermore, taste stimuli interact with the receptor membranes through the taste pore, so that if the seal between the microelectrode and the taste cell membrane is not tight, taste stimuli can leak into the cells, making these experiments vulnerable to artifacts. Because of these and other technical difficulties, investigators interested in taste receptor mechanisms began to use other species, particularly the frog, which has a different type of taste bud. More recently, other investigators have used the mudpuppy taste bud because the cells in this animal are particularly large, permitting stable intracellular penetrations. While these investigations have provided valuable insights into taste receptor mechanisms they also have certain disadvantages. Compared with our knowledge of mammalian taste systems, little is known about the gustatory system and ecology in these lower vertebrates. Hopefully the experience gained from study of these animal models will be used to elucidate receptor mechanisms in mammalian taste systems.

Within the last few years the patch clamp technique has been applied to studies of taste bud cells. This technique makes a very tight seal between the recording electrode and the taste cell membrane, making possible the resolution of small, transmembrane currents. Therefore, activation of single-ion channels in taste cell membranes is being investigated so that mechanisms of taste transduction are now emerging. While the patch clamp technique is very powerful, it too has some drawbacks. Primary among these is the requirement that the taste cells be separated from surrounding cells and structures by the use of selective enzymatic digestion of the tissue, although it is assumed that this process does not damage taste cells and receptor membranes. Moreover, some care is necessary when interpreting results obtained from isolated taste bud cells. Taste bud cells may not operate alone; there is evidence that taste cells within the taste bud are interdependent and possibly also dependent on potentials that exist across the entire gustatory epithelium.

Another important advance in the study of taste receptor mechanisms has resulted from biochemical analysis of taste bud cell membranes. Using techniques that have proved successful in other sensory systems, researchers have made attempts to isolate taste receptor membranes. Two problems have generally impeded progress in the biochemical characterization of taste transduction: the lack of a stimulus that binds tightly to the receptor membrane and the problem of obtaining sufficient quantities of taste cell apical membranes. Because of these problems progress with biochemical analysis of taste receptor membranes has been slow.

Despite these difficulties much has been learned about the membrane properties of taste bud cells. The mean resting membrane potential of mammalian taste cells is about -40 mV when the tongue is adapted to NaCl and -50 mV when

BOX 6-1

Neurophysiological Recording Techniques

The modern era of sensory neurophysiology began when Adrian and Zotterman used vacuum tubes to amplify action potentials from single nerve fibers; this allowed for the first time the study of the relationship between an applied sensory stimulus and the action potential discharge pattern. Adrian described the all-or-none nature of the action potential and discovered that the magnitude of a sensory stimulus was encoded as a frequency of action potentials.[1] The invention of the cathode ray oscilloscope permitted accurate analysis of the time course of the action potential.[2] These early experiments in which the frequency of occurrence of action potentials was measured paved the way for examination of mechanisms of neural coding in all the sensory systems.

Although most studies of peripheral nerve fibers were based on recordings from laboriously dissected single nerve fibers, much information can be gained from studies of whole nerves. In this type of recording, neural activity consisting of asynchronously-occurring compound action potentials is summed, using an electronic circuit that converts the neural activity into a form that can be displayed on a pen recorder.[3] What is measured is the amplitude of the summed neural activity, which increases during simulation as more individual afferent fibers become active.

Once the techniques of electrophysiology had become firmly established, investigators began to apply them to the central nervous system. Extracellular recordings of either populations of neurons using fine insulated wires or of single neurons using sharpened insulated tungsten microelectrodes are now commonly used techniques. These techniques are similar to recordings from the peripheral nervous system. Gerard's invention of the glass microelectrode allowed intracellular recordings and the examination of the biophysical properties of neurons as well as the underlying ionic mechanisms of the action potential and synaptic potentials from single neurons.[4] The intracellular glass recording electrode, fabricated on a special pipette puller, is filled with an electrolyte and, with a high precision micromanipulator, is advanced into areas of the brain under study. The electrode is connected to a specially designed DC amplifier, that measures the electrode potential and is also capable of passing current into the neuron. Once the electrode penetrates the neuronal membrane, the potential shifts abruptly in a negative direction known as the resting membrane potential. Injection of positive and negative currents permits examination of the biophysical characteristics of the neuron. Intracellular recording techniques have also been used to record from sensory receptor cells and the cell bodies of peripheral nerve fibers in sensory ganglia. Although many intracellular studies are conducted by passing current through the electrode and measuring the resulting potential change (often called current clamp), in other experiments, in which investigators are interested in membrane currents, the transmembrane voltage is held constant (called voltage clamp).

BOX 6-1—CONT'D

One of the disadvantages of the glass microelectrode is the relatively poor seal between the electrode and the cell membrane; this prevents measurements of very small transmembrane currents. This was overcome by the development by Neher and Sakmann of a different kind of electrode which seals tightly to the neuronal membrane (the gigaohm seal); the seal allows the resolution of very small currents.[5] This recently developed methodology, called the patch clamp technique, although originally used on isolated neurons, has now been applied to study of neurons in brain slices as well as in the intact nervous system. An additional advantage of the patch clamp technique is that it permits recordings from small neurons that were often damaged by conventional intracellular recording electrodes.

The patch clamp technique was so named because the tight seal between the electrode and the neuronal membrane made it possible to pull off a small patch of membrane for study in isolation. These recordings provided the first information on the activity of single ion channels in the neuronal membrane. There are several other configurations of the patch clamp technique, including a whole cell patch in which, after seal formation, a small hole is made in the membrane by application of suction to the pipette. The contents of the neuron now equilibrate with the pipette solution, allowing manipulation of the internal contents of the neuron. The technique of patch clamping has provided a wealth of new information on neuronal biophysics.

It is apparent, therefore, that neurophysiological techniques have become a very powerful way to study the nervous system. All of these techniques have been applied to studies of sensory and central nervous integrating systems involved in orofacial function, contributing much of the information detailed in this book.

1. Adrian: *The basis of sensation: The action of the sense organs*, London, 1928, Christopher.

2. Erlanger I, Gasser HS: *Electrical signs of nervous activity*, Philadelphia, 1937, University of Pennsylvania Press.

3. Beidler LM: Properties of chemoreceptors of tongue of rat, *Journal of Neurophysiology* 16: 595-607, 1953.

4. Ling G, Gerard RW: The normal membrane potential of frog sartorius fibers, *Journal of Cellular and Comparative Physiology* 34: 383-396, 1949.

5. Neher E: Ion channels for communication between and within cells, *Science* 256: 498-502, 1992.

the tongue is covered with water. When hyperpolarizing and depolarizing current pulses are injected through the recording electrode, the relationship between the applied current and the resulting changes in membrane potential is measured. Results of initial microelectrode recordings indicated that current-voltage relationships were linear, suggesting that taste receptor membranes obey Ohm's law (Fig. 6-5). The slope of the current-voltage relationship gives the input resistance of the cells, which ranges from 17 to 80 $M\Omega$.

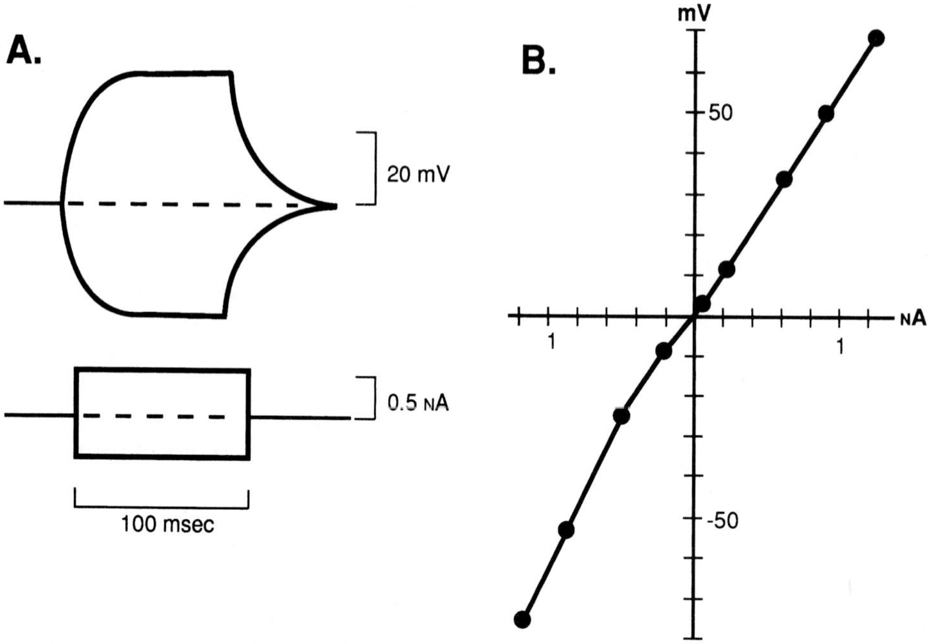

FIG. 6-5
A, Intracellular recordings of the membrane response of a rat taste cell to hyperpolarizing and depolarizing current injections used to measure the basis membrane properties of taste bud cells such as membrane potential and membrane time constants. **B**, Relationship between current and change in membrane potential for a rat taste cell. Slope of line represents input resistance of taste bud cell. (Date from Ozeki M: *Journal of General Physiology* 58:688-699, 1971.)

More recent studies have revealed that taste cell current-voltage relationships are not linear and therefore taste cells do not act as passive transducers. Additionally, taste cells of mudpuppy, frog, salamander, and rat generate single, all-or-none, action potentials when depolarized. The role of these action potentials is not clear, but they may be important in generating the transient portion of the response or possibly be required for transmitter release.

When taste solutions representing the four taste qualities are flowed separately over the tongue, the resting membrane potentials of taste bud cells change slowly (Box 6-2). Stimulation with salty (NaCl), bitter (quinine), sour (HCl), and sweet (sucrose) taste solutions results in three patterns of membrane potential change: depolarization, depolarizaion preceded by hyperpolarization, and hyperpolarization. The composition of the adapting solution influences the pattern of membrane potential change produced by the taste stimuli.

The magnitude of the membrane change produced by applying chemicals to the tongue is related to stimulus concentration. Increasing the concentration of the stimulus results in a greater magnitude of membrane potential change (Fig. 6-6). Since the

BOX 6-2

Taste Qualities

In sensory systems such as vision and audition the relationship between sensation and some physical property of the stimulus has been well established. There is usually a physical continuum such as wavelength that correlates with a systematic change in the sensory quality of the stimulus such as hue or pitch. Although taste is a sensory system responding to chemicals there is no clear continuum of physical properties of taste stimuli and taste sensation. Moreover, since the time of the ancient Greeks, taste sensation has been subdivided into different discrete tastes or qualities now commonly described as sweet, sour, salty, and bitter. Recently a fifth quality of meaty taste or *Umami* has been described. What do these different taste qualities represent? Are there in fact subdivisions of the taste system, each one tuned to respond to these different chemical classes, or is there a continuum of taste sensation waiting to be discovered?

Evidence from a large number of psychophysical studies in animals and humans supports the conclusion that there are least four distinct taste qualities. Nearly all animals are aversive to bitter stimuli and show a preference to sweet stimuli. Behavioral thresholds are much lower to sour and bitter stimuli than sweet and salty stimuli. This and much more evidence supports the existence of different taste qualities with different perceptual properties. However, the physiologic substrate for these behavioral differences remains to be discovered. One of the objectives of the original neurophysiologic analysis of the responses of individual taste fibers by Carl Pfaffmann was to determine if the fibers, and presumably the receptors they innervate, respond specifically to one of the four taste qualities.[1] Pfaffmann found that they did not and had to conclude that taste fibers were relatively specific, responding to more than one of the four taste qualities. Since that pioneering study the same basic question has been reexamined at every level of the taste pathway with essentially the same conclusion. Specific responses to one particular quality have never been found. In recent years the consensus seems to be that chemical stimuli representing one taste quality excite a population of fibers or neurons better than chemical stimuli with different taste qualities, so that specificity is contained in the population response to a particular chemical. Perhaps the only chemical with any degree of specificity is sodium chloride, which seems to excite a set of single afferent fibers that do not respond well to other salts.

Therefore, although it is easy to discriminate between the taste of sodium chloride and sucrose and even between different salts, the underlying mechanisms for discriminating different taste qualities at every level of the taste system have not been fully clarified.

1. Pfaffman C: Gustatory afferent impulses, *Journal of Cellular and Comparative Physiology* 17:243-258, 1941.

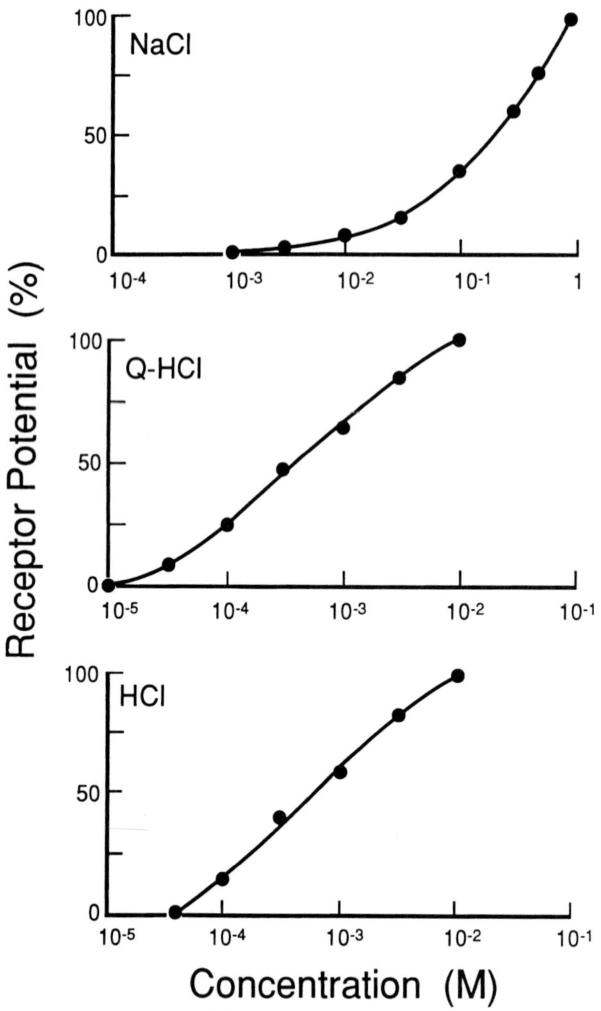

FIG. 6-6
Relationship between concentration of a taste stimulus and change in amplitude of receptor potential of rat taste cells when stimulated with salty (NaCl), bitter (Q-HCl), and sour (HCl) stimuli. (Reprinted from *Comparative Biochemistry and Physiology* 73A, Sato T, Beidler LM: The response characteristics of rat taste cells to four basic taste stimuli, 1-10, Copyright 1982. With kind permission from Pergamon Press Ltd., Headington Hill Hall, Oxford, UK.)

relationships between stimulus concentrations and taste bud cell depolarizations are similar to response concentration functions produced in gustatory afferent fibers, the depolarizations of taste bud cells are considered to be receptor potentials.

The membrane potential of a single taste bud cell changes in response to stimulation with more than one class of taste stimulus. In the same cell some stimuli depolarize the cell, whereas others produce hyperpolarizing potentials. The magnitude and direction of the potential change are different for each particular taste bud cell (Fig. 6-7). It is apparent, therefore, that individual taste bud cells respond to more than one kind of taste stimulus with depolarizing or hyperpolarizing potentials. Taste bud cells responding to only one taste modality have never been described; therefore taste bud cells and taste buds are described as being nonspecific in their

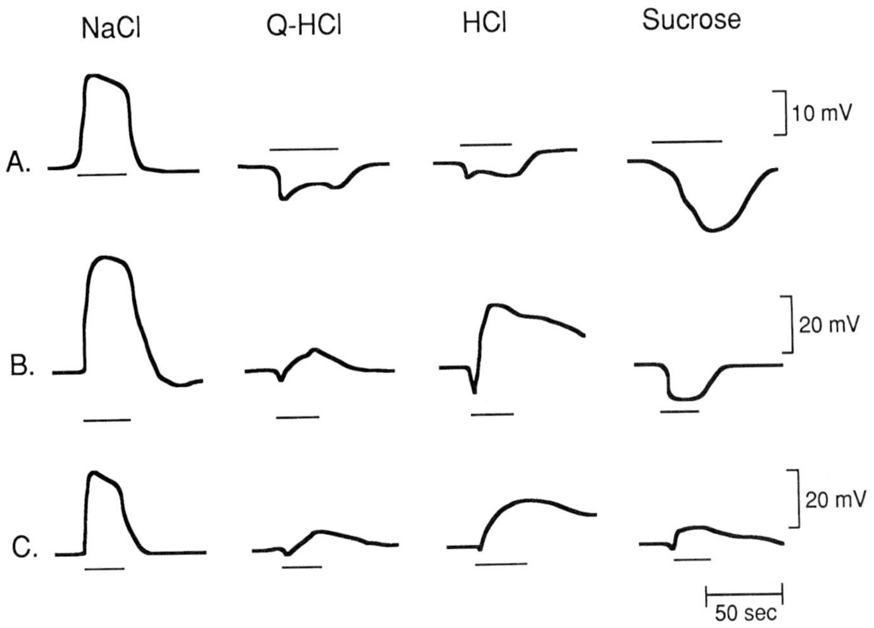

FIG. 6-7
Recordings of responses of three rat taste cells to stimulation with the four taste qualities. Horizontal bars under each recording indicate duration of stimulus application. Note different pattern of response of the three taste cells to same stimuli. (Reprinted from Sato T, Beidler LM: *Comparative Biochemistry and Physiology* 75A, Dependence of gustatory neural response on depolarizing and hyperpolarizing receptor potentials of taste cells in the rat, pp. 131-137, Copyright 1983. With kind permission from Pergamon Press Ltd., Headington Hill Hall, Oxford, UK.)

response to taste stimuli. Moreover, the responses of taste bud cells are similar even when the cells are sampled from taste buds in different mouth areas.

Using the patch-clamp recording technique researchers have described a number of different ion channels in the apical membranes of taste bud cells. In a variety of species, including mammals, taste cells have been shown to possess voltage-gated channels for Na^+, Ca^{2+}, and K^+, and also a Ca-mediated cation channel. The alterations in membrane potential reported from intracellular recording techniques are mediated by activity of these ion channels. Opening or closing of the ion channels results in either depolarization or hyperpolarization of the cells, depending on the nature of the ions involved. Influx of cations (Na^+ or Ca^{2+}) or efflux of anions or stimulus-evoked closure of open K^+ channels would cause depolarization, whereas influx of anions or efflux of cations as well as closure of Na^+ or Ca^{2+} channels would hyperpolarize the cell.

Taste stimuli interact with the apical membranes of the taste bud cells, so that ion channels located on the apical membranes are important in taste transduction. K^+ channels are hypothetically involved in transduction mechanisms for both sour and bitter taste, because K^+ channels are restricted to the apical membranes of taste bud cells and because voltage-gated K^+ currents have been shown to be attenuated by acids and bitter stimuli. A major source of K^+ ions in the extracellular environment of the apical taste cell membranes is saliva. Therefore, salivary K^+ ions are important in taste transduction. The transduction mechanism for Na^+ taste probably involves a voltage-independent Na^+ channel. These passive channels, which transport Na^+ ions into the taste bud cell, contribute to the transepithelial current, which can be measured across the lingual epithelium. The proportion of this current from the Na^+ channels can be demonstrated by the use of amiloride, a drug that specifically blocks passive Na^+ channels. Moreover, evidence linking these amiloride-sensitive channels to taste transductions mechanisms comes from electrophysiological experiments in which the neural response to NaCl but not other salts is markedly reduced after the tongue has been bathed in amiloride. Unlike transduction mechanisms for sour, bitter, and salty tastes, the transduction of sweet tastes appears to involve a specific membrane receptor–mediated stimulation of adenylate cyclase, which in turn causes closure of K^+ channels on the basolateral membrane.

Little is known about membrane receptors in mammalian taste buds. Because catfish have a large number of taste buds that are highly sensitive to various amino acids, this animal has been used to study membrane receptors in taste. Both arginine and proline activate nonselective cation channels in bilayers derived from catfish taste epithelia. This suggests that these channels are directly coupled to membrane receptors involved in initial stages of amino acid transduction. In addition, biochemical studies have identified GTP binding proteins (9-proteins) in taste bud cells that are believed to be involved in sweet and bitter taste transduction in mammals and in amino acid transduction in catfish.

Application of these techniques has resulted in rapid progress in the understanding of taste transduction. Apparently taste buds utilize a number of different mechanisms for sensory transduction, including ionic fluxes through apical ion channels, stimulus block of apical channels, receptor-initiated release of second messengers, and ligand-gated ion channels. Despite this progress much remains to be accomplished, in particular determining the mechanisms by which taste stimuli are discriminated by receptors that respond to many different stimuli.

Recordings from Afferent Taste Fibers

The response properties of peripheral afferent fibers innervating taste buds have been studied in great detail in the chorda tympani nerve (a branch of the seventh cranial nerve) of rats and hamsters. Relatively few studies have been made of taste fiber activity in other species and in other gustatory nerves. To study the response characteristics of the entire population of taste buds innervated by a particular gustatory nerve, investigators record from the whole cut nerve (see Box 6-1).

The response properties of taste buds supplied by different cranial nerves and even different branches of the same cranial nerve are not the same. For example, when the responses of fungiform papilla taste buds (supplied by the chorda tympani branch

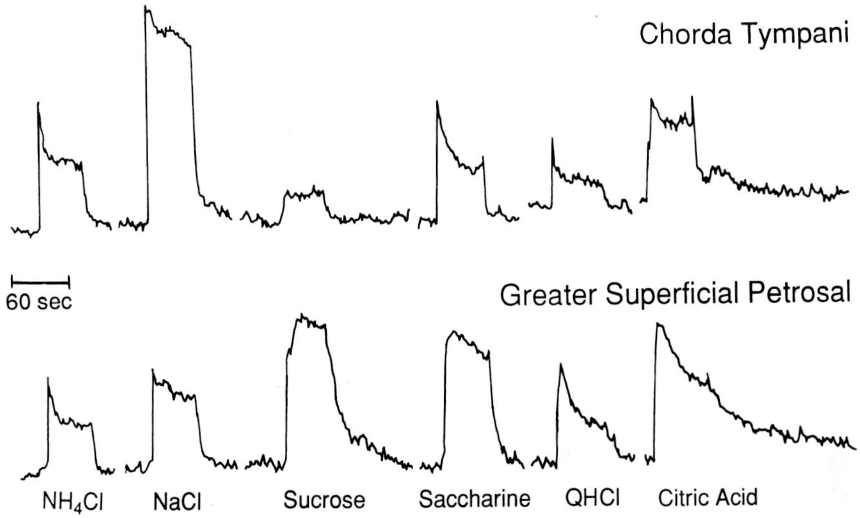

FIG. 6-8
Simultaneous summated whole nerve recordings from greater superficial petrosal and chorda tympani nerves in rat. The chorda tympani supplies taste buds on the anterior tongue, and the greater superficial petrosal nerve supplies taste buds on the palate. Note different relative magnitudes of response to different taste qualities resulting from stimulation of receptive fields of these two nerves. (From Nejad MS: *Chemical Senses* 11:283-293, 1986.)

of cranial nerve VII) of the rat are compared to those in the soft palate (supplied by the greater superficial petrosal branch of the nerve VII) and circumvallate papilla (supplied by nerve IX), NaCl is found to be most effective when applied to the fungiform papillae and sucrose is most effective when applied to the palate (Fig. 6-8). These different response patterns illustrate the importance of considering the entire population of receptors in correlating electrophysiologic response characteristics with behavioral responses to taste stimuli. It is also important to note that no population of taste receptors responds exclusively to a particular taste stimulus or class of taste stimuli.

Increasing concentrations of a taste stimulus result in an increasing response magnitude because of increasing frequency of action potentials in the afferent taste fibers. Response concentration functions are initially linear, but at high concentration become nonlinear. The concentration of a stimulus that produces a maximum response differs depending on the stimulus. Moreover, the magnitude of the response is different for different taste stimuli. Therefore, although there is a limit to the frequency of firing of the afferent taste fiber, the response maximum of a taste bud is determined by receptor processes as well.

The response characteristics of single afferent taste fibers of the chorda tympani nerve to stimulation of the tongue with various stimuli have revealed that single taste fibers do not respond exclusively to any one particular stimulus or group of similarly tasting stimuli (Fig. 6-9). Thus no fibers that respond *only* to sweet, salty, bitter, and sour stimuli have been found.

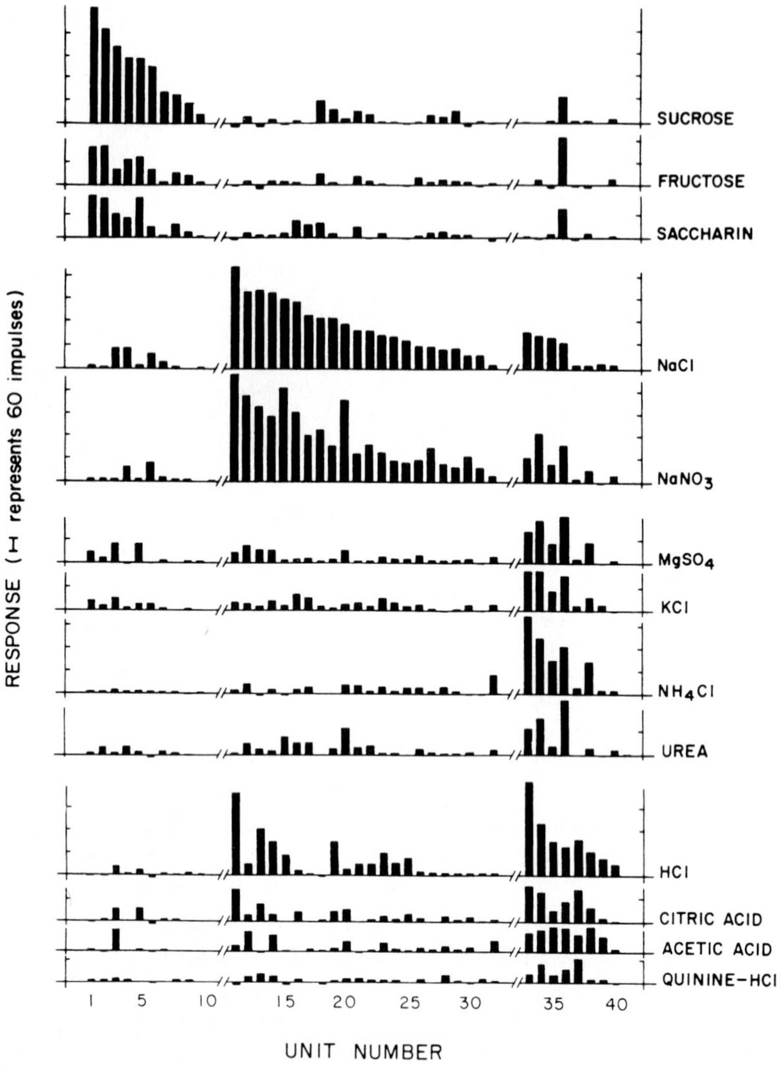

FIG. 6-9

Histograms of the number of impulses per 5 sec initiated in 40 hamster chorda tympani fibers by stimuli representing the four taste qualities. Each row represents the response to the stimulus indicated to the right. The horizontal axis is broken by hash lines to indicate the transition between sucrose best and NaCl best (between fibers 10 and 11), and NaCl best and HCl best (between fibers 32 and 33). (From Frank ME, Beiber SL, Smith DV: *Journal of General Physiology* 91:861-896, 1988. By copyright permission of the Rockefeller University Press.)

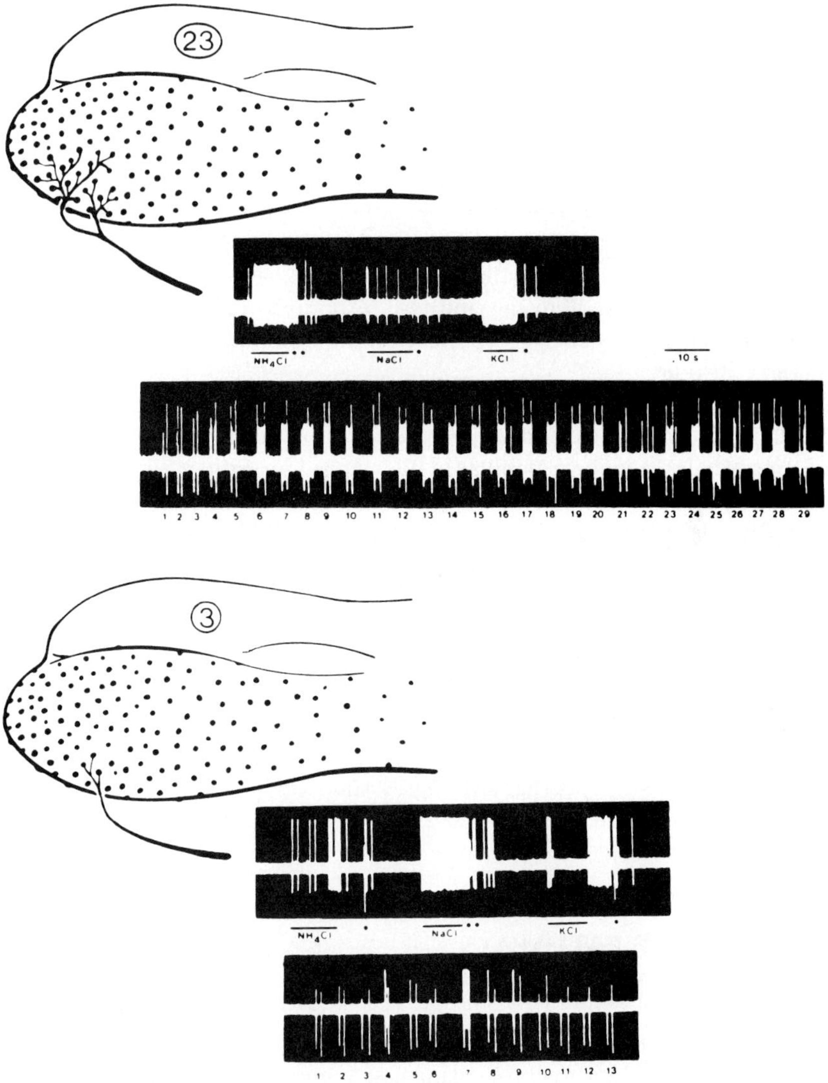

FIG. 6-10
Single fiber recordings from sheep chorda tympani fibers with a large (*top*) and small receptive (*bottom*) fields. In each figure, the response of the fiber to stimulation with NH_4Cl, NaCl, and KCl is shown as top neurophysiological trace. In traces below, the number of papillae innervated by the single fiber was determined by punctate electrical stimulation of fungiform papillae. The fiber with the large receptive field (*top*) was connected to 23 papillae and responded best to NH_4Cl and KCl but not NaCl. Fiber with small receptive field (*bottom*) was connected to three papillae and responded best to NaCl. Receptive field is represented schematically for each fiber. (From Mistretta CM: Developmental neurobiology of the taste system. In Getchell TV, Doty RL, Bartoshuk LM, Snow JBJr, editors: *Smell and taste in health and disease,* New York, 1991, Raven Press, pp. 35-64.)

Analysis of the response characteristics of many chorda tympani fibers has revealed three groups of fibers that respond most effectively to one class of stimulus. One group responds best to sodium salts, a second to salts, acids, and other compounds, and a third to sweet stimuli. Of the three groups the group responding best to sodium salt is perhaps the most specific group and the class responding to salts, acids, and other compounds the most general. These three basic groups are also found in single-fiber recordings from the glossopharyngeal nerve with the addition of a group of fibers that responds best to bitter stimuli. However, the frequency of occurrence of the fiber groups differs. For example, 50% of chorda tympani nerve fibers respond best to sodium salt and few respond to quinine. In contrast, 40% of glossopharyngeal nerve fibers respond best to quinine with considerably fewer responding to sodium salt.

Single chorda tympani fibers branch extensively both below the tongue epithelium and as they ascend the core of the fungiform papillae. By electrically stimulating single fungiform papillae while recording from a single afferent fiber, one can determine the number of papillae innervated by this fiber. In addition, because the rat has one taste bud per fungiform papilla it is possible to count the number of taste buds supplied by a single nerve fiber. With this method the average number of taste buds innervated by a single afferent fiber is 4.5, ranging from one to nine. In sheep, two distinct types of chorda tympani-receptive fields are found. Smaller fields averaging eight fungiform papillae respond best to NaCl whereas much larger fields, averaging 14 papillae, are sensitive to several other monovalent salt stimuli (Fig. 6-10). Nothing is known about the receptive fields of other gustatory nerve fibers, but the anatomical arrangement of the circumvallate and foliate papillae suggests that although a single glossopharyngeal fiber supplies a subset of taste buds in these papillae, these receptive fields probably have little functional significance.

CENTRAL TASTE PATHWAYS

Central Termination of Gustatory Afferent Fibers

Gustatory afferent fibers from the facial (VII), glossopharyngeal (IX), and vagus (X) nerves terminate in a rostral to caudal sequence within the ipsilateral nucleus tractus solitarius. The cell bodies of the gustatory fibers of these three cranial nerves are situated in the geniculate, petrosal, and nodose ganglia respectively (Fig. 6-11). The central sensory branch of the facial nerve formed from the merger of the chorda tympani and greater superficial petrosal nerves is composed almost entirely of gustatory fibers. The central part of the glossopharyngeal nerve contains both gustatory and somatosensory fibers. However, because the glossopharyngeal nerve innervates a large number of taste buds, the number of gustatory fibers in the glossopharyngeal projection is probably larger than in the facial projection. The vagus nerve is the largest nerve terminating in the nucleus tractus solitarius, but only one

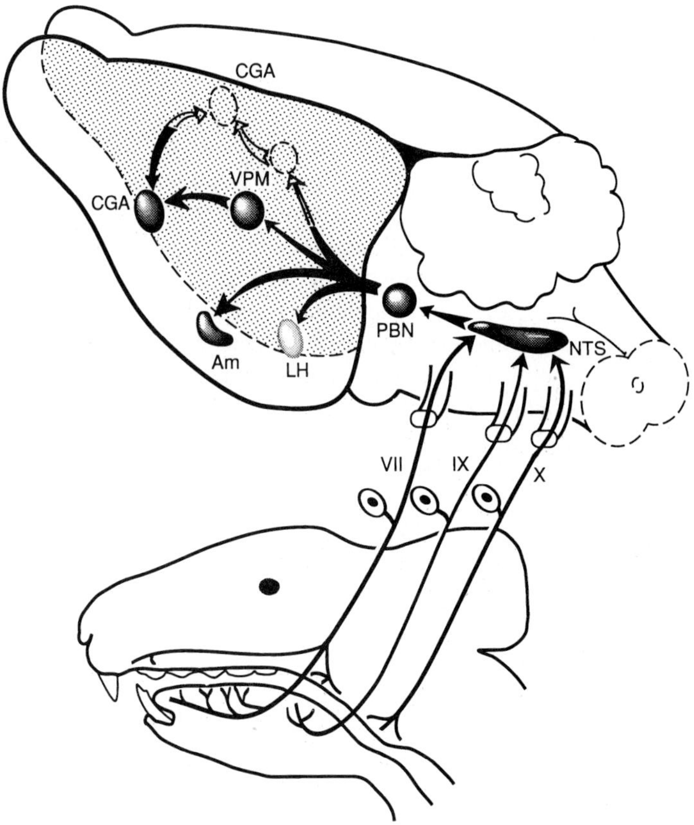

FIG. 6-11
Central taste pathways in a rat with rostral to caudal termination of cranial nerves VII, IX, and X in the nucleus tractus solitarius (NTS). From NTS, the taste pathway next relays in the parabrachial nucleus (PBN). From there pathways diverge, the lemniscal projection relaying in ventroposteromedial nucleus of thalamus (VPM) and terminating in the cortical gusatatory area (CGA). A second path to nuclei in the ventral forebrain and limbic areas (*Am*, amygdala; *LH*, lateral hypothalamus) is also shown.

branch, the superior laryngeal nerve, contains a significant number of chemosensory fibers. Moreover, several studies have indicated that the taste buds supplied by the vagus nerve are principally concerned with initiation of upper airway protection reflexes, so that the vagal chemosensory projection to nucleus tractus solitarius is not part of the central gustatory pathways.

Axons of these three cranial nerves penetrate the lateral border of the medulla in fascicles and pass through the spinal trigeminal tract and nucleus, turning rostrally along the lateral border of the nucleus tractus solitarius to form the solitary tract. Each descending fiber of the solitary tract gives off several collateral branches that enter the nucleus solitarius to terminate on second order neurons.

Nucleus Tractus Solitarius

The nucleus tractus solitarius is usually divided into two functional zones: a rostral zone that processes gustatory information and a caudal zone associated with a number of functions such as swallowing (see Chapter 11), respiration, gastric motility, and cardiovascular reflexes. The two zones are distinguished by cytoarchitectonic features and content of neuropeptides and transmitters.

The gustatory zone of the nucleus tractus solitarius is most frequently divided into lateral and medial subdivisions, although other subdivisions have been described. The medial division contains many unmyelinated axons and neurons smaller than the neurons of the lateral division and can be clearly seen in stained and unstained sections. Three main types of neurons have been described in the nucleus tractus solitarius. Elongate neurons have a fusiform cell body with two primary dendrites that arise from each pole of the soma and then branch caudally and rostrally for considerable distances. Multipolar (or stellate) neurons have a large pyramidal soma with three or four

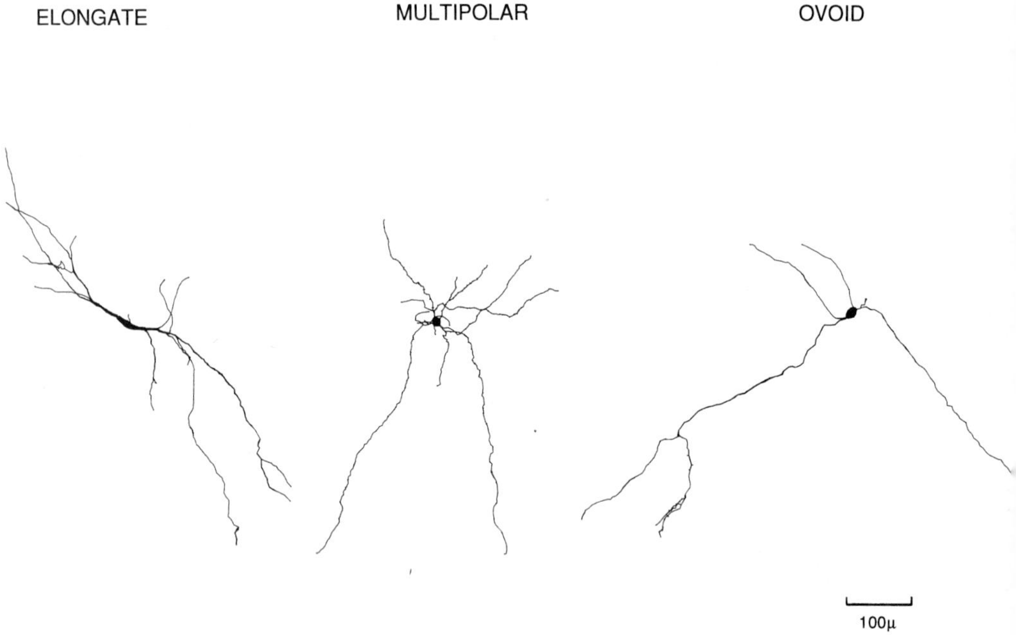

FIG. 6-12
Three major neuron types in gustatory area of nucleus tractus solitarius revealed by intracellular injection of a neural marker. After tissue processing and histochemical staining to reveal filled neurons, the neurons were reconstructed in three dimensions with a computer controlled microscope. Elongated neurons have a fusiform cell body with two primary dendrites arising from each pole of the soma. Multipolar (or stellate) neurons have large pyramidal soma with three or four primary dendrites extending in several directions. Ovoid neurons have a small soma with three or more principal dendrites.

primary dendrites extending in several directions. The third cell type, the ovoid cell, has a small soma with three or more principal dendrites (Fig. 6-12). Studies of projection patterns of neurons in the nucleus tractus solitarius show that the elongate and multipolar neurons send their axons rostrally and to other locations within the medulla. The small ovoid cells connect locally within the nucleus tractus solitarius and are interneurons that contain the inhibitory neurotransmitter gamma-aminobutyric acid.

Electrophysiologic studies of neurons in the nucleus tractus solitarius have been in the form of extracellular recordings from unidentified neurons. Only the general location of the recording site is known, based on electrolytic lesions. There has been limited success with intracellular recordings because of technical difficulties related to stability and problems associated with intracellular recordings from small neurons. Intracellular recordings have been achieved by using an in vitro brain-slices preparation of the gustatory zone of the nucleus tractus solitarius, revealing several types of neurons with different membrane properties. However, this procedure does not permit study of responses of nucleus tractus solitarius neurons to tongue stimulation with chemicals.

Extracellular recordings from gustatory neurons during stimulation of the tongue with taste solutions have revealed that these neurons typically reflect the response characteristics of the peripheral input. For example, the most effective stimuli of hamster chorda tympani fibers are NaCl, HCl, and sucrose and, when recordings are made from second order neurons in the chorda tympani projection zone of nucleus tractus solitarius, the most effective stimuli for these neurons are also NaCl and HCl. Moreover, when the response of a population of these neurons is analyzed, the grouping of the second order neurons is similar to the groups described in peripheral fibers.

There are some differences between the recordings from peripheral fibers and second order gustatory neurons. For example, the second order neurons have a higher level of spontaneous activity and respond to stimulation of their receptive fields with higher frequencies. In addition, the receptive field of the second order gustatory neurons is larger than that of afferent gustatory fibers. Most recordings of nucleus tractus solitarius neurons have been from the chorda tympani nerve projection, and only recently have attempts been made to record from neurons receiving input through other gustatory nerves.

Pontine Taste Relay

Ascending axons arising from the gustatory part of the nucleus tractus solitarius terminate on cells in the parabrachial nuclei of the pons in both rodents and lagomorphs, but not in primates (see Fig. 6-11). In primates the gustatory projection bypasses the pontine relay to connect in the ventroposteromedial nucleus of the thalamus. Therefore, there is a species difference in ascending taste pathways.

Gustatory neurons in the pons are topographically organized along the dorsoventral axis of the brain rather than the rostrocaudal arrangement of the nucleus tractus solitarius. Response characteristics of the pontine neurons are similar to those in the peripheral fibers and the nucleus tractus solitarius. Therefore, for example, like the medullary taste relay of the hamster, pontine neurons respond best to stimulation of the chorda tympani receptive field with NaCl, HCl, and sucrose. The spontaneous rate and evoked response frequency of pontine gustatory neurons are greater than those of second order neurons. Between the periphery and the pons there is a sixfold increase in spontaneous activity and a twofold increase in average evoked response frequencies.

Thalamus and Cortex

The thalamic gustatory relay nucleus is situated at the ventromedial tip of the ventroposteromedial thalamic nucleus, a part of the ventrobasal complex. The gustatory subnucleus contains smaller cells than do the surrounding nuclei and is therefore called the parvocellular subnucleus. Although neurons in the most medial portion respond exclusively to lingual application of taste stimuli, neurons situated more laterally are multimodal, responding to taste, temperature, and tactile stimulation of the oral cavity. Projections from the thalamus ascend to the agranular insular cortex that borders on and overlaps the lingual representation of the primary sensory cortex. Neurons responding to gustatory stimulation as well as multimodal neurons are encountered in the cortical gustatory projection.

Other Projections

Not only do gustatory neurons in the parabrachial nucleus of the pons project to the thalamus, but they also project widely to other brain areas. The densest terminations include the lateral hypothalamus, central nucleus of the amygdala, and the bed nucleus of the stria terminalis (see Fig. 6-11). These structures are responsible for behaviors such as motivation, emotion, reinforcement, and, in particular, food intake. Therefore, there are functional differences between the two rostral projections from the pontine taste relay. The thalamocortical projections probably mediate the sensory discriminative aspects of taste, whereas the ventral forebrain projections are involved in the motivational aspects of taste.

DEVELOPMENT AND AGING

Taste buds appear very early in the tongue of human fetuses, at 7 to 8 weeks of gestation, but mature-appearing taste buds are not observed until later in gestation. Development is not complete at birth and taste bud numbers continue to increase.

Behavioral testing of human newborns reveals that the ability to discriminate between taste stimuli is present at birth, indicating that some attributes of taste preference behavior are innate and do not require any experience for expression (Fig. 6-13). However, other studies have demonstrated that although these taste behaviors

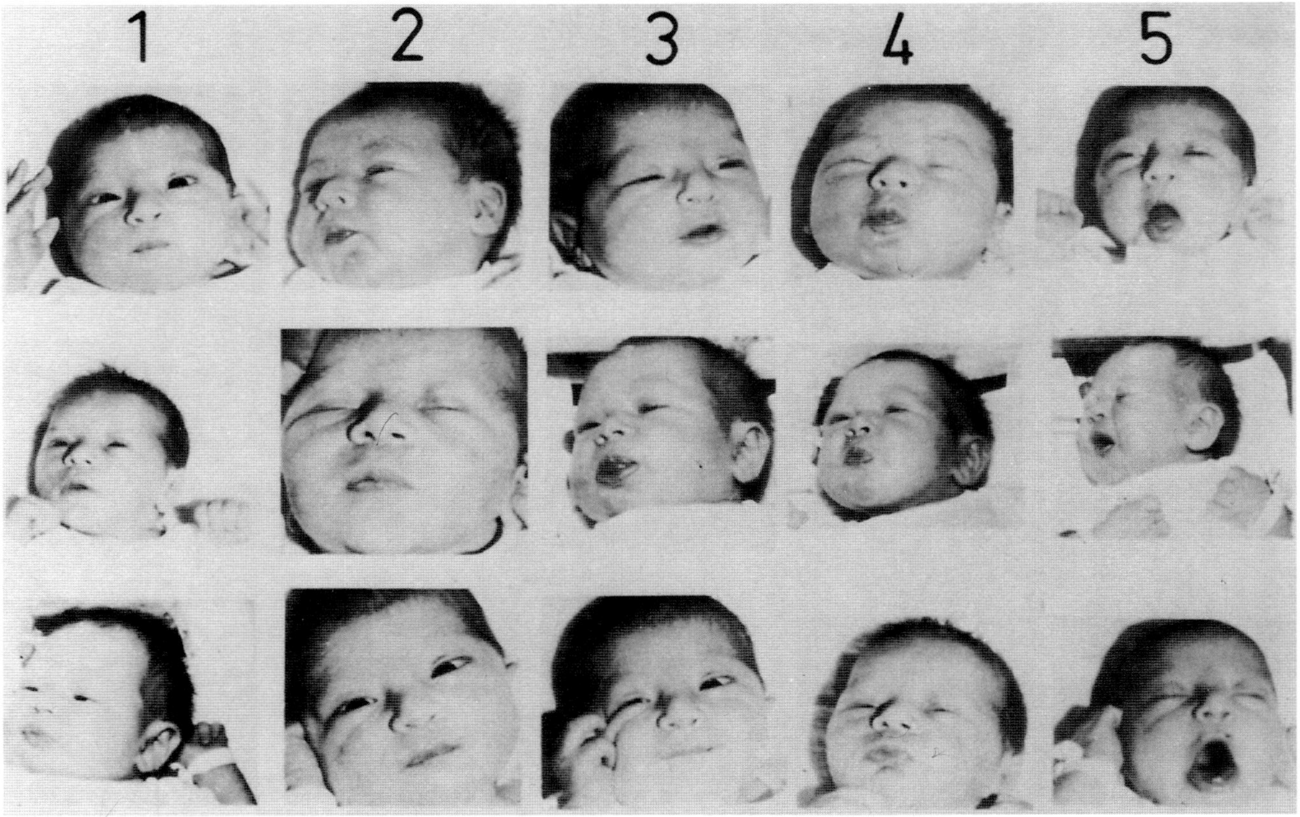

FIG. 6-13
Facial responses to sweet (column 3), sour (column 4), and bitter (column 5) taste stimuli applied to the tongue tip in three human neonates (1 row for each infant) recorded between birth and first feeding. Column 1 is each infant at rest before a stimulus was applied. Column 2 is facial expression after stimulation with distilled water that has no taste. Columns 3-5 are facial expression after taste stimuli have been applied. Note the pleasurable expression with the sweet stimulus (column 3), the pursing of the lips with the sour stimulus (column 4), and the open mouth with tongue protrusion with the bitter stimulus (column 5). (From Steiner JE: Facial expression of the neonate infant indicating hedonics of food-related chemical stimuli. In Weiffenbach JM, editor: *Taste and Development. The Genesis of Sweet Preference*, Bethesda, 1977, US Dept. Health Education and Welfare, pp. 173-189.)

are present at birth they can be extensively modified by postnatal experience.

Electrophysiologic experiments have also demonstrated changes in taste responses during development. In two species, the sheep with a long gestation and rat with a very short gestation, similar changes take place during development of the taste system. Of particular significance are the functional changes that occur in responses to NaCl. In both immature sheep and rat no responses are recorded to stimulation with NaCl, but other salts are effective stimuli. As development takes place there is a gradual increase in the frequency of response of afferent fibers to NaCl (Fig. 6-14). A second characteristic of the developing taste system is the acquisition of small receptive fields that are highly responsive to stimulation with NaCl.

The emerging sensitivity to NaCl can be manipulated by restriction of NaCl in the diet during development; this prevents the development of responses to NaCl but not to other nonsodium salts. This demonstration that dietary sodium can influence the development of the taste system has important implications for salt intake

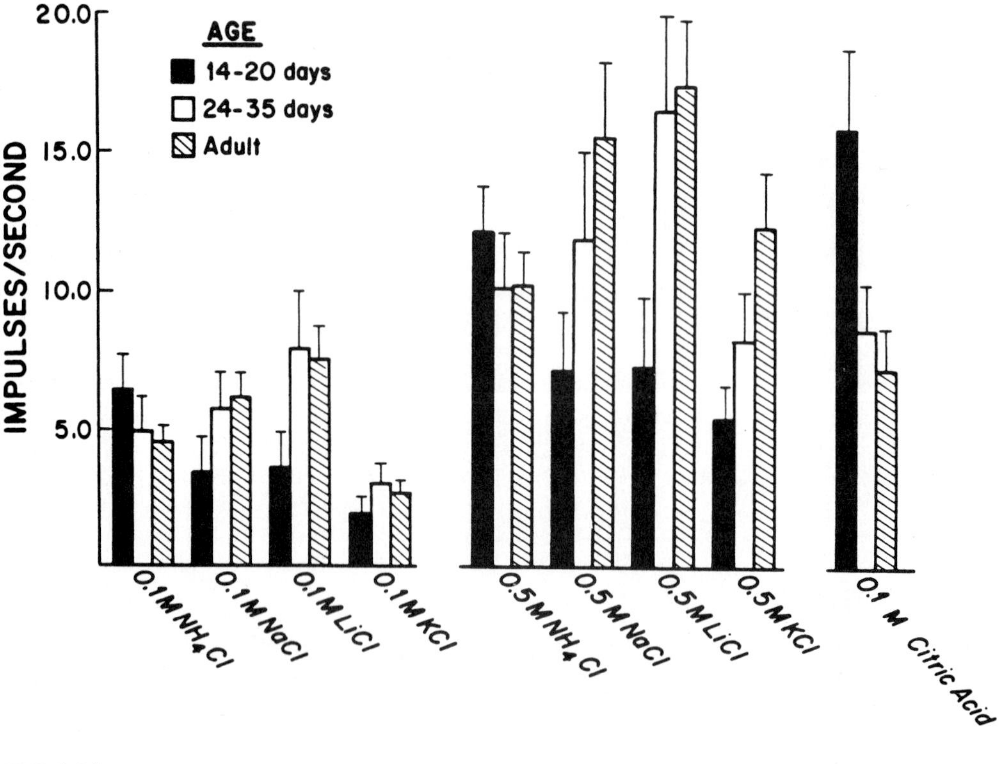

FIG. 6-14

Mean response frequencies of rat chorda tympani fibers in three age groups to stimulation of tongue with 0.1M and 0.5M salts and 0.1M citric acid. Frequencies in response to NH_4Cl remain constant during development, whereas response frequencies to NaCl and LiCl increase and those of citric acid decrease. (From Hill DL, Mistretta CM and Bradley RM: *Journal of Neuroscience* 2:782-790, 1982.)

in humans, especially in relation to the role of sodium intake in hypertension.

In contrast to these anatomic and functional changes during development, aging has very little effect on the taste system. Counts of taste buds in carefully controlled experiments have revealed little or no reduction in taste bud numbers. Behavioral studies have also shown that in a healthy population of individuals the decline in behavioral measures of taste sensitivity is small and relatively insignificant. Moreover, although significant changes are observed in neurophysiologic response to taste stimuli, they are relatively small. Recent data from quantitative studies of taste buds in old humans, rhesus monkeys, and rats compliment the neurophysiologic data on taste responses from aged rats and lead to the general conclusion that the peripheral taste system is maintained structurally and functionally across the life span.

ROLE OF SALIVA IN TASTE FUNCTION

Saliva is essential for normal taste function. It is usually difficult to taste food with a dry mouth. Saliva not only acts as a solvent for chemical stimuli in food, but also transports these stimuli to the taste receptors. At rest gustatory receptors are covered with a layer of fluid that extends into the taste pores and bathes the receptor surface of the microvilli. Little is known about this surface layer. For taste buds in the fungiform papillae it presumably consists of pooled saliva from all the salivary glands. Taste buds in the circumvallate and foliate papillae are bathed in saliva derived from von Ebner's glands. Taste buds on the palate, larynx, and pharynx are covered in fluid secreted by a large number of small salivary glands draining onto the surface of the epithelium. However, the composition of the microenvironment within the taste pore might be different from the layer of fluid that overlies the epithelial surface. Moreover, because gustatory stimulation alters salivary flow and composition, the fluid environment may alter during transduction. Although this microenvironment, acting as a transport system, may merely play a passive role in taste mechanisms, it may have a more active role. Components within the taste pore may control access and removal of stimuli and interact with tastants during the initial events in receptor-stimulus interactions.

Stimulus Transport by Saliva

During feeding and drinking, muscles controlling the jaws, tongue, and face working in concert move food and fluid around the mouth and facilitate access of solubilized taste stimuli to the whole population of taste receptors. This may be particularly significant for taste receptors situated in the clefts of the circumvallate and foliate papillae, because muscle movements may be essential to transporting the taste stimuli into the clefts. These muscle movements determine the rate and direction of stimulus delivery to the taste receptors. The importance of stimulus delivery rate has been demonstrated in electrophysiologic experiments in which stimulus flow was shown to control the magnitude of the dynamic portion of neural responses recorded in primary afferent taste fibers. In these experiments on anesthetized animals, stimulus delivery parameters were controlled, permitting accurate measures of response latency (time between stimulus application and the beginning of the neural response). For example, the latency of the neural response to 0.2M NaCl has been reported to be 26 msec. This latency includes the time necessary for transduction, synaptic delay, and conduction of the action potential to the recording electrode as well as transport of the stimulus to the receptor sites. The latency is influenced by flow rate, which determines the number of stimulus molecules delivered to the receptor environment to reach threshold concentration.

Saliva as Adapting Solution

Since saliva contains various ions that are themselves gustatory stimuli, taste receptors are continuously stimulated by salivary components. Normally this stimula-

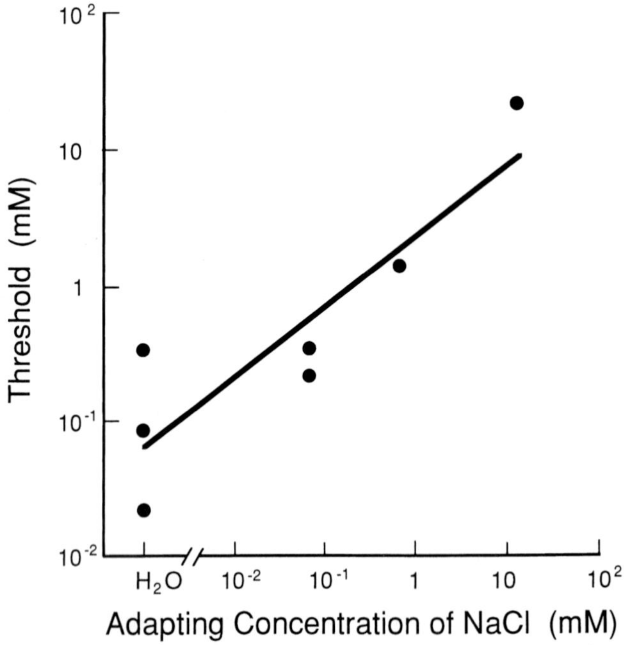

FIG. 6-15
Effect of adapting lingual taste buds to different concentrations of NaCl on taste detection thresholds. Lowest thresholds (highest sensitivity) are obtained when the tongue is adapted to water. (Data from McBurney D and Pfaffmann C: *Journal of Experimental Psychology* 65:523-529, 1963.)

tion is not apparent, and the taste system is said to be adapted to the normal salivary environment. The interactions between salivary composition and taste perception have been studied principally for NaCl, although other salivary constituents such as urea and potassium are present in saliva at concentrations that could potentially stimulate taste receptors and, therefore, influence taste responses. Behavioral experiments have demonstrated that to detect the presence of a stimulus such as sodium that is normally found in saliva, its concentration must exceed salivary levels (Fig. 6-15). Thus, detection and recognition thresholds for NaCl are influenced by the sodium concentration in the oral cavity. Detection thresholds are lowest when the mouth is rinsed with distilled water, and become higher as the adapting solution contains greater concentrations of NaCl. It is, therefore, important to rinse the mouth before making behavioral measurements of taste threshold and to rinse between stimulus presentations to return taste receptors to control levels of adaptation.

Role of Saliva in Taste Transduction

Of the many organic constituents of saliva, the proline-rich proteins have been associated with the ability to taste bitter compounds such as quinine, raffinose undecaacetate, and cyclohexamide. The connection was established when gene maps for proline-rich proteins were compared with the genes encoding the characteristics of bitter taste responses in mice. In 19 different inbred strains of mice the distribution pattern of the two genes was identical. This suggests that the proline-rich proteins may act as carriers of molecules in bitter taste transduction.

Saliva from the major salivary glands bathes taste receptors that are contained in fungiform papillae. However, the majority of the lingual taste buds are situated in the epithelium that lines the clefts of the circumvallate and foliate papillae. The saliva bathing these taste buds is supplied by the lingual salivary (von Ebner's) glands that drain into the base of these clefts. Presumably these glands control the access of taste stimuli to the circumvallate and foliate papillae taste buds. They provide a diffusion path for stimuli to gain access to the taste buds, and they remove stimuli by active secretion. Taste stimuli must, therefore, traverse this salivary layer before interacting with receptor membranes. Ebner's glands could play an important role in taste transduction in most lingual taste buds.

Recently it has been shown that von Ebner's glands secrete a protein that is structurally similar to the odorant-binding proteins isolated in nasal glands. This protein is not found in other salivary glands, and because of the relationship between von Ebner's glands and taste receptors situated in the circumvallate and foliate papillae, it is thought that this protein may be important in transporting lipophilic stimuli to the taste receptor membranes. Because many bitter substances are highly lipophilic, this protein could be important in bitter taste transduction mechanisms. It is possible, therefore, that these glands do not serve merely to rinse the clefts of the foliate and circumvallate papillae but play an active role in the transduction process.

Effect of Reduced Salivation of Taste Perception

Because saliva has a major role in transport of taste stimuli to the receptors, reduction in saliva production should have an effect on taste perception. It is not surprising, therefore, that patients with reduced salivation following head and neck irradiation often report taste disturbances and, when tested, show a decrease in taste acuity. Although irradiation could also effect turnover of the taste buds and possibly damage nerve terminals, the xerostomia (dry mouth) is thought to be a major factor in the altered taste perception.

In animal experiments xerostomia can be produced either by removing all the major salivary glands or by using a parasympathetic antagonist to block synaptic transmission controlling salivary flow. This experimentally induced xerostomia has been reported to result in altered taste perception. Interpretation of the results of these experimentally induced xerostomias is complicated because even though the major salivary glands are removed all the minor glands are still present so that the residual pooled saliva is different in composition from that normally present. It is also significant that the salivary supply to the majority of the oral taste buds secreted by von Ebner's glands remains intact so that only a minority of the oral taste buds are affected by xerostomia produced by removal of the major salivary glands. On the other hand, xerostomia produced by parasympathetic blockage affects all the salivary glands and reduces saliva associated with all the oral taste buds. However, using a drug that blocks the parasympathetic synapse at the gland leaves the sympathetic system; salivary flow is therefore present at a lower rate and different composition, complicating the interpretation of such data. Using experimentally induced xerostomia to explore the role of reduced saliva production in taste function is problematic and requires caution when interpreting the conclusions drawn from these studies.

Removal of the salivary glands has a marked effect on oral health, including the structural integrity of taste buds. Electron microscopic examination of taste buds after removal of the major salivary glands reveals the presence of macrophages within the taste buds and large numbers of bacteria invading the taste pore. The taste buds are, therefore, invaded by bacteria and become pathologic. Their ability to function is then altered leading to changes in taste perception.

Dry mouth is characteristic of the condition known as Sjögren's syndrome which results from pathology of the salivary glands. Many patients with this syndrome complain of reduced enjoyment of food and decreased sense of taste. Behavioral testing of patients with Sjögren's syndrome revealed significant reductions in taste sensitivity for the four basic taste qualities. Although Sjögren's syndrome has not been reported to involve taste receptors, the reasons for altered taste perception can probably be associated with problems in stimulus transport and a reduction in oral hygiene.

CLINICAL CONSIDERATIONS

Disorders of taste and smell are often classified according to the type of sensory loss. Complete loss of the sense of smell is called anosmia and loss of taste is called ageusia; partial loss is termed hyposmia and hypogeusia respectively. Often patients have distortions of taste and smell called dysgeusia and parosmia respectively, in which a chronic taste or smell is present in the absence of any stimulus. When an aberrant taste or smell is experienced because of abnormal stimulation within the central nervous system, the disorder is called a phantom. Although these terms are used by clinicians who diagnose chemosensory disorders, patients usually describe their disorder in different terms.

Patients with a chemosensory disorder often complain that "I cannot taste," or "I have a bad taste all the time." Often these individuals have no obvious clinical cause for these complaints and treatment is difficult. Until recently, information regarding the causes of chemosensory disorders consisted of an extensive clinical literature with more than 200 conditions and many medications linked to alterations in taste and smell. Fortunately, several clinical centers have now been established specifically for diagnosis, treatment, and research into chemosensory disorders, and for the first time patients with disorders of the chemical senses have been studied intensively. There is now some consensus regarding causes of chemosensory disorders.

Although patients examined at clinical centers devoted to chemosensory disorders often complain of altered taste perception, they are in fact referring to changes in the flavor of food. Flavor consists of a combined sensory experience derived from olfactory, thermal, tactile, and taste receptors. Other sensory systems may also participate in the overall flavor of food. Therefore, when patients are actually tested there seems to be little correlation between the patient's complaint and the results of the sensory testing to determine the actual sensory loss. Even though the patient complains of a taste problem, the measured sensory loss frequently occurs in the olfactory system (Fig. 6-16).

Olfactory disturbances result most commonly from nasal and/or sinus disease, upper respiratory infection, or head trauma, but they can also be associated with a variety of disease states, chemical exposures, and congenital syndromes. Although true taste disorders are much less common that olfactory dysfunctions, they may also arise from upper respiratory infections or head trauma, as well as numerous medications, oral pathology, and radiation therapy. In some cases treatment of the underlying condition (for example, nasal disease) can relieve associated chemosensory symptoms, or the symptoms may resolve spontaneously within a few months (for example, in cases of head trauma). Although these are the most common causes of chemosensory disturbances, other factors can affect taste and olfaction.

Vitamin A deficiency increases keratinization of the tongue, including the pore area of the taste buds and adjacent epithelial and glandular tissue. Rats made deficient of vitamin A gradually lose their normal preference for NaCl and aversion to

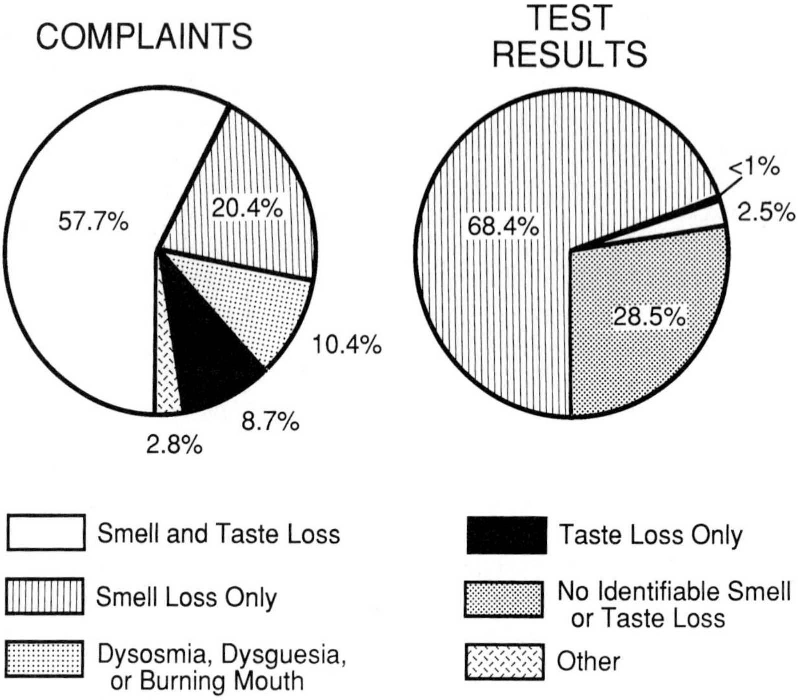

FIG. 6-16
Comparison of complaints of 750 patients who had chemosensory disorders and the results of sensory testing on same individuals. (From Deems DA, and others: *Archives of Otolaryngology and Head and Neck Surgery* 117:519-528, 1991.)

quinine solutions. Vitamin A repletion tends to restore normal preference or aversion behavior. Significant reductions also occur in the neural response of the chorda tympani to tongue stimulation with NaCl. Loss of gustatory sensitivity from vitamin A deficiency presumably results from blocking of the taste pore with keratin plugs, which prevents access of stimuli to the receptor membranes. However, other factors could be involved such as possible alterations in quantity and composition of salivary secretion, since glandular tissue is also affected by the deficiency.

Gustatory hallucinations are sometimes reported by patients with epilepsy as one manifestation of parietal, temporal, or temporoparietal seizures. A brief gustatory hallucination can be induced by electrical stimulation of the parietal area as well as the amygdala and hippocampus in patients with gustatory seizures. The hallucinations are reported as, "The taste was bitter and dry;" "I tasted something in my throat;" "It's starting again, the taste starts in the stomach, it rises and falls." The taste is usually not described in detail but rather in more general terms such as "bitter," "unpleasant," or "a taste."

Familial dysautonomia affects children of Jewish ancestry and is transmitted by an autosomal recessive trait. A smooth tongue with decreased papillae and devoid of taste buds is an important feature of familial dysautonomia and is clinically associated with marked reduction in taste sensitivity. Patients with this disorder are unable to taste. Even concentrated sucrose solutions are identified as "not water" by the subject who is uncertain whether it is sweet or sour.

Numerous studies in humans and animals have demonstrated that taste declines after head and neck irradiation. Examination of the tongues of irradiated animals reveals that after a single radiation dose the number of taste buds declines. This decrease leads to taste loss as well as reduction in salivary flow rate.

Many patients with malignancy become anorexic and their food intake declines so that they lose weight: this results in increased mortality. The hypothesis is that this anorexia is possibly caused by alterations in taste sensation, because taste is important in guiding food intake. In an attempt to examine this hypothesis a number of studies testing taste sensitivity have been conducted on cancer patients and have found taste threshold abnormalities for one or more of the four taste qualities. However, when study results were carefully analyzed, no abnormalities of taste perception could be demonstrated among patients grouped by tumor site, therapy, or appetite. Preference for sweet stimuli is altered in a manner that might reduce ingestion of sweet foods in some anorexic cancer patients and some patients receiving chemotherapy. Therefore, most studies to determine the role of taste disorders in the anorexia experienced by cancer patients have produced equivocal results, and the alteration in taste sensitivity reported by cancer patients is likely from multiple causes, including the radiation or chemotherapeutic drugs used in treatment.

Many drugs have been reported to alter taste sensitivity. Some drugs influencing the peripheral and central nervous system presumably produce their effect by altering the transmission of neural information through central taste relays. Other drugs may be excreted in saliva and produce their effect by a persistent taste. The reason that other drugs influence chemosensitive responses is not known. Caution has to be observed when evaluating this literature. The reports may be anecdotal, lacking any systematic investigation. Drugs may have general effects. For instance d-penicillamine has been reported to produce hypogeusia in 20% to 40% of patients taking this drug, and, when it is administered to experimental animals, it produces altered taste preferences. However, electrophysiologic recordings from peripheral taste nerves revealed no differences in response characteristics between control and experimental animals, suggesting that the drug was having its effect centrally.

The association of taste and smell dysfunction with zinc deficiency has led to studies of zinc therapy in such disorders. Claims for therapeutic benefits in ameliorating taste and smell disorders have been made. The results of a double blind study (neither the investigator not the subjects know whether they are in placebo or treatment groups) did not substantiate the benefit claimed in earlier studies for zinc treatment of taste disorders. The results of this double blind study leave little doubt that at present there is no scientific basis for administering zinc sulfate therapeutically for ordinary taste and smell dysfunction.

A further condition with associated chemosensory disorders is called burning mouth syndrome, which is an intraoral pain condition occurring primarily in postmenopausal females. Although the oral cavity appears normal in patients with burning mouth syndrome, there is an apparent change in sensory perception. The cause of these changes is not known but may be a peripheral or central dysfunction of small afferent nerve fibers.

In conclusion, chemosensory disorders are not uncommon and can be very debilitating. Individuals with abnormalities of taste and smell are unable to appreciate food and lose the ability to detect spoiled food, fumes, and gas leaks. Moreover, persons with certain occupations that use the chemical senses, such as chefs, perfumers, and firefighters, may be unable to continue their profession. It is important to recognize that these patients do have a disorder that, once accurately diagnosed, may be treatable.

SUMMARY

Taste buds are epithelial structures distributed throughout the oral cavity and pharynx. On the tongue taste buds are contained in specialized structures called papillae. Taste buds contain several types of cells that make contact with the oral cavity by specialized apical projections through a taste pore. At the basal end of the taste bud taste cells contact primary afferent nerve fibers. Taste buds are dynamic structures that are renewed and are capable of regenerating if their nerve supply is interrupted. Only gustatory nerves will support the regeneration of taste buds.

Several receptor mechanisms including ion channels and receptor-coupled second messenger systems are involved in taste transduction processes. Taste cells, and therefore taste buds, respond to more than one of the four basic taste qualities of sweet, sour, salty, and bitter. Single afferent taste fibers innervating taste buds also respond to more than one of the four basic taste qualities. However, even though taste fibers do not respond to a single taste quality, they respond best to two or more of the taste qualities.

Afferent chemosensory information is carried over cranial nerves VII, IX, and X, which terminate in a rostral to caudal direction in the nucleus tractus solitarius in the medulla. The rostral end of this nucleus is the gustatory relay nucleus while the caudal end is responsible for control of several visceral functions. Neurons of the nucleus tractus solitarius respond to chemical stimulation of the tongue in a similar way to peripheral fibers. In rodents and lagomorphs the next relay in the taste pathway is in the pons, but in primates it is in the thalamus. From the thalamus the gustatory pathway projects to the agranular insular cortex. Recordings at the pontine, thalamic, and cortical areas do not reveal any change in the specificity of gustatory responses, although there are changes in receptive field characteristics and in response frequencies.

At birth humans respond differentially to bitter, sweet, and sour stimuli but are indifferent to salty taste. During growth and development there are major changes in responses to NaCl and in receptive field properties of taste fibers and relay neurons. Aging has little biological effect on the taste system.

Saliva plays an important role in taste perception. Saliva acts as a transport medium for taste stimuli, is an adapting solution, provides ions important in transduction, and provides the microenvironment for transduction for taste buds in the circumvallate and foliate papillae. Loss of saliva because of disease or irradiation results in a marked reduction in taste acuity.

Many individuals experience alterations or complete loss of the sense of taste and smell. Often this is because of nasal obstruction or other condition involving the nasal cavities and sinuses. Other causes of chemosensory disorders are more obscure, although a patient's report of chemosensory loss may not correlate with the actual cause of the disorder. Several conditions such as epilepsy, burning mouth syndrome, and familial dysautonomia are all associated with chemosensory disorders.

SELECTED READINGS

Bradley RM, Mistretta CM: Neurophysiology of the developing taste system. In Cagen RH, editor: *Neural mechanisms in taste*, Boca Raton, 1989, CRC Press.

Bruch RC, Kalinoski DL, Kare MR: Biochemistry of vertebrate olfaction and taste, *Annual Review of Neuroscience* 8:21-42, 1988.

Doty RL, Bartoshuk LM, Snow JB Jr: Causes of olfactory and gustatory disorders. In Getchell TV and others, editors: *Smell and taste in health and disease*, New York, 1991, Raven Press.

Kinnamon SC: Taste transduction: diversity of mechanisms, *Trends in Neuroscience* 11:491-496, 1988.

Kurihara K, Yoshii K, Kashiwayanagi M: Transduction mechanisms in chemoreception, *Comparative Biochemistry and Physiology* 85A:1-22, 1986.

Mistretta CM: Anatomy and neurophysiology of the taste system in aged animals. In Nutrition and the chemical senses in aging: recent advances and current research needs, vol 561, *Annals of the New York Academy of Sciences*, 1989.

Mott AE, Leopold DA: Disorders in taste and smell, *Medical Clinics of North America* 75:1321-1353, 1991.

Norgren R: Central neural mechanisms of taste. In Darian-Smith I, editor: *Handbook of physiology; the central nervous system*, vol 3, Bethesda, 1984, American Physiological Society.

Oakley B: Trophic competence in mammalian gustation. In Pfaff DW, editor: *Taste, olfaction, and the central nervous system*, New York, 1985, Rockefeller University Press.

Roper SD: The cell biology of vertebrate taste receptors, *Annual Review of Neuroscience* 12:329-353, 1989.

Sato T: Recent advances in the physiology of taste cells, *Progress in Neurobiology* 14:25-67, 1980.

Sato T: Receptor potential in rat taste cells. In Autrum H and others, editors: *Progress in sensory physiology*, vol 6, Berlin, 1986, Springer-Verlag.

Teeter JH, Brand JG: Peripheral mechanisms of gustation: physiology and biochemistry. In Finger TE, Silver WL, editors: *Neurobiology of taste and smell*, New York, 1987, Wiley.

7 Smell

LEARNING OBJECTIVES

At the end of this chapter you should be able to:

1. Describe the location of the olfactory mucosa in the nasal cavities.
2. Describe the structure of olfactory receptors.
3. Describe the turnover properties of the olfactory mucosa
4. Describe the process of transduction in olfactory receptors.
5. Describe the response properties of afferent olfactory fibers.
6. Describe the central termination of afferent olfactory fibers in the central nervous system.
7. Describe the structure of the olfactory bulb.
8. Describe the ascending neural pathways transmitting olfactory information to olfactory cortex.
9. Describe the changes taking place in the olfactory system during development and aging.

The sense of smell is basic to all animals. It is important in food recognition and in detection of predators and prey for survival, and plays an essential role in reproductive behavior. Many animals communicate with each other by a specialized olfactory system in which chemicals called pheromones are released by the female and detected by the male as part of the mating process. These pheromones are often species specific and aid in species identification as well. Olfactory receptors are exquisitely sensitive molecular detectors capable of responding to more than 10,000 different odor molecules at very low concentrations. Until recently the mechanisms underlying this molecular recognition were largely unknown but with the techniques of molecular biology they are beginning to be understood. However, much further work is required to understand how we can discriminate so many odors.

Although the focus of most investigations into smell has been confined to olfactory receptors, other receptor systems exist that respond to chemicals in inspired air. For example, in addition to the olfactory system the nasal cavity of many vertebrates contains the neuroepithelium of the vomeronasal and septal organs and is richly innervated with trigeminal endings that respond to chemicals in inspired air. Of these sensory systems that respond to odor only the olfactory system will be described in this chapter.

SMELL RECEPTORS

Olfactory receptors are located in two patches of mucosa, one on each side of the nasal septum (Fig. 7-1). The receptor patches are situated out of the main nasal airstream in the most superior part of the nasal cavity. Odors reach the mucosa by turbulence in the flow of air within the nasal cavity. Gross examination of the olfactory mucosa reveals that the receptor patches are a faint yellowish color, in contrast to the pinkish color of the surrounding respiratory mucosa.

Structure of Olfactory Mucosa

The olfactory mucosa is 100 to 200 μm thick and consists of an olfactory epithelium overlying a lamina propria. The pseudostratified columnar epithelium is sensory in function and contains olfactory receptors, sustentacular (supporting) cells, and basal cells (Fig. 7-2). The lamina propria contains bundles of olfactory receptor cell axons, Bowman's glands, and blood vessels. The olfactory mucosa is covered by a 35 μm-deep layer of mucus secreted by sustentacular cells and Bowman's glands.

Olfactory receptor cells are bipolar neurons with cell bodies in the olfactory epithelium. A single small diameter unmyelinated axon arises from the basal end of the soma of the olfactory receptor neuron, penetrates the basal lamina, and aggregates with other olfactory receptor axons to form the olfactory (I) cranial nerve. A single dendrite extends from the apical end of the soma to the epithelial surface, terminating in an apical dendritic knob. Several motile cilia, ranging in length from 20 to 200 μm, arise from the knob and extend into the overlying mucus layer. A second

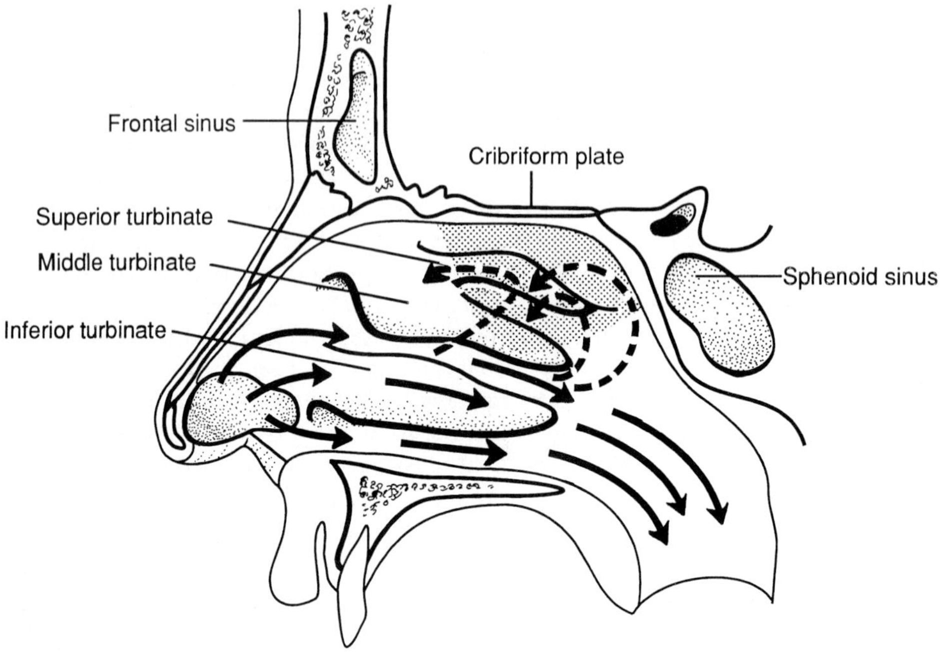

FIG. 7-1
Lateral wall of nasal cavity with location of olfactory mucosa (stippled area) immediately below cribriform plate. Arrows indicate direction of main stream of inspired air over turbinate bones. Olfactory epithelium is outside of main airflow and probably receives odorous molecules by turbulent flow (*dashed arrows*).

type of olfactory receptor with apical microvilli instead of cilia has also been described. The olfactory receptive apparatus is believed to be localized on olfactory cilia. Although the area of the olfactory mucosa is relatively small, it contains a very high density of receptors, estimated at 60 to 100 million depending on the species.

The olfactory epithelium contains high concentrations of olfactory marker protein, a high molecular weight protein found predominantly in olfactory neurons including their axons and dendrites. Besides olfactory marker protein, olfactory receptor cells contain carnosine. The significance of olfactory marker protein and carnosine in the function of olfactory receptors is unknown.

Olfactory receptor cells are separated from each other by columnar sustentacular cells that extend from the basal lamina of the epithelium to the epithelial surface. These cells have a series of irregular microvilli on their apical surface. Besides providing mechanical support for the slender receptor neurons, sustentacular cells contribute secretions to the olfactory mucus. The supranuclear part of the cell contains mucopolysaccharides that are released into the overlying mucus layer. Other functions have been suggested for the sustentacular cells, such as maintenance of an

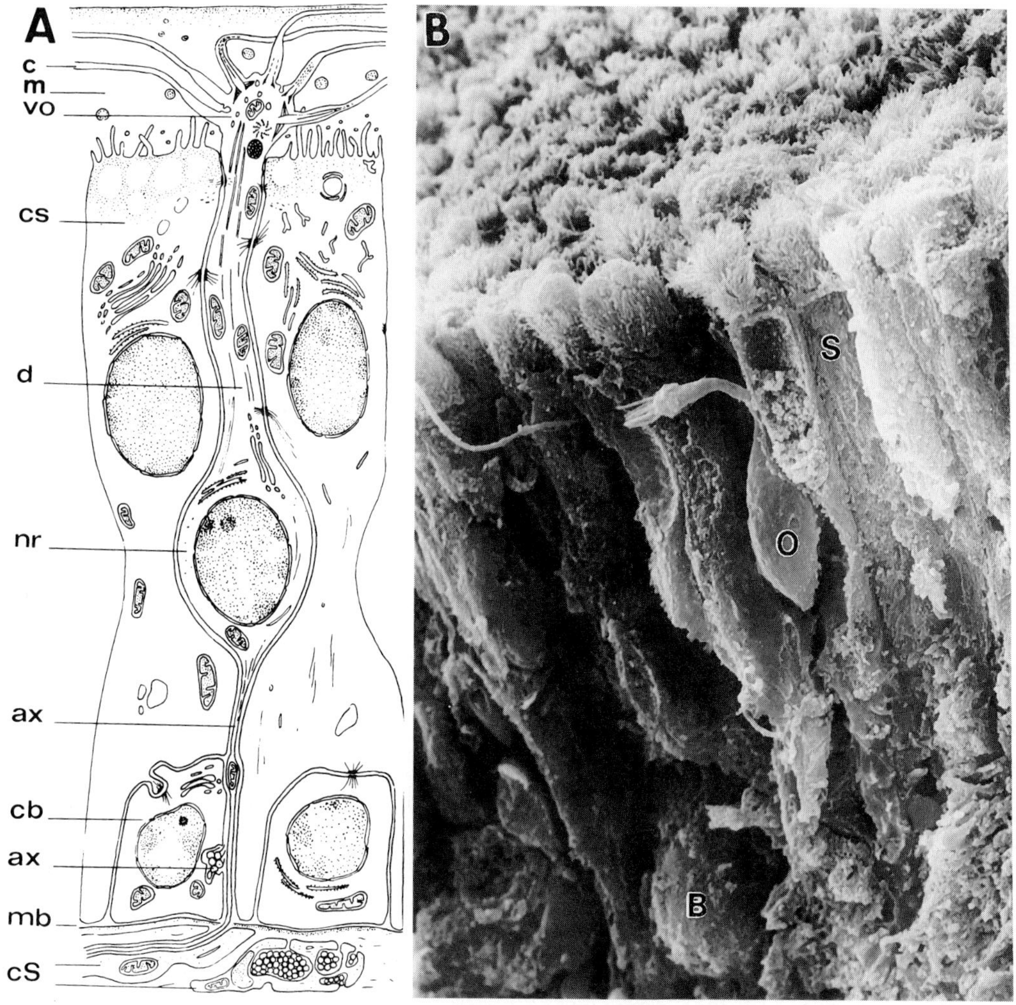

FIG. 7-2

A, Cellular components of the olfactory epithelium: *c*, cilia; *m*, mucus; *vo*, olfactory vesicle; *cs*, supporting cell; *d*, dendrite of olfactory receptor cell; *nr*, nucleus; *ax*, axon; *cb*, basal cell; *mb*, basement membrane; *cS*, Schwann cell. From Holley A, MacLeod PJ: *Journal de Physiologie [Paris]* 73:725-828, 1977). **B**, Scanning electron micrographs of freeze fractured human olfactory epithelium showing the ciliated surface, an olfactory neuron (*O*), supporting c (*S*) and a basal cell (*B*). (From Morrison EE, Costanzo RM: *Journal of Comparative Neurology* 297:1-13, 1990. Reprinted by permission of Wiley-Liss, a division of John Wiley and Sons, Inc.)

ionic reservoir for the electrical activity of the receptor neurons and uptake and transport of odorants.

Prism-shaped basal cells are located close to the basal laminae arranged between basal ends of the sustentacular cells. Basal cells are progenitor cells that replenish the population of receptor neurons.

Dynamic Properties of Olfactory Neurons

Olfactory receptor neurons undergo continual renewal and are the only neurons in mature mammals to do so. Certain cells in the basal region of the epithelium function as progenitor cells. After mitosis, migration, and maturation, they become functionally mature olfactory receptors. Under normal conditions, an olfactory receptor neuron has a life span of 4 to 8 weeks, depending on the species. The senescent receptors are sloughed off from the surface of the epithelium to be replaced by newly formed receptor cells (Fig 7-3).

Receptor Mechanisms

The initial action in odor perception is the inhalation of a mixture of air and the odor. The odor molecules distribute over the epithelial receptor sheet as determined

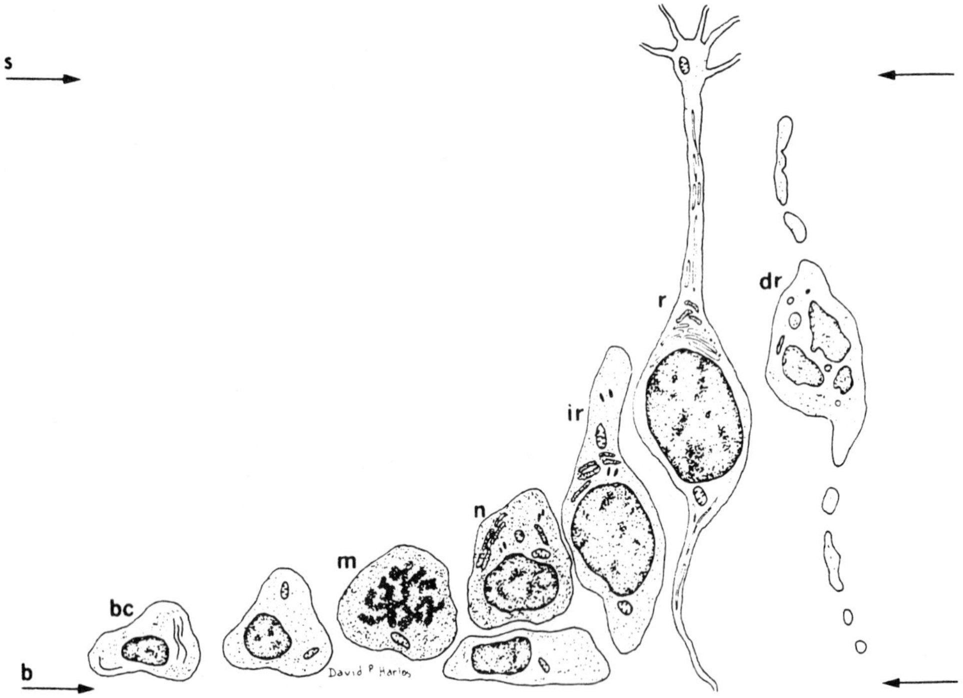

FIG. 7-3
Stages in life cycle of an olfactory neuron. *bc*, Basal cell; *m*, basal cell undergoing mitosis; *n*, neuroblast; *ir*, immature neuron; *r*, receptor neuron; *dr*, degenerating receptor neuron. Arrows indicate suface (s) and basal lamina(*b*) of the epithelium. (From Costanzo RM, Graziadei, PPC: Development and plasticity of the olfactory epithelium. In Finger TE, Silver WL [editors]: *Neurobiology of taste and smell*, New York, 1987, Wiley, pp.233-250, copyright © 1987. Reprinted by permission of Wiley-Liss, a division of John Wiley and Sons, Inc.)

by the turbulence of the airflow, the shape of the nasal cavity, and the differential adsorption of the compound with the muscosal surface. Thus, odorant molecules with different chemical properties are distributed over the receptor sheet in an irregular pattern before any neural events take place.

Because the surface of the olfactory mucosa is covered with mucus, odorants have to cross this layer to reach the olfactory receptors. The mucus layer moves across the surface of the olfactory mucosa at 10 to 60 mm/min toward the internal nares. Study of olfactory mucus has revealed that several events take place during passage of the odorants to the receptors. These include differential sorption of the odorants across the mucosal surface, diffusion of the odorants to the receptor neurons, and interactions of odorants with the chemoreceptive membranes.

The mucus is an aqueous solution of electrolytes and proteins. Many odorants in air occur in low concentrations of hydrophobic molecules that must traverse the hydrophilic mucus layer. The access of hydrophobic odorants to the olfactory recep-

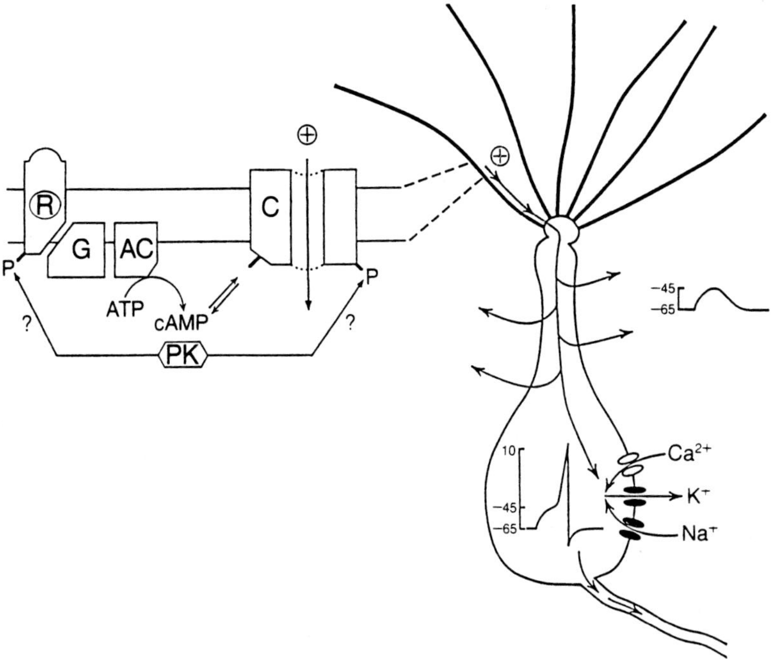

FIG. 7-4
Early events in olfactory transduction. Odorants interact with membrane receptors (*R*) on the cilia coupled by a GTP-binding protein (*G*) to a second messenger system that uses cyclic AMP as well as other second messengers. Activation of cyclic AMP by adenylate cyclase (*C*) opens ion channels to depolarize the neuron resulting in the production of action potentials. Both the receptor protein and the ion channel have phosphorylation sites, and protein kinase A (*PK*) has been identified in the cilia. Receptor-coupled events are diagrammed on left and olfactory neuron on right. (From Firestein SA: *Trends in Neuroscience* 14:270-272, 1991.)

tors is thought to be enhanced by an odorant binding protein. By binding and solubilizing hydrophobic odorants, olfactory binding protein is thought to increase the odorant concentration in the mucus layer and, therefore, in the environment of the olfactory receptors. It is also possible that odorant binding proteins may function to remove odorants from the receptor environment as well.

Once the odorants cross the mucus layer they interact with the olfactory receptor neurons to begin the process of molecular detection, odorant discrimination, and sensory transduction. Based on electrophysiologic, biochemical, and morphologic studies, odorants are believed to interact with cellular membrane proteins in the ciliary membranes and apical dendritic knob. The interaction of an odorant with the chemosensory membrane initiates a series of membrane events associated with sensory transduction and subsequent electrical changes. Most odorants bind reversibly to the receptor, which is essential in preventing continued olfactory stimulation once the odorant has been removed. It is known that binding of an odorant to a receptor molecule activates a guanosine triphosphate (GTP) binding protein or G-protein, which modulates the activity of adenylate cyclase, an enzyme that produces the sec-

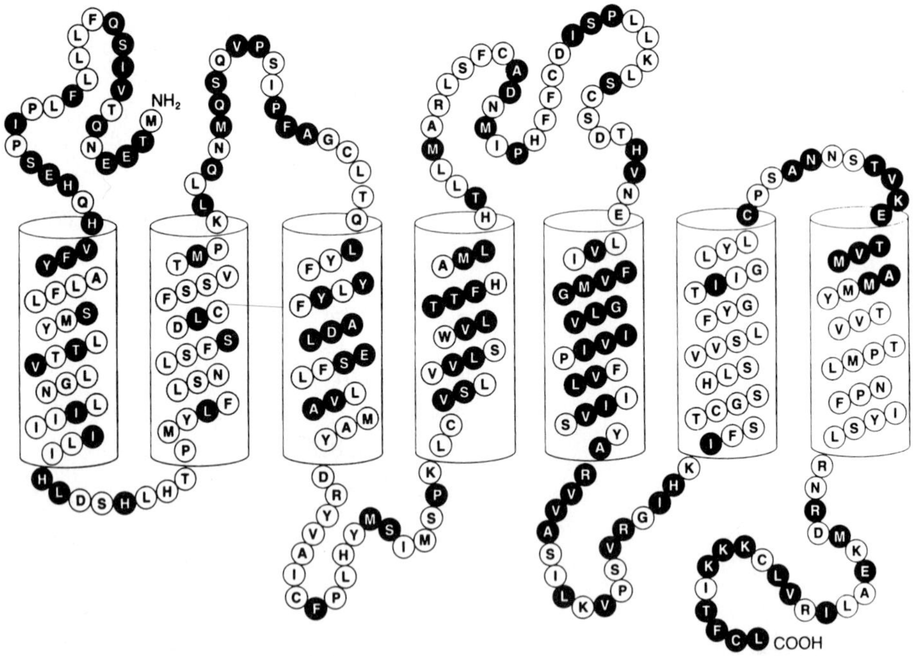

FIG. 7-5
Proposed structure of an olfactory receptor protein. Seven transmembrane regions are indicated by cylinders. Amino terminus is located extracellularly and carboxy terminus intracellularly. Residues in black are those showing most variability in the different clones isolated. By analogy with β-adrenergic receptor, length of intracellular residues linking transmembrane domains V and VI (the fifth and sixth cylinders from the left) is believed to include the site of interaction with the G protein. (From Buck L, Axel R: *Cell* 65:175-187, 1991. Copyright by Cell Press.)

ond messenger cyclic adenosine monophosphate (AMP). The latter molecule activates cyclic AMP-dependent protein kinase to cause phosphorylation of ion channel peptides, thereby opening ion channels to produce changes in membrane potential (Fig. 7-4).

G-proteins in other receptor systems, such as the β-adrenergic receptor, link membrane spanning receptors with enzymes inside the cell. All of these receptors share certain parts of their amino acid sequences, and are members of a "superfam-

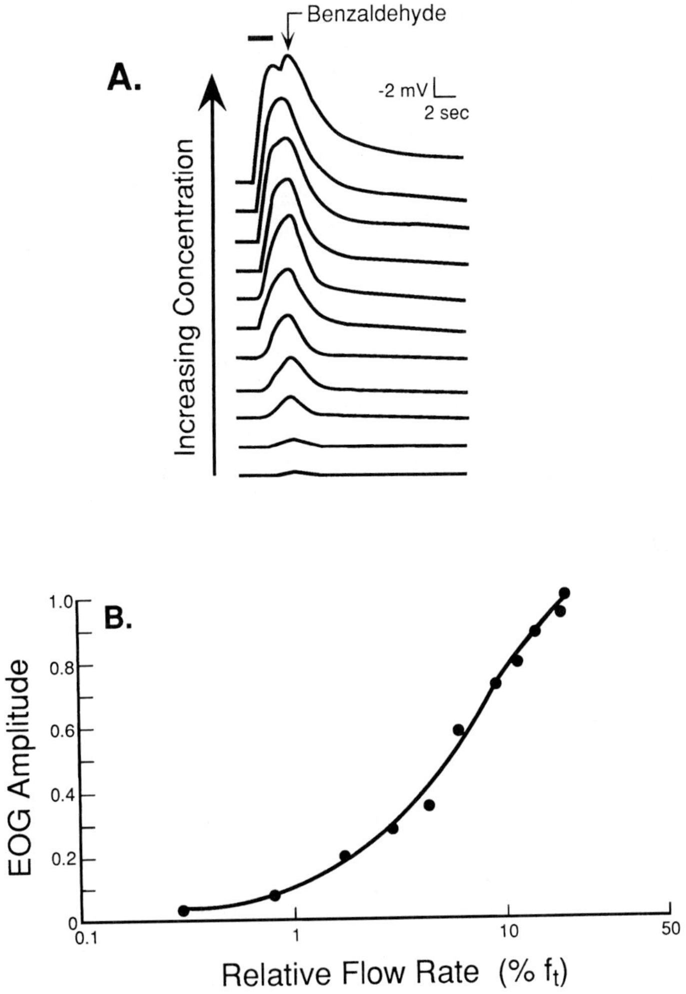

FIG. 7-6
A, Electroolfactograms (EOG) in response to increasing concentrations of benzaldehyde. Horizontal bar indicates time of stimulus application. **B,** Relationship of magnitude of the EOG as a function of odorant concentration. Odorant concentration was manipulated by increasing the flow rate of odorant. (From Getchell TV: *Journal of Neurophysiology* 6:1115-1130, 1974.)

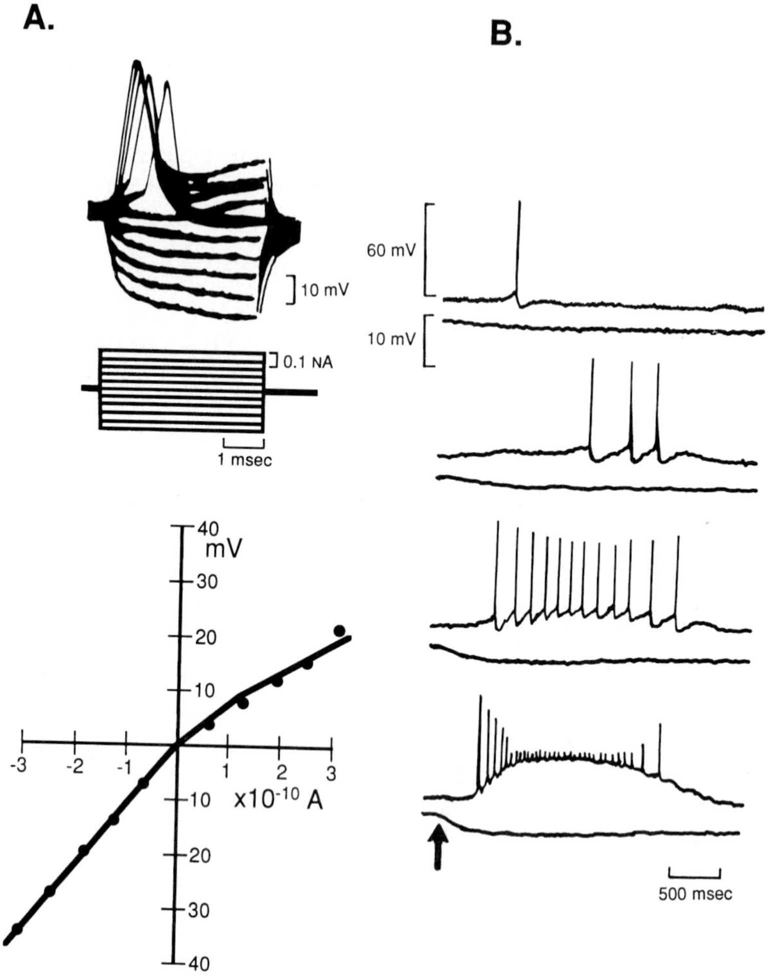

FIG. 7-7

A, *Top*. Response of lamprey olfactory receptor neuron to hyperpolarizing and depolarizing current injections through intracellular recording electrode. *Bottom*. Plot of the steady state membrane response to injected currents. (From Suzuki N:Intracellular responses of lamprey olfactory receptors to current and chemical stimulation. In Katsuki Y, Sato M, Takagi S, Oomura Y, editors: *Food Intake and the Chemical Senses*, Tokyo, 1977, Japan Scientific Societies Press, pp. 13-22.) **B**, Responses of olfactory receptor neuron to stimulation with increasing concentrations of amyl acetate. Top record shows action potentials superimposed on membrane depolarizations. Bottom trace is the EOG, which starts at the arrow. (From Trotier D, Macleod P: *Brain Research* 268:225-237, 1983.)

ily," with seven transmembrane regions. Molecular cloning techniques have revealed that olfactory receptors belong to this superfamily (Fig. 7-5). Each olfactory receptor probably expresses a subset of the large (estimated more than 100) receptor repertoire. While there is little doubt that these recently discovered receptors are involved in olfaction, it is not known how they actually bind odor molecules nor is it known if they are capable of binding one or a range of odors. However, the size of the family implies that there are many different receptors distributed over the millions of olfactory neurons and this suggest that a considerable amount of sensory process takes place at the level of the olfactory epithelium.

Several types of ion channels have been characterized in isolated olfactory neurons with the patch clamp technique. These include two types of Ca^{2+}-activated K^+ channel, a K^+ channel that opens and then is inactivated by rapid depolarization, a Cl^- channel, and voltage-gated Ca^{2+} channels. There is no major difference in the types of channels found on the dendritic knobs and somatic membranes so that the exact role of these channels in olfactory transduction remains unknown.

A slow voltage transient caused by receptor current flow occurs in response to odorant interaction with the olfactory receptors. This monophasic-negative transient mucosal potential is called the electro-olfactogram (EOG). The amplitude and rise time of the EOG increase with increasing odorant concentration (Fig. 7-6). The EOG is a summation of the initial receptor events taking place in olfactory transduction and cannot be recorded from a nasal mucosa that does not contain olfactory receptors.

Intracellular recordings have been obtained from nonmammalian olfactory receptor neurons. Olfactory receptor neurons have membrane potentials ranging from -33 to -65 mV, a high input resistance that ranges from 75 to 600 MΩ, with action potentials superimposed on membrane depolarization. Increased injections of current through the recording electrode or odorant application result in increased levels of membrane depolarization and the number of superimposed action potentials (Fig. 7-7). Analysis of the current voltage plots indicates that the receptor membrane obey Ohm's law in the hyperpolarizing direction but is nonlinear in the depolarizing direction exhibiting rectification.

Recordings from Afferent Olfactory Fibers

Spontaneous action potentials ranging from 3 to 60 impulses per second can be recorded from individual axons of the olfactory nerve. In response to short pulses of odorants, receptor neurons initiate action potentials after a short latency with a frequency that is concentration-dependent. The initial frequency of the response is high, adapting to a lower frequency that returns to spontaneous levels after the stimulus is removed.

When a large number of olfactory stimuli are used, approximately 50% of the olfactory neurons sampled respond to at least one odorant. Many receptor neurons respond to more than one odorant, but individual neurons respond to a different

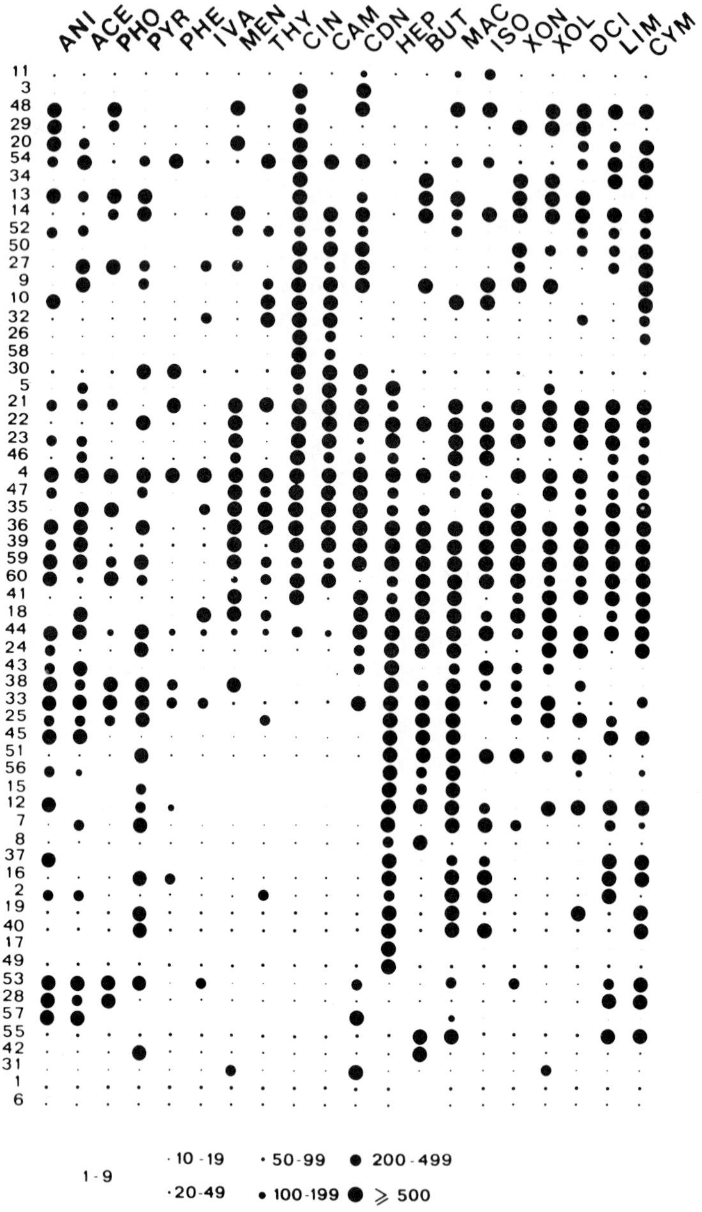

FIG. 7-8
Extracellularly recorded response of 60 frog olfactory neurons. Size of each dot is proportional to impulse's discharge frequency (impulses/min). Abbreviations along top of figure indicate 20 odorants used to stimulate each receptor. Receptor cells are indicated by numbers on the left. Note that there is no apparent response pattern, and olfactory receptor neurons do not respond exclusively to any one odorant. (From Sicard G, Holley A: *Brain Research* 292:283-296. 1984.)

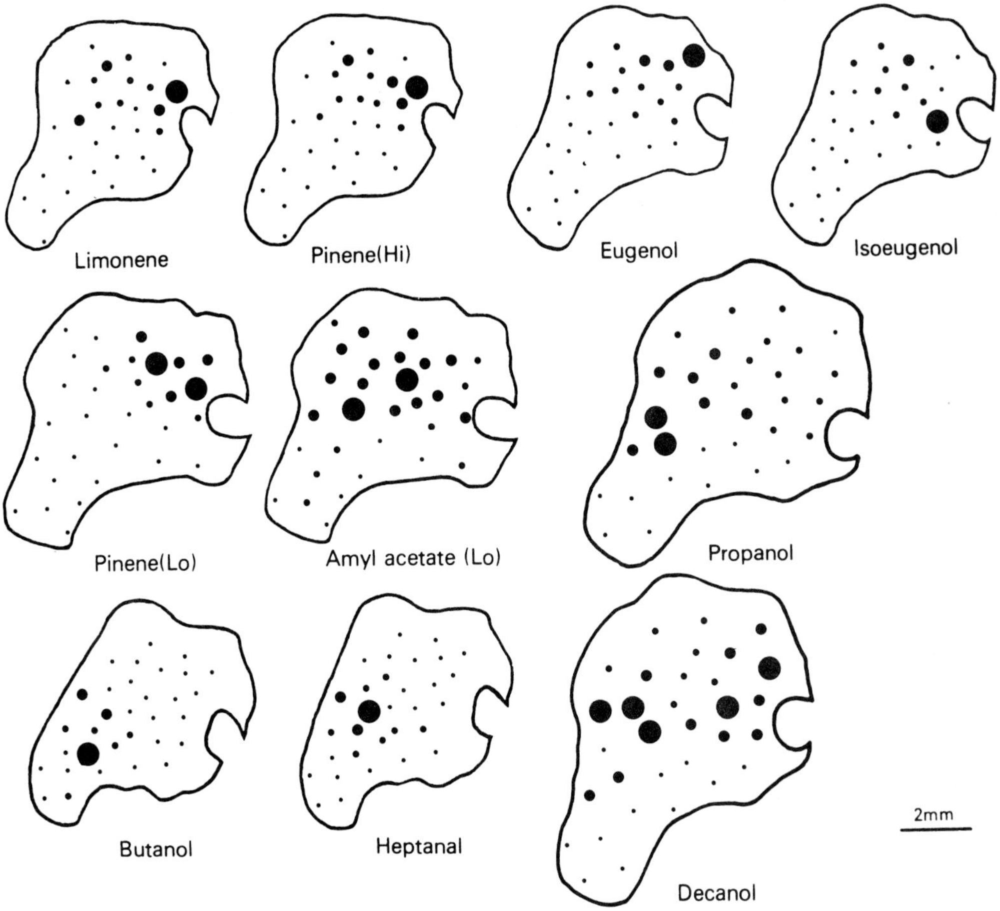

FIG. 7-9

Average amplitudes of EOG response to different odors recorded at different location on the olfactory epithelium of a salamander. Size of dots represents relative EOG amplitudes. Largest dot represents 95% to 100% of maximum, the next largest represents 60% to 94% of maximum, third largest 30% to 35%, and the smallest dots represent 0% to 29% of maximum. Note that different odorants have different spatial patterns of activity. (From Mackay-Sim A, Shaman P, Moulton DG: *Journal of Neurophysiology* 48:548-596, 1982.)

subset of the total battery of odorant stimuli (Fig. 7-8). This suggests that a different distribution of molecular receptors exists in the chemoreceptive membranes across the population of olfactory receptor cells.

Examination of neural activity over the whole area of the olfactory mucosa to applied odorants has revealed a spatial pattern of activity characteristic of each odorant. This suggests that the spatial pattern of activity of the whole olfactory mucosa might be important in coding odor quality (Fig. 7-9).

CENTRAL OLFACTORY PATHWAYS

Central Termination of Olfactory Afferent Fibers

In most mammals axons of olfactory receptor neurons aggregated into bundles pass through foramina in the bone immediately above the olfactory mucosa. This bone is called the cribriform plate. The axons then distribute over the surface of the olfactory bulb, a layered structure that is the site of the first synaptic interactions in the olfactory pathway. Electrophysiologic, degeneration, and central tracing studies have revealed a topographic projection of the olfactory mucosa onto the olfactory bulb. Moreover, spatial pattern of activity observed in the olfactory mucosa to odorant stimulation is preserved at the olfactory bulb level.

Olfactory bulb

The layered appearance of the olfactory bulb results from the arrangement of different neuronal types in each layer (Fig. 7-10). From the surface of the bulb inward the layers of the bulb are the olfactory nerve layer, the periglomerular region, the glomerular layer, the external plexiform layer, the mitral cell layer, the internal plexiform layer, and the granule cell layer (Fig. 7-11, *A*). Afferent axons of the olfactory nerve enter the bulb to form the olfactory nerve layer. Many of these axons connect with the dendritic tree of mitral cells to form spherical structures called glomeruli which are the most prominent feature of the bulb (see Fig. 7-10). The granule cell layer contains the output axons from the bulb and substantial numbers of centrifugal fibers originating in various forebrain structures.

Several different neuron types are distributed within the layers of the olfactory bulb. Neurons with axons that leave the bulb, called principal cells (Fig. 7-11, *A*), are mitral and tufted cells. A number of other neuron types are intrinsic to the bulb (Fig. 7-11, *B*). These interneurons, scattered throughout the bulb, comprise perglomerular cells, short axon cells, and several types of granule cells.

Cell bodies of mitral cells form a single layer within the bulb. Mitral cells send smooth, apical dendrites into the glomeruli where they branch and connect with primary afferent axons. The axons of the mitral cells form the lateral olfactory tract, the main output path of the olfactory bulb. The cell bodies of the tufted cells are scattered throughout the external plexiform layer, and, based on their location and on dendritic arbors, are subdivided into three different morphologic types referred to as external, middle, and internal tufted cells (Fig. 7-11). Tufted cells situated in the middle and deeper external plexiform layers send their axons to join the lateral olfactory tract, while the axons of superficial tufted cells are intrinsic to the bulb. Both tufted and mitral cells have long secondary dendrites that run laterally within the bulb.

Periglomerular cells, as their name suggests, are situated between and interconnect the glomeruli. Granule cells, which do not have axons, have apical dendritic trees extending into the external plexiform layer and basal dendrites localized in

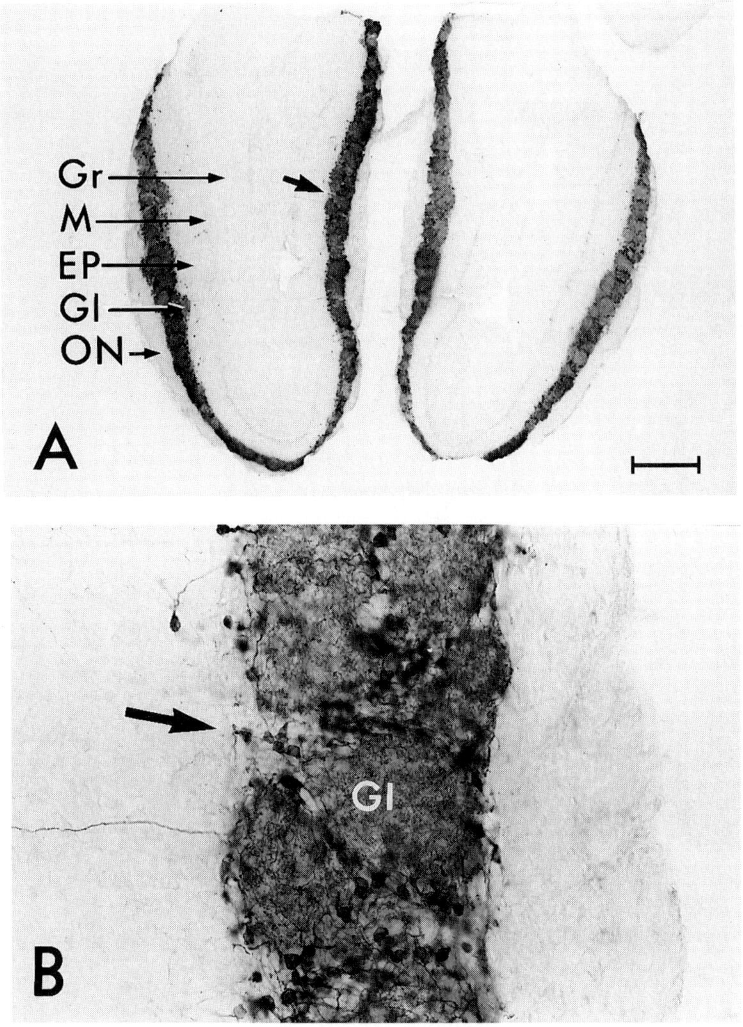

FIG. 7-10
Horizontal section of mouse olfactory bulbs stained for tyrosine hydroxylase immunoreactivity. This stains the glomerular layer (*Gl*) intensely as seen at the higher power in the lower panel. Laminar structure of the olfactory bulb can be clearly seen. Granule cell layer (*Gr*); mitral cell layer (*M*); olfactory nerve layer (*ON*); external plexiform layer (*EP*). Scale bar in **A** = 400 μm and in **B** = 40 μm. Large arrow in **A** indicates region shown at higher magnifiaction in **B**. (Photomicrographs kindly supplied by Dr. Harriet Baker.)

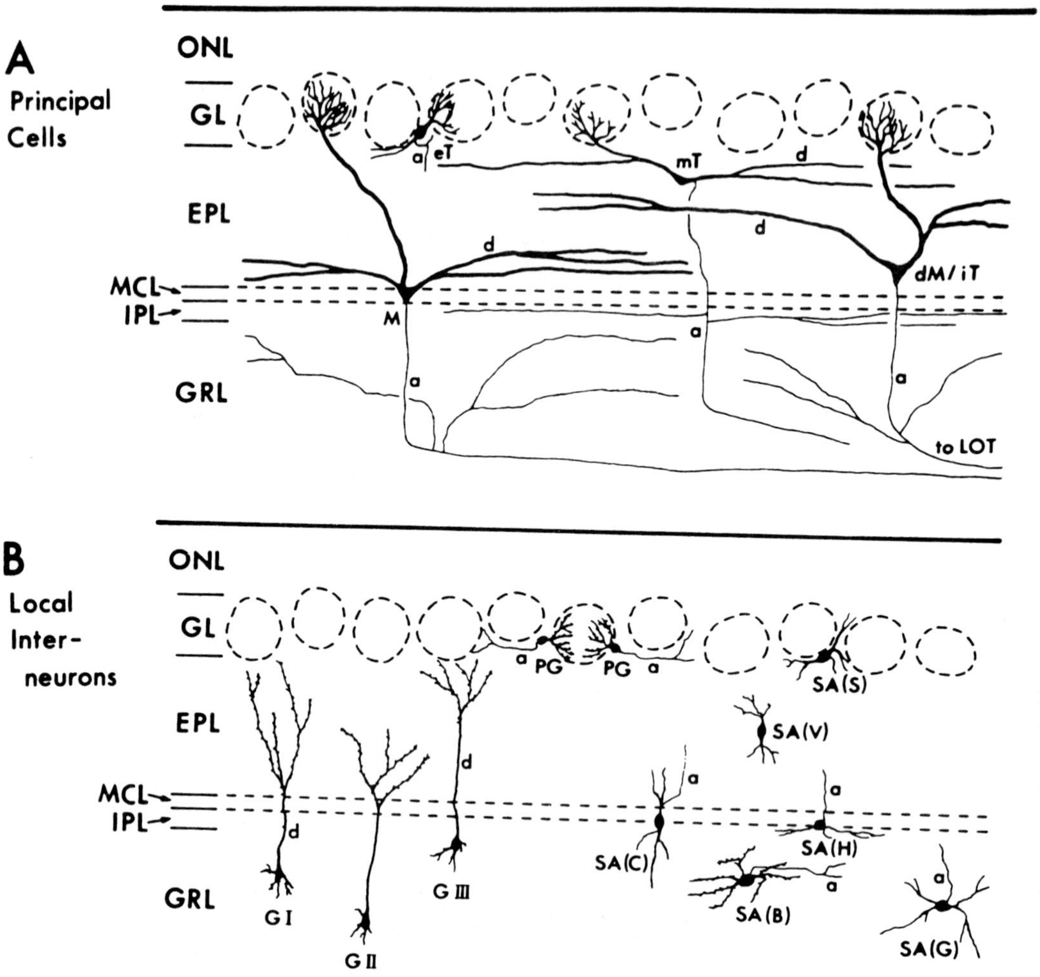

FIG. 7-11
Laminar distribution of principal cells (**A**) and local interneurons (**B**) in mammalian main olfactory bulb. *ONL*, olfactory nerve layer, *GL*, glomerular layer; *EPL*, external plexiform layer; *MCL*, mitral cell layer; *IPL*, internal plexiform layer; *GRL*, granule cell layer; *LOT*, lateral olfactory tract; *M*, mitral cell soma; *d*, dendrites; *a*, axons; *mT*, middle tufted cell; *dM/iT*, displaced mitral or internal tufted cell; *GI*, *GII*, *GIII*, three types of granule cell, *PG*, periglomerular cell; *SA(V)*, *SA(S)*, *SA(H)*, *SA(B)*, *SA(G)*, *SA(C)*, various types of short axon cells. (Reprinted from Mori K: *Progress in Neurobiology* 29:275-320, copyright 1987, with permission from Pergamon Press Ltd., Headington Hill Hall, Oxford, UK.)

the granule cell layer. Various types of short axon cells are located in the external plexiform and granule cell layers.

Tens of millions of olfactory afferent fibers terminate within approximately 2000 glomeruli associated with 70,000 mitral cells and 160,000 tufted cells. Therefore, there is a considerable degree of convergence/divergence between the periphery and within the olfactory bulb. The presence of two output neurons in the bulb suggests parallel circuits for processing olfactory information and the number and variety of interneurons indicate that the bulb is responsible for considerable processing of the olfactory information.

Since there is considerable convergence/divergence between the periphery and the mitral cells plus interactions between glomeruli mediated by periglomerular cells, it is not surprising to find that odor responses of mitral cells are complex. Response patterns are composed of temporal sequences of depolarization and

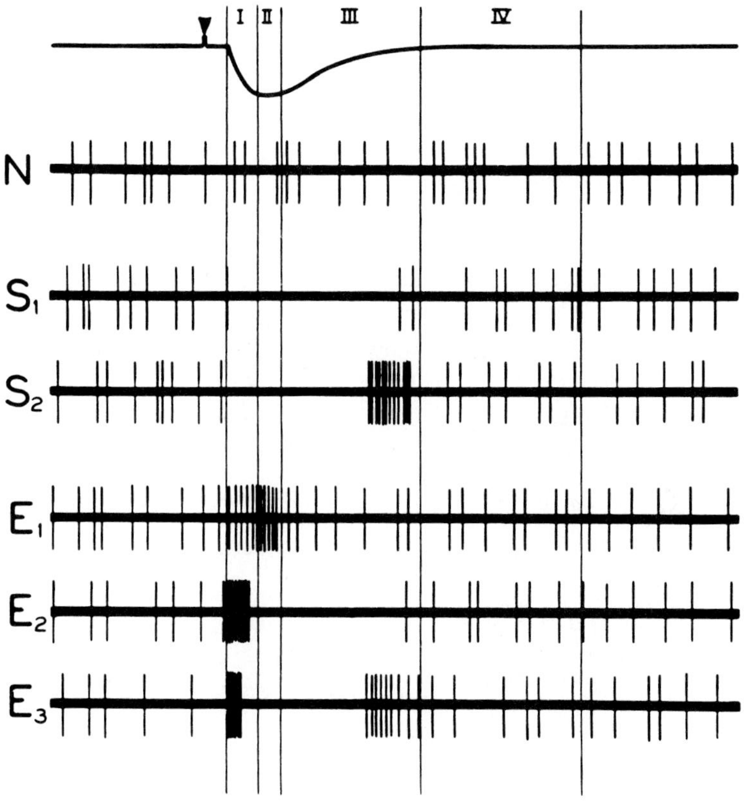

FIG. 7-12
Extracellular recordings from olfactory bulb mitral cells to show different responses to odors. Time of odor application is shown by arrow in the top trace, which represents the EOG recorded from surface of olfactory epithelium designated I-IV. Response patterns are as follows: N shows no response; S_1 and S_2 are responses in which odor application suppresses the ongoing spontaneous activity; E_1-E_3 are responses in which odors increase frequency of action potentials. In E_2 there is a pronounced burst of action potentials, called an "on response," at the time the odor reaches the receptors. In E_3 there is a pronounced burst of action potentials at the time odor reaches receptors as well as when odor pulse ends, called an "off response." (From Kauer JS: *Journal of Physiology [London]* 243:695-715, 1974.)

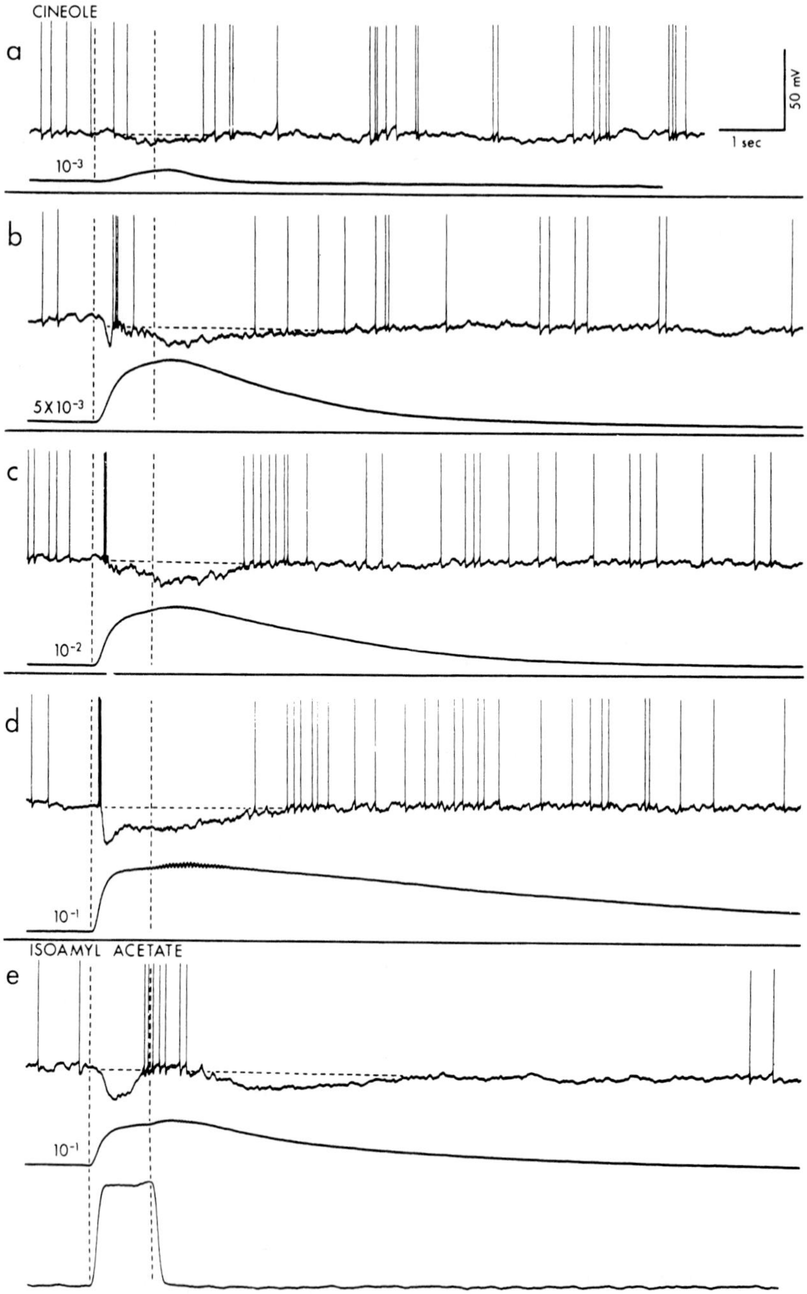

FIG. 7-13
Intracellular recordings of responses by a salamander mitral/tufted cell to four concentrations of cineole (*a-d*) and one concentration of amyl acetate (e). Both of these odors were applied to the olfactory epithelium. Bottom trace indicates the time course of the odor pulse application. Under each action potential trace is shown the EOG for each odor application recorded at the olfactory mucosa. Response to cineole shows sequences of excitation and suppression similar to E response of Fig. 7-12. Suppression of activity followed by excitation at end of the stimulus is similar to the S_2 pattern of Fig. 7-12. (From Hamilton KA, Kauer JS: *Brain Research* 338:181-185, 1985.)

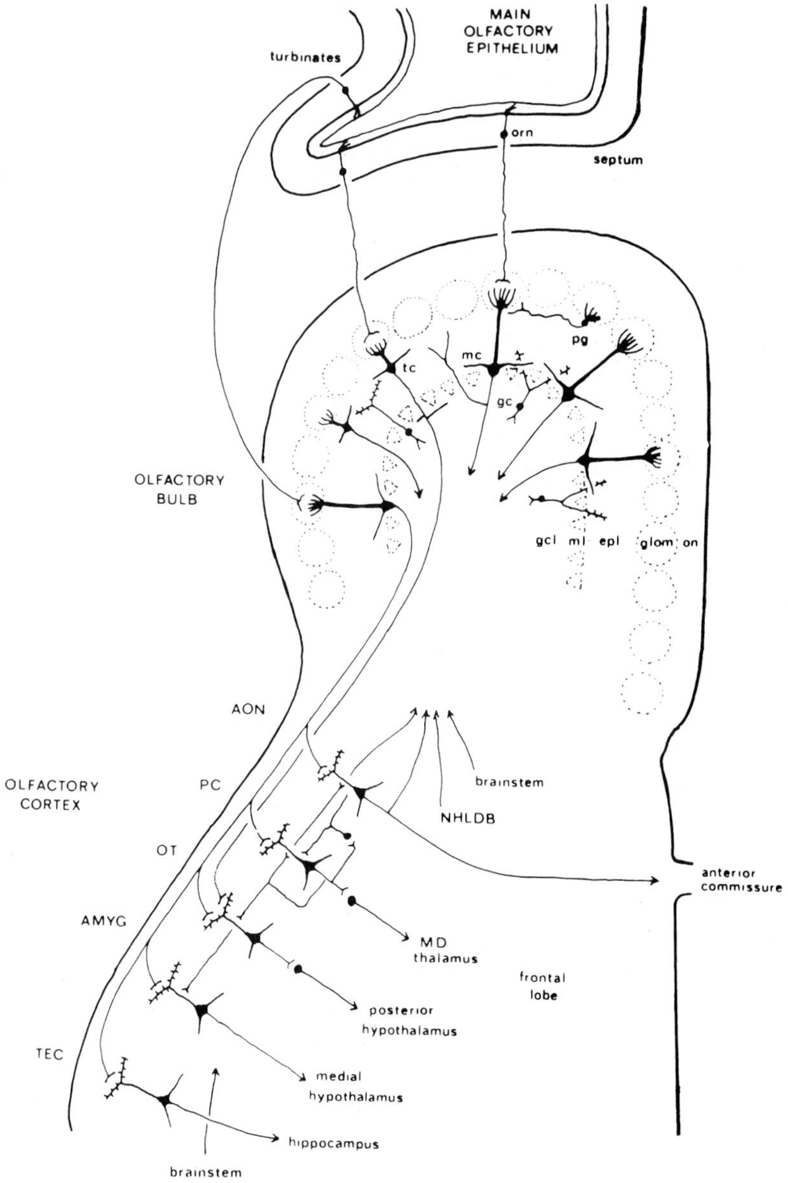

FIG. 7-14
Olfactory pathways. Olfactory bulb receives input from olfactory receptors and projects to olfactory cortex, with connection to other brain areas. *AON*, anterior olfactory nucleus; *PC* piriform cortex; *OT*, olfactory tubercle; *AMYG*, amygdala, *TEC*, temporal entorhinal cortex; *on*, olfactory nerve layer; *glom*, glomerula layer; *epl*, external plexiform layer; *mi*, mitral cell layer; *gcl*, granule cell layer; *tc*, tufted cell; *mc*, mitral cell; *pg*, periglomerular cell; *gc*, granule cell; *orn*, olfactory receptor neuron. (From Greer CA: Structural organization of the olfactory system. In Getchell TV, Doty RL, Bartoshuk LM, Snow JB Jr, editors: *Smell and taste in health and disease*, New York, 1991, Raven Press, pp. 65-91.)

hyperpolarization that presumably result from interactions of excitatory and inhibitory synapses in the bulb. With both extracellular and intracellular recording techniques, mitral cells either do not respond to an odor, their spontaneous activity is suppressed by an odor, or they are excited by an odor (Fig. 7-12). These basic types of response can be subdivided based on other criteria such as the occurrence of a burst at the beginning of odor stimulation. Moreover, a single mitral cell can respond with one pattern to one odorant and a second pattern to another odorant, indicating the complexity of the integration taking place at the second order neuron (Fig. 7-13).

Projections to olfactory cortex

The olfactory cortex is a region of the cortex that receives direct axonal input from the olfactory bulb. This projection area is subdivided into the anterior olfactory nucleus, the piriform cortex, the olfactory tubercle, the cortical surface area of the amygdala, and the temporal entorhinal cortex (Fig. 7-14). Most parts of the mammalian olfactory cortex have three prominent layers. Layer I is a superficial molecular layer containing apical dendrites of the cells in deeper layers. The axons from the olfactory bulb terminate in the superficial part of this layer. Layer II is a densely packed cellular layer composed primarily of the cell bodies of pyramidal cells. Layer III contains a high density of larger pyramidal cell soma and polymorphic cells.

Mitral and tufted cell axons from all parts of the olfactory bulb are distributed diffusely across the cortex, and there is no clear topographical arrangement in the central olfactory pathways. Although the terminal fields of mitral and tufted cells are generally intermingled, tufted cells do not appear to project to caudal piriform cortex or entorhinal cortex. Neurons in the olfactory cortex respond to a large number of odors, and there is no indication of any neurons responsive to specific odors.

Olfactory information is sent from the olfactory cortex to several other parts of the brain, including the orbital neocortex, the mediodorsal and submedial nuclei of the thalamus, the lateral hypothalamus, and the limbic area such as the amygdala and hippocampus. The neocortical projections are very close to the gustatory cortical area, and it has been suggested that these two areas overlap and thus form the neurobiological substrate responsible for flavor. However, physiologic recordings indicate that the gustatory and olfactory regions of the cortex are separate and it is, therefore, still unclear whether there is a specific brain region devoted to flavor. The olfactory projection to hypothalamic areas is important in reproductive behavior and, if lesioned, interrupts mating behavior in male hamsters. Other projections probably function in the emotional and motivational aspects of odor stimuli as well as contributing to odor memory. Often an odor can arouse a memory of an event that has taken place many years ago through these limbic system connections.

DEVELOPMENT AND AGING

The olfactory epithelium originates from paired thickenings of the cranial ectoderm called the olfactory placode. During development, these placodes invaginate to form the olfactory pits, which then develop into the olfactory cavities. This ectoderm of the placode consists of two layers—a superficial nonnervous layer and a deeper nervous layer. The nervous layer gives rise to the olfactory receptors; the sustentacular cells and Bowman's glands originate from the nonnervous layer. In rodents the olfactory system is functional during the latter stages of gestation and prenatal rats respond behaviorally to odorants.

In humans the olfactory system shows a decreased sensitivity over the lifespan. Estimates of the magnitude of the threshold changes associated with aging vary, but range from a twofold to tenfold decrease in sensitivity depending on the odor used for testing and the age of the individual. These age-related changes in the olfactory system are probably the most significant factor in complaints regarding food in the elderly.

SUMMARY

Olfactory receptors are highly sensitive molecular detectors situated in the olfactory epithelium. The receptors are neurons with cell bodies in the epithelium. Odors interact with the olfactory receptor cilia situated on dendritic knobs. The axons of the olfactory neurons form the olfactory nerve. Two other cell types are found in the olfactory epithelium. They are the sustentacular cells, which contribute secretions to a layer of mucus overlying the olfactory epithelium, and the basal cells, which by division form new olfactory receptors. Olfactory receptors turn over and are capable of regeneration. Below the epithelium are numerous glands, called Bowman's glands, which also contribute their secretions to the olfactory mucus.

To gain access to the olfactory receptors odorants have to cross the mucus layer. Several events take place during this passage, including differential sorption of the odorants across the mucosal surface, diffusion of the odorants to the receptor neurons, and interactions of odorants with the chemoreceptive membranes. Many odorants are hydrophobic and their access to the olfactory receptors is enhanced by an odorant-binding protein.

Odorants are believed to interact with the cellular membrane, which initiates a series of membrane events involving binding of an odorant to a receptor molecule. This activates a G-protein–coupled adenylate-cyclase cascade causing ion channels to open, with changes in the membrane potential.

When a large number of odorants are used to stimulate olfactory receptors, olfactory neurons respond to at least one odorant. Many receptor neurons respond to more than one odorant, but individual neurons respond to a different subset of odorant stimuli. Examination of neural activity over the whole area of the olfactory mucosa reveals a spatial pattern of activity of the olfactory receptors that is related to the applied odorant. This spatial pattern of activity might be important in coding odor quality.

Olfactory axons terminate in a layered structure, called the olfactory bulb, and form synapses with the dendrites of mitral and tufted cells in glomeruli. The olfactory bulb contains many different kinds of interneurons and is responsible for considerable sensory processing. Recordings from mitral cells in the olfactory bulb reflect the complexity of the neural processing, because these neurons respond with one pattern of neural discharge to one odorant and a second pattern to another.

From the olfactory bulb the axons of mitral and tufted cells project to several areas of the olfactory cortex. Neurons in the olfactory cortex respond to a large number of odors, and there is no indication of any neurons responsive to specific odors.

The olfactory system shows a decreased sensitivity over the lifespan. These age-related changes in the olfactory system are probably the most significant factor in complaints of changes of food flavor from aging individuals.

SELECTED READINGS

Buck LB: The olfactory multigene family, *Current opinion in neurobiology* 2:467-473, 1992.

Carr WES, Gleeson RA, Trapido-Rosenthal HG: The role of perireceptor events in chemosensory processes, *Trends in Neuroscience* 13:212-215, 1990.

Firestein, S: A noseful of odor receptors, *Trends in Neuroscience* 14:270-272, 1991.

Getchell TV: Functional properties of vertebrate olfactory neurons, *Physiological Reviews* 66:772-818, 1986.

Kauer JS: Contributions of topography and parallel processing to odor coding in the vertebrate olfactory pathway, *Trends in Neuroscience* 14:79-85, 1991.

Lancet D: Vertebrate olfactory reception, *Annual Review of Neuroscience* 9:329-355, 1986.

Mori K: Membrane and synaptic properties of identified neurons in the olfactory bulb, *Progress in Neurobiology* 29:275-320, 1987.

Shepherd GM: Current issues in the molecular biology of olfaction, *Chemical Senses* 18:191-198, 1993.

8 Thermal Receptors

LEARNING OBJECTIVES

At the end of this chapter you should be able to:

1. Describe the distribution of warm and cold spots on the body surface.
2. Describe the variation of thermal sensitivity over the body surface.
3. Describe the variation of thermal sensitivity in the oral cavity.
4. Give a classification of thermal receptors.
5. Describe what is known about the structure of thermal receptors.
6. Describe the process of transduction in thermal receptors.
7. Describe the response characteristics of cold receptors.
8. Describe the response characteristics of warm receptors.
9. Describe the ascending neural pathways transmitting thermal information in the central nervous system.

Temperature or thermal sensation originating in the oral cavity is important in the appreciation of flavor, and many different foods must be served at a particular temperature in order to be appreciated. For example, ice cream has an optimum flavor when eaten cold but if served hot is not very palatable. Receptors in the oral cavity called thermal receptors (sometimes referred to as thermoreceptors) respond to food temperature and transmit it to the central nervous system.

In the physical world temperature is a continuous variable extending from the extreme cold of outer space to the intense heat at the center of the sun. Humans are exposed only to a very narrow range of this physical temperature continuum. Moreover, when behavioral measures are made of human temperature experience, it is found that thermal sensation is not a continuous variable but is divided into sensations we call warm and cold. Between the temperature ranges that give rise to sensations of warm and cold is a range that produces neither sensation. This range of indifference in which we are neither warm nor cold is the temperature at which we are most comfortable.

Given these dual behavioral expressions of thermal sensation, it is not surprising to find that the body surface and oral cavity are not uniformly sensitive to temperature but are divided into areas of sensitivity that respond to temperatures we call cold or warm. These areas consist of small spots of heightened thermal sensitivity that respond to either warm or cold stimulation separated by areas insensitive to thermal stimulation. When the density of these spots was measured it was found that cold-sensitive spots are more numerous than warm-sensitive spots, with the highest density of both cold and warm spots found on the face (Table 8-1). Because the face has a higher density of warm and cold spots than any other area of the body it has the highest sensitivity to warm and cold stimulation. This was tested by measuring the rate of sweating on thigh skin when various body surfaces such as the face

TABLE 8-1

Number of cold and warm spots per square centimeter of human skin

	Cold spots*	Warm spots†
Forehead	5.5-8.0	
Nose	8.0	1.0
Lips	16.0-19.0	
Other parts of face	8.5-9.0	1.7
Chest	9.0-10.2	0.3
Abdomen	8.0-12.5	
Thigh	4.5-5.2	0.4
Sole of foot	3.4	

*Strughold H, Porz R: 1931. Die Dichte der Kaltpunkte auf der Haut des menschlichen Korper, *Z Biol* 91:16-17, 1931.

†Rein FH: Über die Topographie der Warmempfindung, Beziehungen zwischen Innervation und receptorischen Endorganen, *Z Biol* 82:515-535, 1925.

were heated. Areas with the highest sensitivity to warm stimuli produced the highest rate of sweat production. When the different areas of the body were exposed to equal intensities of warm stimulation, the sweat rate varied according to the stimulated region; warming the face produced the highest rate of sweating on the thigh skin. Similar experiments with the application of cold stimuli to various body areas showed that the facial region was most sensitive to cooling also, the measure here being the decrease in sweating rate of thigh skin when different parts of the body are cooled (Fig. 8-1).

Measurement of sweating rate is an indirect method of measuring thermal sensitivity. Recently the thermal sensitivity of the face and oral cavity has been measured with magnitude estimation in which the subjects assigned a number representing

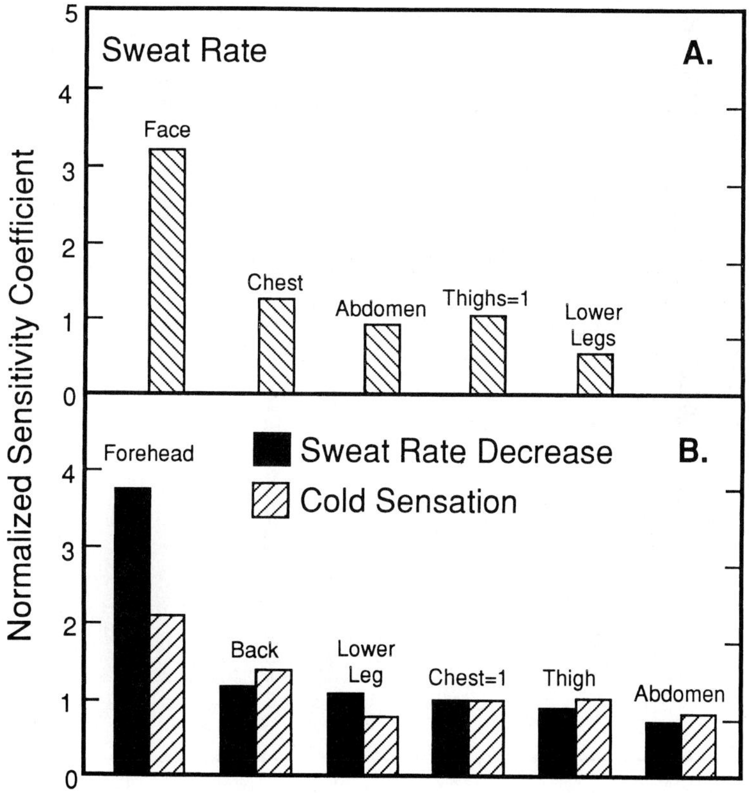

FIG. 8-1
Sensitivity coefficients of various body surfaces. **A**, Sensitivity to warming measured by reflex sweat rate. (From Nadel ER, Mitchell JW, Stolwijk JAJ: *Pflügers Archiv* 340:71-76, 1973.) **B**, Sensitivity to cooling measured by decrease in reflex sweat rate and perceived cold sensation. (From Crawshaw LI, and others: *Pflügers Archiv* 354:19-27, 1975.)

their perception of the intensity of an applied thermal sensation. The measured sensitivities to warm varied substantially across oral and facial areas, whereas values of sensitivities to cold were more uniform (Fig. 8-2). Except for the vermilion lip and tongue tip, oral regions are significantly less sensitive to warming than other facial regions. In contrast, the sensitivity to cooling of the posterior hard palate is equal to or better than that of most locations tested on the face. Of all the intraoral regions tested the tongue tip has the highest sensitivity to both cooling and warming.

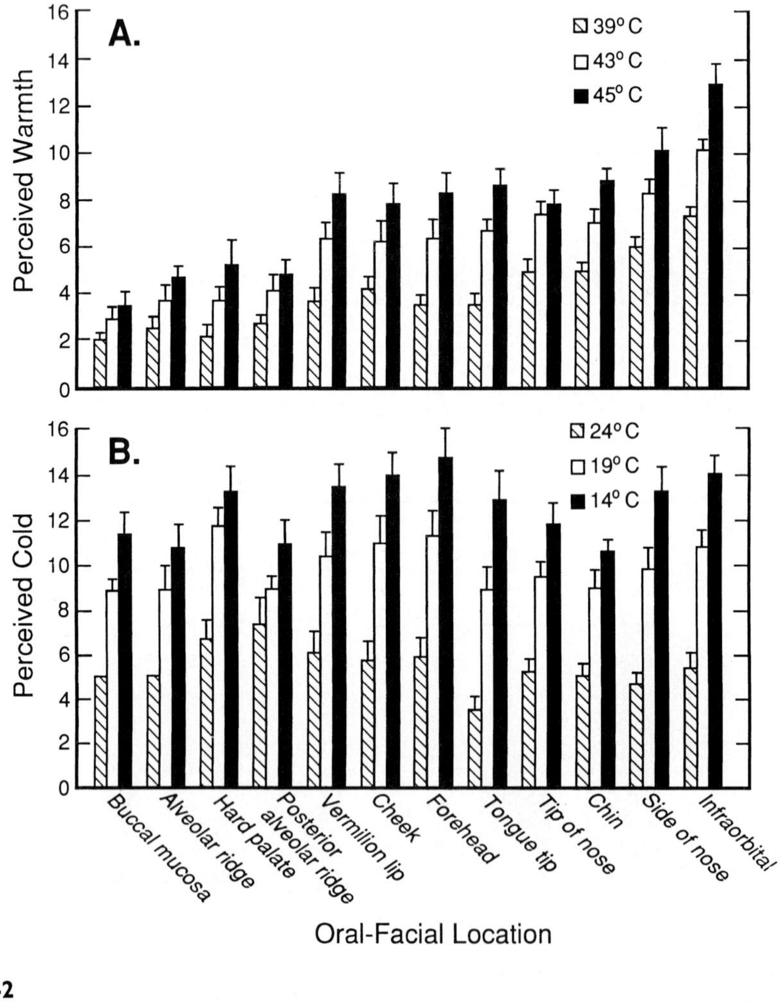

FIG. 8-2

A, Mean values of magnitude estimates of warmth at various locations in the oral cavity for three applied temperatures. **B,** Mean values of magnitude estimates of cold at various locations in the oral cavity for three applied temperatures. (From Green BG, Gelhard B: *Somatosensory Research* 4:191-200, 1987.)

The reasons for these spatial variations in sensitivity probably include density of thermal receptors, epidermal thickness, epidermal composition, and receptor depth. Compared with the rest of the body the orofacial area is somewhat unique in that there are relatively large differences in thermal sensitivity between close sites. For example, the difference in warm sensitivity between the forehead and the chin is equal to the difference in warm sensitivity between the forehead and the lower leg.

THERMAL RECEPTORS

Classification

Neurophysiologic recordings from cutaneous and oral mucosal afferent fibers have revealed that there are two distinctly separate groups of thermal receptors. Based on their dynamic response to a step change in temperature, thermal receptors can be divided into warm and cold receptors. These receptors form the underlying biological structure responsible for the cold and warm spots described previously and are the neurobiological reason that we divide temperature experience into warm and cold. Irrespective of the initial temperature, a warm receptor always responds with an increase in its discharge frequency on sudden warming and a transient inhibition on cooling. On the other hand a cold receptor responds in the opposite way, with an inhibition on warming and excitation on cooling. Besides these dynamic properties there are also differences in response to steady-state skin temperature usually called the static response frequency. These thermal receptors are responsible for responding to ambient temperatures and they respond to food temperature in the oral cavity. As will be discussed below, thermal receptors are always actively responding to environmental temperature. They are therefore important receptors in the maintenance of body temperature, and, depending on their response to environmental temperature, can initiate reflex sweating or shivering. They are particularly sensitive to sudden changes in temperature such as when a person takes a mouthful of hot coffee or steps out of a warm room into a cold winter day. Based on the information provided below it might be constructive to think about what your own thermal receptors are doing as you read this page or drink an ice-cold beverage.

Structure

By using measurements of electrophysiologic response latency and thermal conduction of the skin, cold receptors have been estimated to be 0.18 mm deep while warm receptors are located 0.22 mm below the skin surface. Therefore, cold receptors are more superficially located than warm receptors. The structure of a cold receptor has been determined by histologic examination of the receptive field of a neurophysiologically isolated cold fiber. A single, small-diameter, myelinated axon divides into several unmyelinated axons. These axons, covered by Schwann cells, penetrate the basement membrane and invaginate into the basal

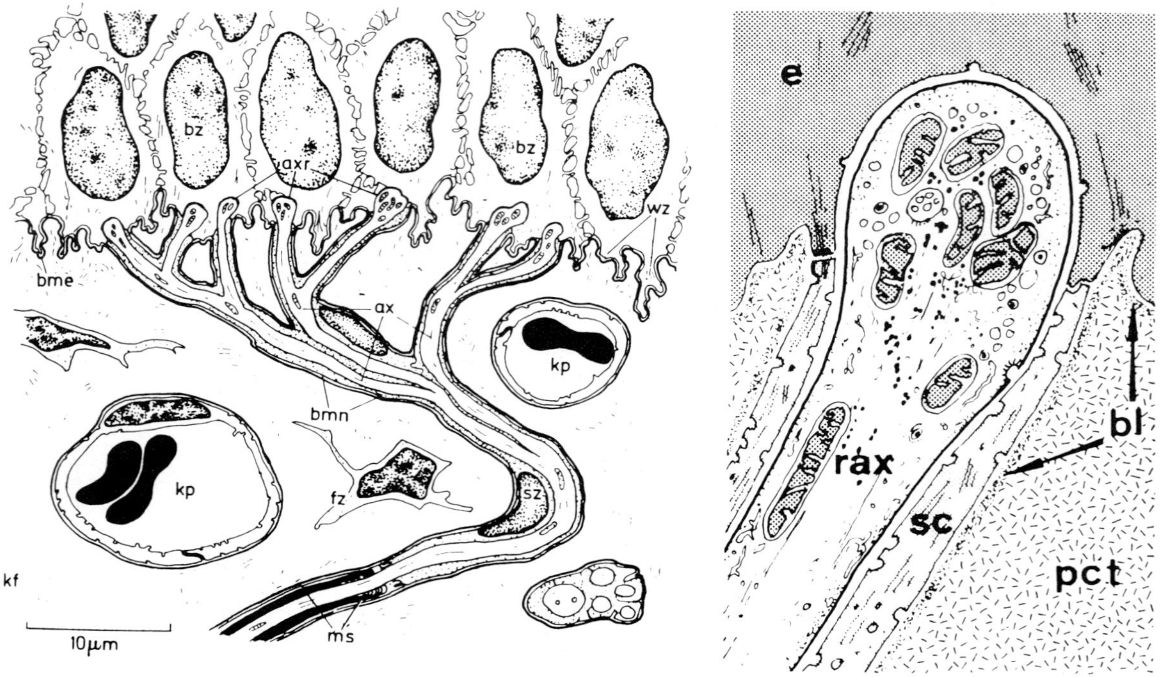

FIG. 8-3
Left, Cold receptor. *ms*, Myelin sheath; sz, nonmyelinated Schwann cell accompanying terminal axon (*ax*) to basement membrane (*bme*) of epidermis; *bmn*, basement membrane of nerve terminal; *axr*, axoreceptive endings with mitochondria; *bz*, basal cells; *wz*, root feet of basal cells; *kp*, capillaries; *fz*, fibrocyte; kf, collagen fibers. *Right*, Cold receptor terminal. Terminal bulges into a basal epidermal cell; *rax*, receptor axon; *sc*, Schwann cell; e, epidermis; *pct*, papillary connective tissue; *bl*, basal lamina. (From Hensel H, Andres KH, von During M: *Pflügers Archiv.* 352:1-10, 1974.)

cells of the epidermis. The terminals contain mitochondria, vesicles, and filaments (Fig. 8-3). The structure of a warm receptor has not been elucidated.

Transduction

The smallness and inaccessibility of thermal receptors have prevented direct study of their transduction mechanisms. However, by the use of topically applied drugs both in vivo and in isolated skin/nerve preparations, some insight into potential transduction mechanisms has been obtained. It is possible that alterations in receptor temperature change the operation of the highly temperature-sensitive sodium/potassium (Na/K) pump that is responsible for maintaining the difference in concentration of potassium and sodium ions across the cell membrane. A fall in temperature would decrease pump activity and therefore depolarize the membrane giving rise to a receptor current. Support for the role of the Na/K pump in thermal receptor transduction comes from experiments in which the activity of the pump is inhibited. Increasing K^+ concentration, which is known to influence the Na/K pump, decreases the static sensitivity of cold receptors. The cardiac glycoside ouabain, which inhibits the Na/K pump, also results in thermoreceptors becoming insensitive to temperature.

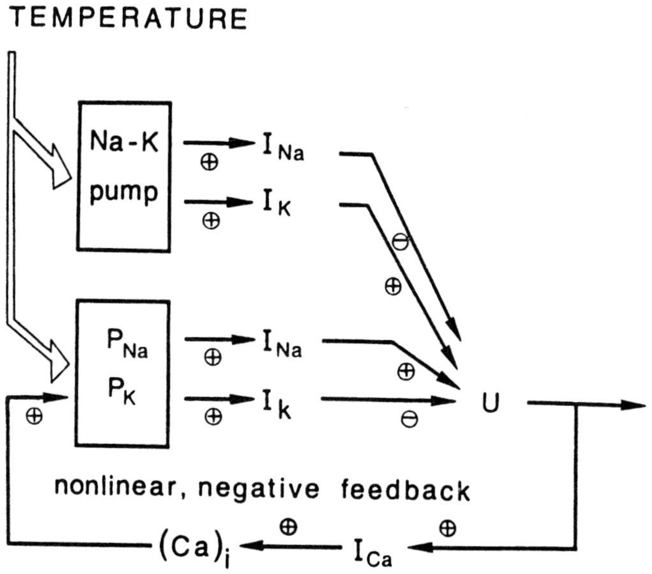

FIG. 8-4
Hypothetical transduction mechanisms involved in thermoreception. I_{Na}, sodium current; I_K, potassium current; I_{Ca}, calcium current; *Na-K pump*, sodium/potassium membrane pump; P_{Na} and P_K refers to membrane permeability to these ions; $(Ca)_i$, intracellular concentration of calcium ions. From Braun HA, Schäfer K, Wissing H: Theories and models of temperature transduction. In Bligh J, Voigt K, editors: *Thermoreception and temperature regulation.* Berlin, 1990, Springer Verlag, pp. 1-306.)

The characteristic bursting discharge pattern of cold fibers (see below and Fig. 8-5) reflects oscillation of the receptor membrane potential resulting from changes in Ca^{2+} dependent K^+ conductances. Addition of Ca^{2+} or Ca^{2+} chelators has a marked influence on the response of thermal receptors supporting the involvement of Ca^{2+} in the transduction mechanism. The cooling taste of menthol is partly caused by its action on cold receptors reflected in alterations in the bursting discharge pattern. Application of Ca^{2+} completely abolished the effect of menthol; this provides further evidence for the role of Ca^{2+} in thermal receptor transduction mechanisms (Fig. 8-4).

Response Characteristics of Cold Receptors

Cold receptors are innervated by small-diameter, myelinated Aδ fibers and unmyelinated C fibers. Their receptive field is small, usually less than 1 mm^2. When the temperature of the receptive field of a cold receptor is kept constant, the cold receptor is usually active, displaying a static frequency of discharges related to the applied skin temperature (Fig. 8-5). The temperature range over which cold recep-

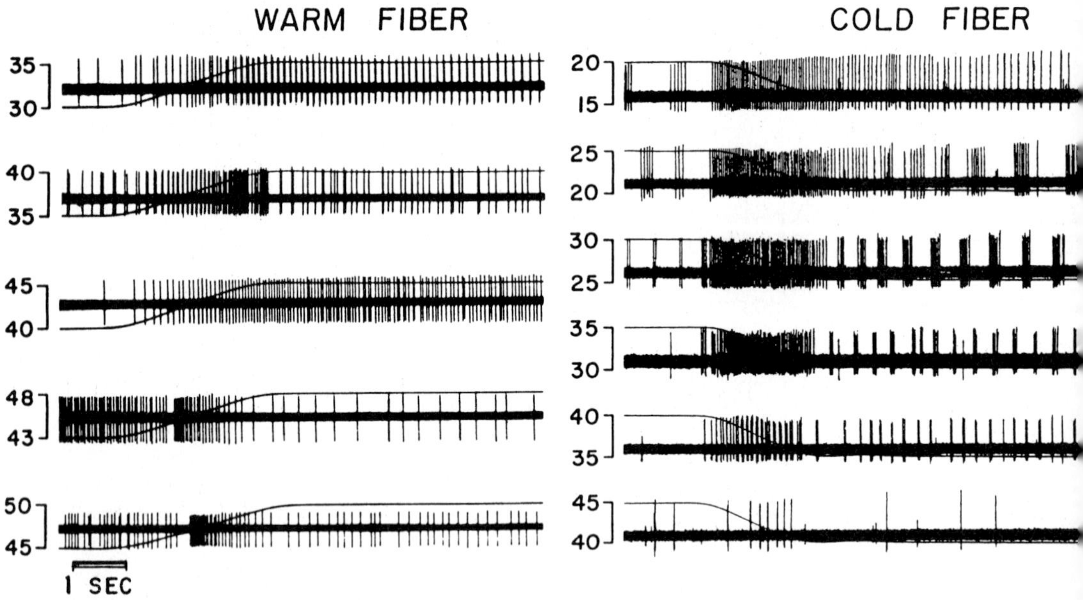

FIG. 8-5
Neurophysiological recordings from rhesus monkey warm and cold afferent fibers. Fibers innervating a warm or cold receptor are usually called warm or cold fibers, although response specificity of these fibers is not intrinsic to the fibers but to receptors they innervate. Superimposed on each record is recording of temperature applied to receptive field of fibers. For each fiber the temperature of the receptive field is changed from one constant temperature to a new one. (From Kenshalo DR: Correlations of temperature sensitivity in man and monkey, a first approximation. In Zotterman Y, editor: *Sensory functions of the skin.* New York, 1976, Pergamon Press, pp. 305-330.)

tors are active varies for different cold receptors, the extremes being ⁻5° and 43° C. These extremes represent the temperature applied to the skin surface. The temperature at the receptor membrane is probably different because the thermal stimulus must conduct across the skin to stimulate the cold receptor. The static impulse frequency of individual cold receptors rises with temperature, reaches a maximum, and then falls again at higher temperatures. The shape of the static discharge curve for cold receptors is roughly symmetrical (Fig. 8-6). For a large population of cold receptors in different species the temperature giving rise to the maximum static discharge frequency is highly variable, ranging from ⁻5° and 40° C with maximum frequencies between 5 and 10 impulses per second. Therefore, a large cold receptor population will cover a broader span of temperatures than a single receptor. The temperatures between which the average static maximal neural discharge frequency occurs for a large population of cold receptors range from 25° to 30° C. Therefore, when we are exposed to the steady temperature of the home or workplace, cold receptors are active, relaying information to the central nervous system on ambient environmental temperatures between ⁻5° and 40° C.

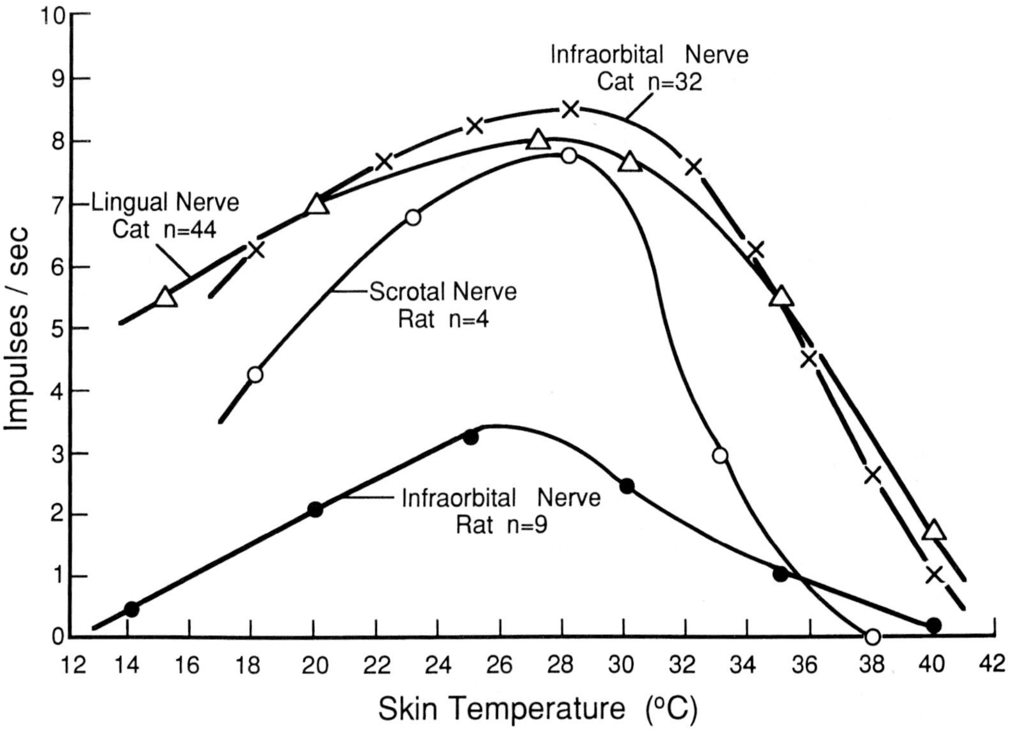

FIG. 8-6
Mean static impulse frequencies of various cutaneous cold fibers as a function of steady skin temperature. (From Hensel H. Wurster RD Static properties of cold receptors in nasal area of cats. *Journal of Neurophysiology* 33:271-275, 1970.)

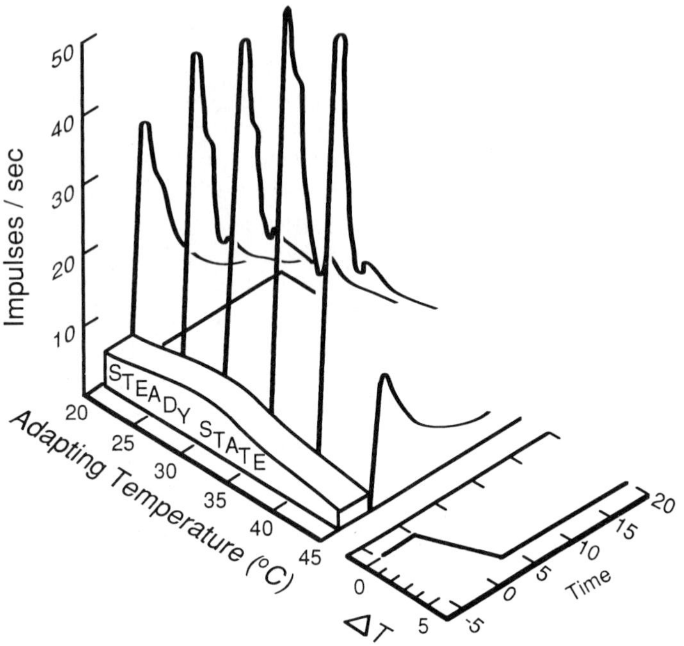

FIG. 8-7
Mean impulse frequencies of 15 cold fibers as a function of time afer stimulus application. For each function, receptive field of fiber was adapted to a different skin temperature and then rapidly cooled to −5° C. The time course of the cooling stimulus is indicated to the right of the figure. (From Kenshalo DR, Duclaux R: *Journal of Neurophysiology* 40:319-332, 1977.)

When the receptive field of a cold receptor is cooled, the receptor responds with a transient high frequency burst of action potentials (see Fig. 8-5). If the receptive field is then returned to its initial temperature, there is a transient decrease in frequency, or silent period, after which the frequency returns to its initial static value. The higher the rate of cooling for a given adapting temperature, the higher the frequency of the dynamic response (Fig. 8-7). Cold receptors are therefore important in signalling sudden cooling of the body.

Cold receptors often show a temporal pattern of impulse discharges. This pattern consists of bursts of activity separated by intervals when the fiber is inactive (Fig. 8-8; see also Fig. 8-5). If the intervals between action potentials is measured, they comprise two groups: short intervals occurring between the action potentials of the burst and long intervals between bursts. The length of these intervals and the number of action potentials within a burst are related to stimulation temperature. The bursting pattern usually appears at the temperature of the highest static average frequency and continues to temperatures as low as 20° C. At low temperatures, the burst discharge becomes irregular with variable interval lengths (Figs. 8-5 to 8-8). As mentioned previously, the bursting pattern of cold receptors is caused by oscillation of the receptor membrane potential. Although cold receptors display this bursting pattern, the sensation that results is not an oscillating temperature sensation, because, as will be discussed later, the bursting pattern is not transmitted across the first synapse in the central nervous system.

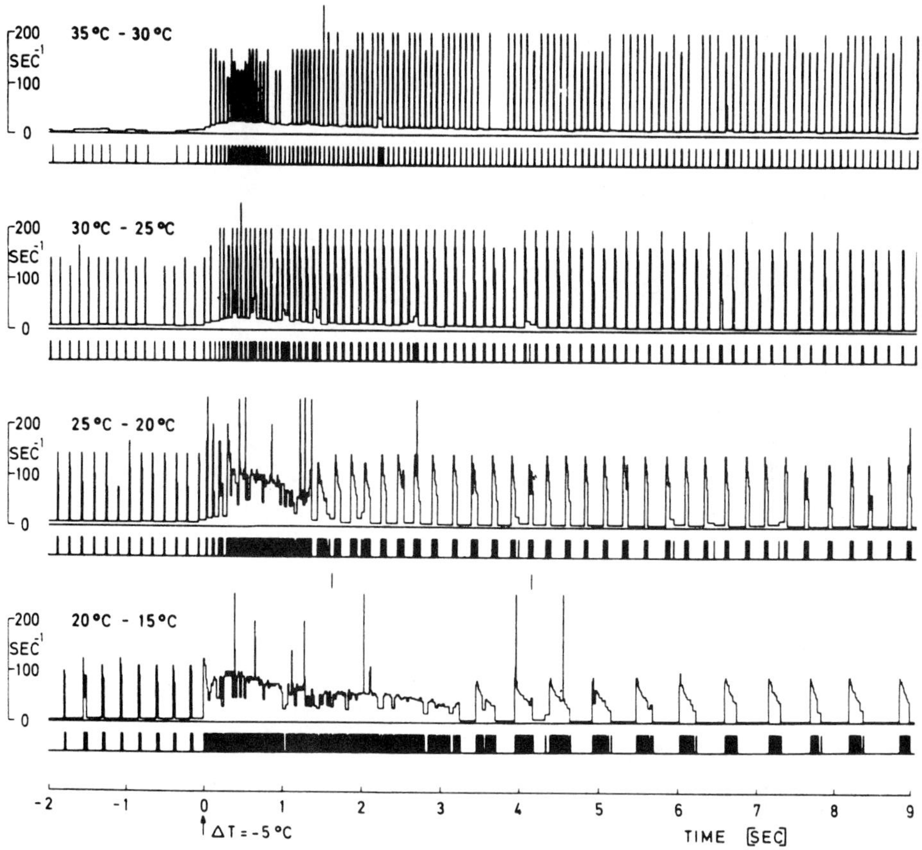

FIG. 8-8
Dynamic response of a single cold fiber to cooling steps of 5° C from different adapting temperatures. For each cooling step, upper trace represents instantaneous frequency of action potentials, and lower trace the pattern of impulses produced by the cooling step. Note that a bursting patern becomes apparent when the receptive field is cooled from adapting temperatures below 30° C. (From Braun HA, Bade H, Hensel H: *Pflügers Archiv* 386:1-9, 1990.)

Response Characteristics of Warm Receptors

Warm receptors are innervated by small-diameter, unmyelinated C fibers with receptive field areas of less than 1 mm^2. Like cold receptors, warm receptors have a static discharge at constant skin temperatures. The static discharge range for warm receptors begins above 30° C, increases in frequency with rising temperature, and decreases again at still higher temperatures. The shape of the static discharge curve for warm receptors is asymmetrical and falls off steeply after the static maxima (Fig. 8-9). The maximum static discharge frequency occurs between 41° and 47° C and is generally much higher than cold fibers ranging from 10 to 35 impulses per second.

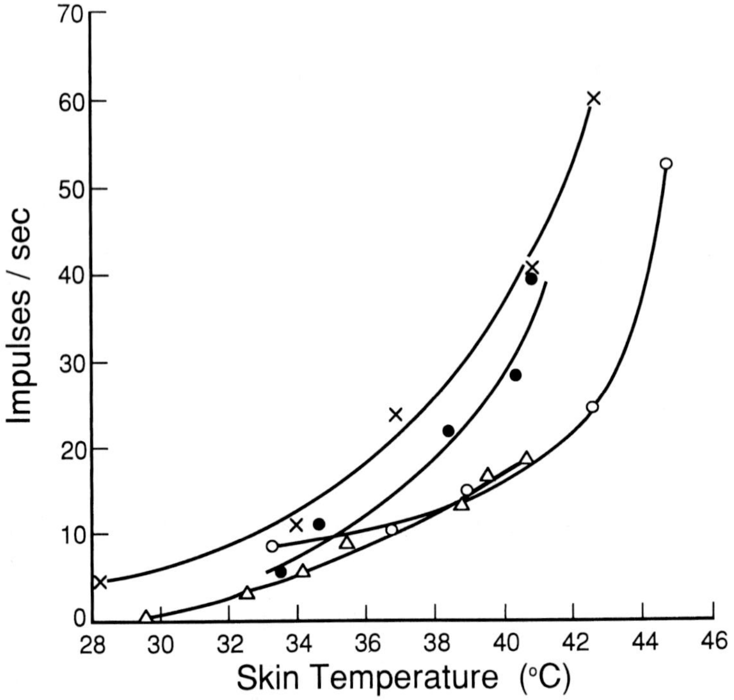

FIG. 8-9
Static impulse frequencies of four cutaneous warm fibers as a function of steady skin temperature. (From Hensel H, Kenshalo DR: *Journal of Physiology [London]* 204:99-112, 1969.)

There is some overlap in the static discharge ranges of warm and cold receptors, which is in the range of thermal sensation described as neutral.

Responses of warm receptors to dynamic changes in applied temperatures are opposite to responses recorded from cold receptors. Sudden cooling of the receptive field of a warm receptor inhibits the impulse discharge while warming results in increase in impulse discharge frequency (see Fig. 8-5). Transient increases in frequency in response to warming can attain levels of 200 impulses per second, more than 5 times higher than the static maximum. The higher the adapting temperature, the higher the dynamic response to the same step increase in skin temperature. Warm receptors do not show a bursting discharge.

CENTRAL PATHWAYS

Spinal Cord

Cutaneous thermal receptor fibers with cell bodies in the dorsal root ganglion enter the spinal cord by way of the dorsal root. The fibers terminate in lamina I and are therefore intermingled with nociceptive-specific axons (see Chapter 2). Second-order cold neurons in lamina I respond to moderate cooling of the peripheral receptive field that is larger than the receptive fields of cold receptors. The bursting discharge of the peripheral afferent fiber is not present at the central level presumably because of desynchronization when several fibers converge onto a second-order neuron, preventing the preservation of the bursting pattern. In addition, spinal cord-wide dynamic range neurons (see Chapter 2) respond to both noxious heat and nonnoxious (warm) thermal stimulation, so that these neurons receive input from cutaneous thermal receptors as well as heat nociceptors.

Trigeminal Nucleus

Thermosensitive afferent fibers from the oral cavity and face form a synapse with second-order neurons in the trigeminal nucleus. The second-order neurons are located in subnucleus interpolaris and the marginal layer (lamina I) of the medullary dorsal horn. The receptive fields of both the warm and cold second-order neurons are ipsilateral and large, covering an area of 10 to 100 mm^2. Trigeminal cold units show a steady discharge depending on the temperature applied to the receptive field. The

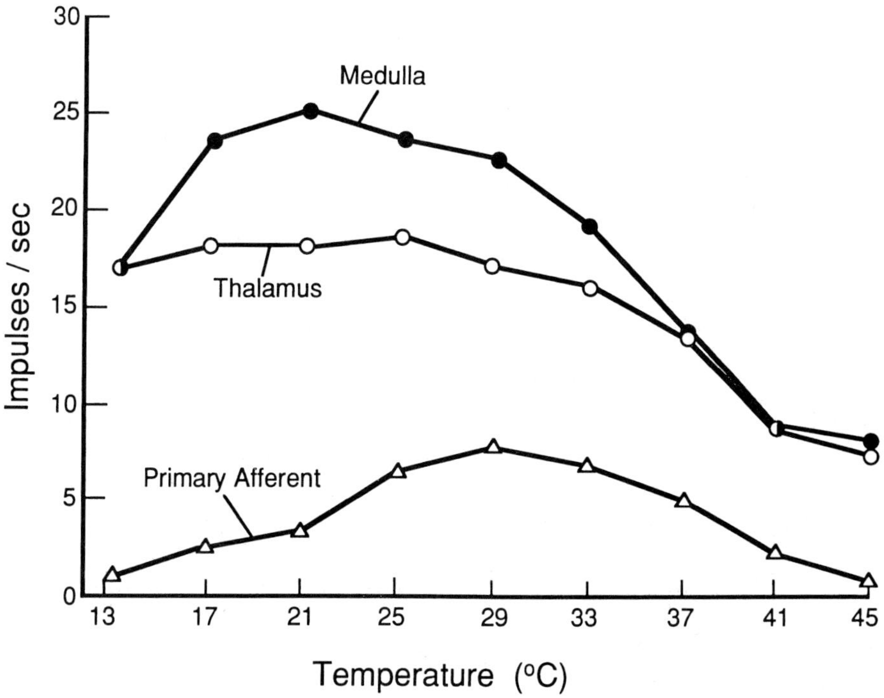

FIG. 8-10
Mean static impulse frequencies of cold fibers, trigeminal neurons, and thalamic neurons as a function of steady skin temperature. (From Poulos DA: *Federation Proceedings* 40:2825-2829, 1981.)

discharge pattern is irregular and no burst patterns are observed. The static maximal frequency occurs between 10° and 35° C and the static frequency curve is similar in shape and range to the static curve of peripheral cold receptors (Fig. 8-10). Trigeminal cold neurons respond to sudden cooling in the same way as cold receptors.

Trigeminal second-order warm neurons have a similar response pattern to peripheral warm receptors. With increasing skin temperature, both the static frequency and the dynamic response to warming steps increase (Fig. 8-11).

It can therefore be concluded that there is little processing of peripheral thermal activity in the second-order neurons of the trigeminal nucleus. However, the bursting pattern of cold receptors is lost and the receptive field size of the second-order neurons is considerably larger than the thermal receptors. The response characteristics of the second-order neurons are very similar to those of facial cold and warm receptors.

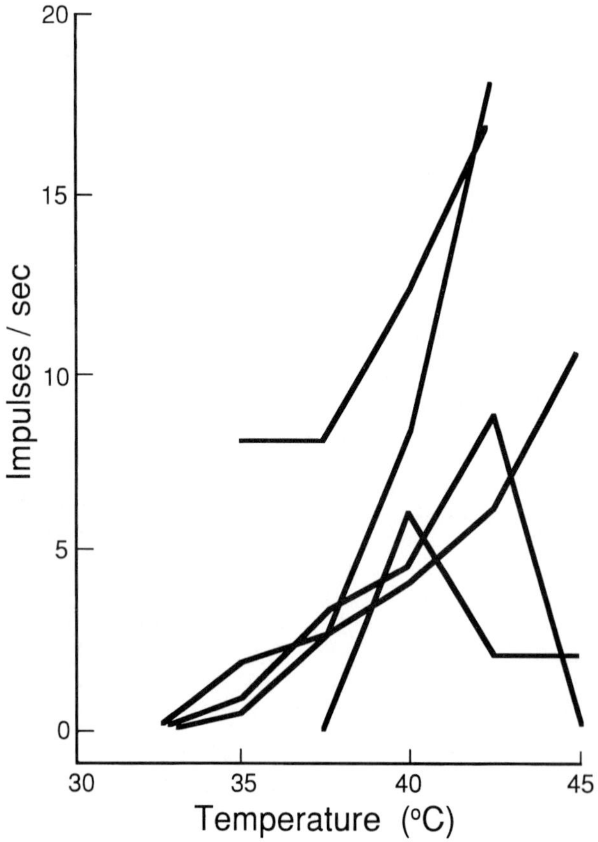

FIG. 8-11
Static impulse frequency of five warm neurons in medullary dorsal horn of the cat. (From Dostrovsky JO, Hellon RF: *Journal of Physiology [London]* 277:29-47, 1978.)

Thalamus

The axons of spinal cord thermosensitive second-order neurons ascend in the ventrolateral spinothalamic tract. Trigeminal thermal neurons ascend in the trigeminothalamic tract. Both of these tracts terminate in the ventrobasal complex of the thalamus. A proportion of the neurons in this thalamic area respond specifically to cooling, but the remainder are multimodal and respond to touch and taste. Once again the response characteristics of the peripheral thermal receptors are preserved at the thalamic level (Fig. 8-10).

Cortex

Even at the level of somatosensory cortex the specificity of peripheral thermal receptors is maintained. Recordings from single cortical cells that receive input from the tongue have revealed a number of specific cold units not excited by other stimuli.

Although the static response functions of thermal fibers and neurons observed at different synaptic levels of the central nervous system are generally similar, there are some notable differences. The range of activity over which central nervous system units respond is wider than that seen in primary afferent fibers, and medullary cold neurons display static response frequencies that are greater than either those of primary afferent fibers or thalamic neurons (see Fig. 8-10).

SUMMARY

The skin and oral mucosa are not uniformly sensitive to temperature. Small areas or spots are sensitive to thermal stimuli separated by areas of insensitivity. These sensory spots are either sensitive to warm or cold temperatures. The density of these sensory spots varies depending on the body area. Thermal sensitivity of the body skin is also variable with the face and oral cavity being one of the body areas most sensitive to temperature.

Receptors in the skin and oral mucosa that respond to temperature consist of two distinct groups called warm and cold receptors. These receptors respond over different ranges of temperature. At constant applied temperatures they produce a static discharge of action potentials. In response to alterations in applied temperature, warm and cold receptors respond by changes in impulse frequency that are related to the direction of the temperature change. Thermal receptors are not excited by mechanical stimuli and only respond to temperatures considered nonnoxious.

Thermoreceptive fibers from the skin terminate in the dorsal horn of the spinal cord. Those from the face and oral cavity terminate in the trigeminal sensory nucleus. Generally the terminations are intermingled with terminations of nociceptive fibers. From the spinal cord and medulla, thermosensitive projections relay in the thalamus and then to the somatosensory cortex. Although the static response functions of thermal fibers and neurons observed at different synaptic levels of the central nervous system are generally similar, there are some indications of synaptic processing. The range of activity over which central nervous system units respond is wider than that seen in primary afferent fibers. Medullary cold neurons display static response frequencies that are greater than either those of primary afferent fibers or thalamic neurons.

SELECTED READINGS

Bligh J, Voigt K: *Thermoreception and temperature regulation*, Berlin, 1990, Springer-Verlag.

Hensel H: *Thermoreception and temperature regulation*, London, 1981, Academic Press.

Hensel H: *Thermal sensation and thermoreceptors in man*, Springfield, Ill, 1982, CC Thomas.

Poulos DA: Central processing of cutaneous temperature information, *Federation Proceedings* 40:2825-2829, 1981.

Spray DC: Cutaneous temperature receptors, *Annual Review of Physiology* 48:625-638, 1986.

9 Salivary Secretion

- *Structure of Salivary Glands*
- *Composition of Saliva*
  - *Inorganic Components*
  - *Organic Components*
- *Glandular Mechanisms of Secretion*
  - *Factors Affecting Composition*
  - *Secretion of Water and Electrolytes*
  - *Secretion of Proteins*
- *Control of Salivary Secretion*
  - *Parasympathetic Control*
  - *Sympathetic Control*
  - *Distribution of Nerve Fibers in Glands*
  - *Excitation Secretion Coupling*
  - *Myoepithelial Cells*
  - *Salivary Reflexes*
- *Buffering Action of Saliva*
- *Effects of Aging on Salivary Secretion*

LEARNING OBJECTIVES

At the end of this chapter you should be able to:

1. List the functions of saliva.
2. Describe the characteristics of saliva.
3. Describe the characteristics of salivary glands.
4. Describe the structure of a salivary gland.
5. Describe a salivary gland secretory unit.
6. Describe the composition of saliva.
7. Describe the factors that influence salivary composition.
8. Describe the process of secretion of electrolytes in salivary glands.
9. Describe the process of secretion of proteins in salivary glands.

10. Describe the central nervous system salivatory nuclei.
11. Describe the control of salivary secretion by the sympathetic nervous system.
12. Describe the process coupling neural activity to secretion of saliva.
13. Describe the reflex control of salivary secretion.
14. Describe the role of saliva as a buffer system in the oral cavity.
15. Describe the influence of aging on salivary secretion.

A critical component of the oral environment is saliva, a dilute aqueous solution containing both inorganic and organic constituents. Saliva plays an essential role during mastication in bolus formation and acts a lubricant in swallowing and speech production. Substances solubilized in saliva during mastication are transported to and stimulate taste receptors. Salivary amylase is a digestive enzyme responsible for the initial stage in starch and glycogen breakdown, and salivary lipase secreted by the lingual salivary glands (von Ebner's glands) may be significant in fat digestion. In many animals evaporation of saliva spread on fur or while panting is important in temperature regulation during heat stress. Another important function of saliva is revealed when saliva flow is diminished or stopped altogether for any length of time, producing a dry mouth (xerostomia). Because the cleansing and antimicrobial actions of saliva has an essential buffering action on acids produced by the action of bacteria on food materials, reduction in salivary flow can lead to a lowering of mouth pH resulting in etching and even complete dissolutions of the crowns of the teeth. Thus, an important function of saliva is to protect the teeth and buccal mucosa from bacterial attack (see Box 9-1).

Recently additional functions of salivary glands have been uncovered. Salivary glands have been shown to contain, and possibly secrete, a large number of physiologically active substances, such as nerve growth factor, vasoactive peptides, and regulatory peptides. Thus salivary glands may have a role in functions not normally associated with their traditional alimentary function.

BOX 9-1
Major Functions of Saliva

- Lubrication
- Digestion
- Solvent action
- Antibacterial action
- Antifungal action
- Buffering action
- Remineralization
- Temperature regulation
- Production of growth factors and other regulatory peptides

A considerable volume of saliva is produced in one day. An estimated 0.5 to 0.75L of fluid is produced by the salivary glands, about one fifth the total plasma volume. Since most of this fluid is swallowed and reabsorbed by the gut it is not lost. Some salivary components are derived from blood plasma, and others are synthesized within the salivary glands. Therefore, the basic action of salivary glands is to translocate components from one fluid compartment to another, adding some synthesized components in the process.

Three large paired salivary glands, the parotid, the submaxillary (sometimes called the submandibular), and the sublingual, are responsible for the bulk of saliva production. These glands, characterized by large glandular masses, drain into the oral cavity through a system of ducts that terminate in a final major duct. Lingual salivary glands, contained in the tongue (von Ebner's glands), are similar in structure to the paired salivary glands and are of comparable size to the sublingual glands. These glands drain into the clefts of the circumvallate and foliate papillae. Numerous other glands, lying beneath the mucous membrane of the lips (labial glands), palate (palatine glands), and cheek (buccal glands), consist of small glandular masses that open by way of many individual ducts onto the surface of the mucosa. It has been estimated that in humans the parotid, submandibular, and sublingual glands contribute about 90% of the total saliva volume.

Salivary glands are remarkably diverse in structure and function. Much of the information on salivary secretion has been derived from investigations of the rat parotid gland, which has taken on the role of the archetypical salivary gland. However, parotid glands in other species have different morphologies and physiologies. Despite this diversity in structure and function there are a few general rules that are common to most salivary glands. First, secretomotor autonomic nerves invariably control flow. Second, the osmotic pressure (tonicity) exerted by saliva is usually lower than that of serum. Third, tonicity increases as flow rate of saliva increases. Fourth, saliva contains potassium ions at 2 to 10 times the concentration of serum potassium. Finally, the saliva in many animals contains a high level of the digestive enzyme amylase and other macromolecules.

STRUCTURE OF SALIVARY GLANDS

Salivary glands are made up of a large number of individual secretory units which consist of an acinus, an intercalated duct, and a striated duct. Many thousands of these secretory units converge on a main excretory duct that extends from the gland mass to drain into the oral cavity (Fig. 9-1). The terminology applied to the different parts of the secretory unit reflects differences in cytoarchitecture. Saliva forms at the proximal end of the duct in pyramid-shaped acinar cells arranged in spherical collections called acini. Acinar cells are by far the most numerous of the cell types and account for the bulk of the tissue making up a salivary gland. Several acini converge on a single intercalated duct which con-

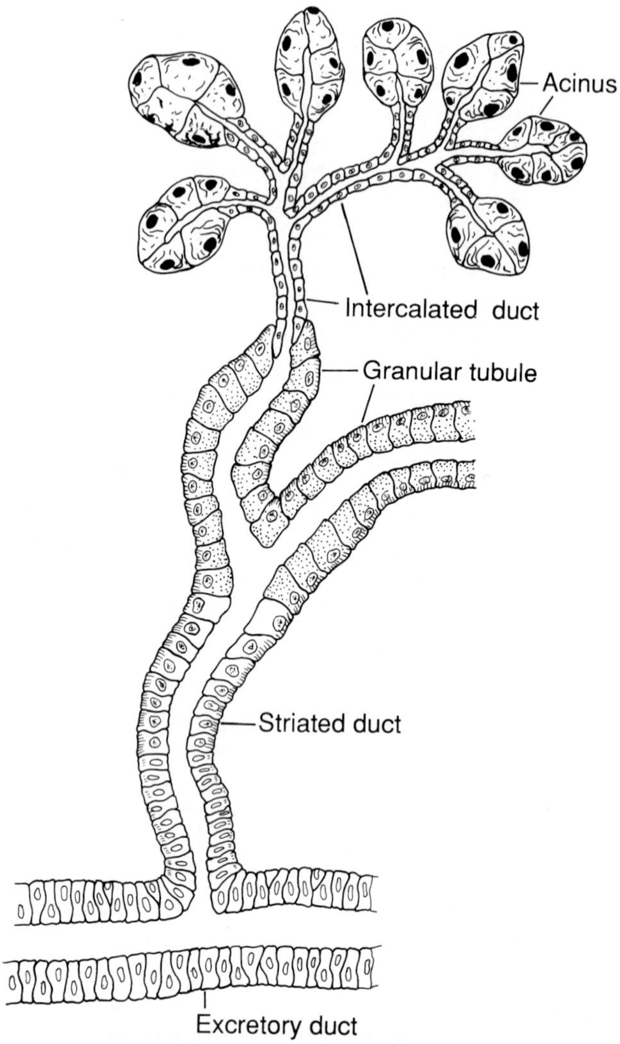

FIG. 9-1
Components of a salivary secretory unit. Each salivary gland consists of a large number of these units all converging on a main excretory duct. There is wide diversity in the structure of secretory units, depending on type of gland and species of animal.

nects to other intercalated ducts, which in turn converge on a striated duct or directly into the granular segments of the striated ducts if present. Many striated ducts connect to a few excretory ducts which all merge to form a single main excretory duct.

In addition to the secretory units other structures are found in salivary glands. Most notable are the myoepithelial cells, which envelop acini and intercalated ducts in long cytoplasmic extensions containing filaments that have contractile properties. Salivary glands possess a rich blood supply important not only in nutrient supply, but also as a major source of many components of saliva that are directly derived

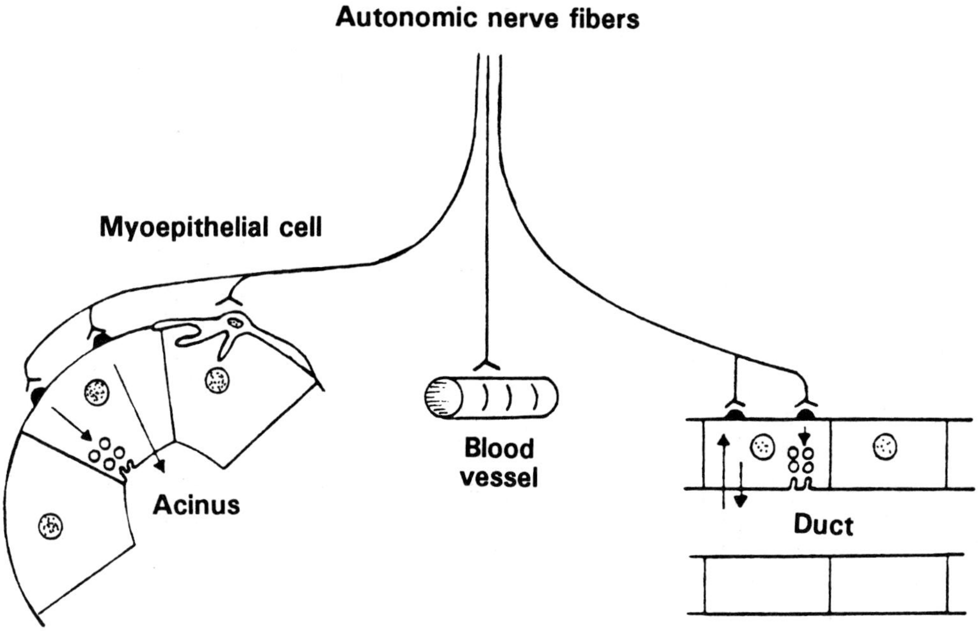

FIG. 9-2
Distribution of nerves to different effector systems of a salivary gland. (From Emmelin N: *Philosophical Transactions of the Royal Society of London*, Series B, 269:27-35, 1981.)

from the blood. Associated with the acinar and duct cells are neural elements responsible for the control of salivary secretion, blood flow, and the contraction of myoepithelial cells (Fig 9-2).

COMPOSITION OF SALIVA

Saliva is usually a dilute aqueous solution that is hypotonic when compared to serum. However, saliva can be isotonic or even hypertonic relative to serum. Only 1% of saliva is made up of ions and organic components, the rest being water.

Inorganic Components

The most important cations of saliva are sodium and potassium; the major osmotically active anions are chloride and bicarbonate. Other electrolytes that are present include calcium phosphate, fluoride, thiocyanate, magnesium sulfate, and iodine. Water and the ionic constituents of saliva are derived by translocation from blood plasma. However, although salivary electrolytes are derived from the blood

TABLE 9-1
Electrolyte composition of human submandibular saliva compared with plasma

	Saliva		Plasma(mEq/L)
	*Resting**	*Stimulated†*	
Na^+	2.6 mM	54.8 mM	143.3
K^+	14.4 mM	13.7 mM	4.1
Cl^-	11.9 mM	32.3 mM	100.9
HCO_3^-	2.2 mM	35.3 mM	27.5
Mg^{2+}	70.4 μM	36.0 μM	1.85
Ca^{2+}	1.56 mM	2.13 mM	2.47
P(inorganic)	3.6 mM	1.57 mM	3.5 mg/100 ml
pH	6.47	7.62	7.4

From Dawes, C.: *Archives of Oral Biology* 19:887-895, 1974

* 0.26 ml/min
† 3.0 ml/min

TABLE 9-2
Electrolyte composition of human parotid saliva compared with plasma

	Saliva		Plasma (mEq/L)
	*Resting**	*Stimulated†*	
Na^+	2.7 mEq/l	63.3 mEq/l	143.3
K^+	46.3 mEq/l	18.7 mEq/l	4.1
Cl^-	31.5 mEq/l	35.9 mEq/l	100.9
HCO_3^-	0.6 mEq/l	29.7 mEq/l	27.5
Mg^{2+}	0.45 mg/100 ml	0.04 mg/100 ml	1.85
Ca^{2+}	4.16 mg/100 ml	3.78 mg/100 ml	2.47
P(inorganic)	31.9 mg/100 ml	9.7 mg/100 ml	3.5 mg/100 ml
pH	5.82	7.67	7.4
Osmolality	85.7 mOsm/kg	132.0 mOsm/kg	296.0 mOsm/kg

From Shannon IL, Suddick RP, Dowd FJ: Saliva: composition and secretion, *Monographs in oral science* vol 2, Basel, Karger, 1974.

* <0.011 ml/min
† >1.0 ml/min

supply, their ionic concentrations are not identical to plasma, so that saliva is not merely an ultrafiltrate of plasma (Table 9-1 and 9-2).

Organic Components

Saliva contains many organic components with diverse functions, such as enzymatic action, coating of tissue surfaces, protection of dental tissues, and control of tissue growth (Box 9-2). The digestive enzyme amylase is the organic component found in highest concentration in saliva. Amylase consists of two families of isoen-

BOX 9-2

Organic components of saliva

Proteins of acinar cell origin	*Proteins of nonacinar cell origin*
Amylase	Lysozyme
Lipase	Secretory immunoglobulin A
Mucous glycoproteins	Growth factors
Proline-rich glycoproteins	Regulatory peptides
Basic glycoprotein	
Acidic protein	
Tyrosine-rich protein (statherin)	
Histadine-rich protein	
Peroxidase	

From Ellison SA: The identification of salivary components. In Kleinberg I, Ellison SA, Mandel ID: *Saliva and dental caries,* New York, 1979, Information retrieval, pp. 13-29.

zymes, glycosylated and nonglycosylated. Doubt has always existed concerning the function of salivary amylase, since there is little time for the enzyme to be active before the food bolus is swallowed and exposed to stomach pH that would inactivate the enzyme. It has been argued, however, that salivary amylase remains active in the stomach, because it is protected inside the food bolus.

Lipase secreted by the lingual (von Ebner's) salivary glands probably has a very significant role in digestion. Lingual lipase is the enzyme responsible for the first step in fat digestion and is active at stomach pH. This enzyme is particularly important when pancreatic levels of lipase are low, as in the newborn or immature animal or in diseases such as cystic fibrosis of the pancreas, since it then becomes the sole source of digestive lipase.

Mucous glycoproteins secreted in saliva have a high molecular weight and consist of multiple oligosaccharide chains attached to a peptide core. All oral soft tissues are coated with mucous glycoproteins, which are thought to act as a trap for bacteria and a regulator of interaction and interchange between surface epithelial cells and the oral environment. Some of these glycoproteins bind strongly to the tooth surface and are, therefore, an important constituent of enamel pellicle.

There are two groups of proline-rich glycoproteins in saliva. The basic group binds lipids and may preferentially adsorb to membranes, while the acidic group comprises calcium binding proteins and attaches to the tooth surface. Some of these proteins may have a role in stabilizing the tooth surface or promoting remineralization of enamel. A tyrosine-rich peptide, called statherin, may play a role in stabilizing supersaturated solutions of calcium and phosphate and therefore prevent calcium precipitating from saliva. The functions of other peptides such as histadine-rich peptide are unknown, although it has been suggested that they have a role in pellicle formation. Other possible functions for these proteins include aggregation of bacteria, which contributes to oral clearance of the microorganisms.

Numerous other proteins found in saliva are not secreted by the acinar cells. Secretory immunoglobulin A (IgA) is synthesized by plasma cells. Lysozyme in concert with other salivary bactericidal agents is probably important in oral protective functions. The salivary duct cells are capable of secreting complex molecules such as nerve growth factor and kallikrein, but, although the functions of these macromolecules are well established, they are probably of little importance if secreted into the oral cavity, unless some undiscovered function emerges.

GLANDULAR MECHANISMS OF SECRETION

Factors Affecting Composition

Salivary composition is highly variable depending on a number of factors, including the type of gland, species of animal, time of day, and degree and type of stimulation. Perhaps the most studied aspect of salivary secretion is the effects of flow rate on composition. During sleep salivary flow is almost zero, a finding with clinical implications since all the protective functions of saliva are virtually eliminated. It is, therefore, important to cleanse the mouth thoroughly before sleep to remove substrates that could be fermented by oral microorganisms and lead to oral diseases.

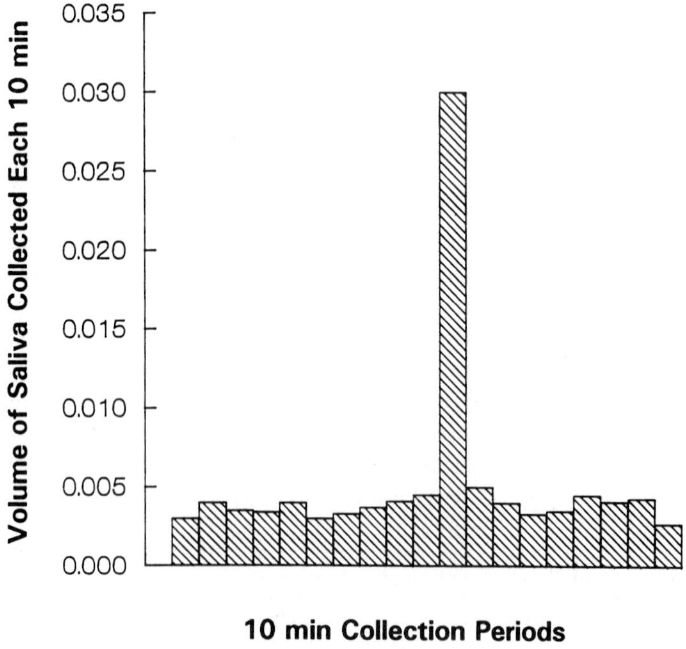

FIG. 9-3
Effect of feeding on salivary secretion. Saliva was collected every 10 minutes and volume was measured. After 100 minutes feeding occurred and salivary flow rate increased. Feeding evoked a marked increase in salivary flow rate. After feeding, salivary flow rate returns to basal levels. (Data from Emmelin N: *Acta Physiological Scandinavica* [Suppl] 111:34-58, 1953.)

TABLE 9-3
Protein composition of human parotid saliva

	Resting*	Stimulated†
Total protein	134.0 mg/100ml	302.0 mg/100ml
Amylase units	340.6	528.0

From Shannon IL, Suddick RP, Dowd FJ: Saliva: composition and secretion, *Monographs in Oral Science*, vol 2, Basel, Karger, 1974.

* <0.011 ml/min
† >1.0 ml/min

If salivary flow is measured over a 24-hour period in the absence of any apparent stimulation (for example, chewing, feeding), a circadian variation in flow becomes apparent, indicating that salivary glands produce saliva at a varying basal or resting level throughout a 24-hour period. This basal flow can be eliminated by appropriate pharmacologic agents indicating that a chronic level of gland stimulation is responsible for resting secretion. In some species such as ruminants, however, there is a persistent spontaneous secretion that cannot be stopped even by extensive experimental manipulation. Superimposed on these spontaneous or resting rates of secretion are periods of higher flows (Fig. 9-3), usually associated with feeding or anticipation of feeding.

With an increase in flow the composition of saliva changes (sometimes called Heidenhain's law). As can be seen in Tables 9-1 to 9-3, the concentrations of all salivary components in resting and stimulated saliva are not the same. As flow increases

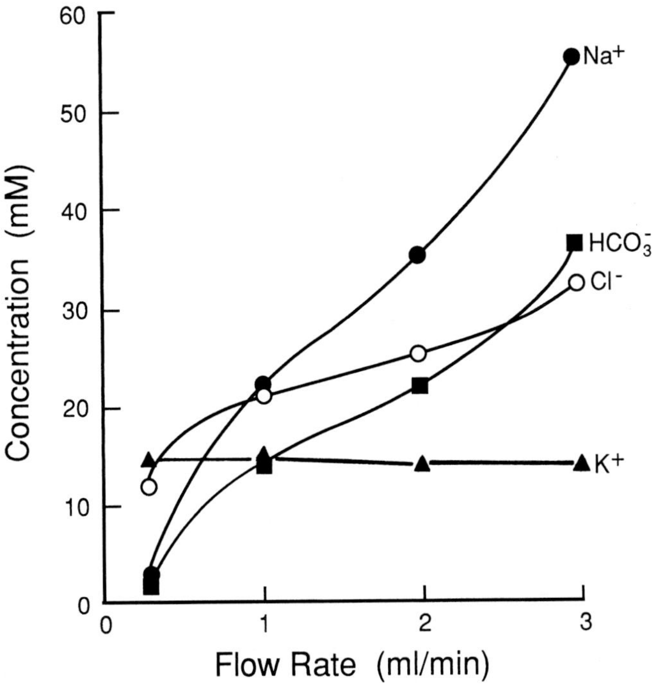

FIG. 9-4
Variations in the concentrations of ions in human parotid gland saliva as flow rate is increased. (Data from Sahnnon IL, Suddick RP, Dowd FJ: Saliva: *Composition and Secretion, Monographs in Oral Science*, vol. 2, Basel, 1974, Karger.)

there are nonlinear changes in the concentration of most major salivary components (Fig. 9-4). For certain components such as Na^+ the concentration increases with increasing flow, whereas other ions such as K^+ fall in concentration as flow rate rises. The effect of flow rate on concentration of salivary constituents varies depending on the gland being studied and the type of stimulation producing the increase in flow. For all salivary glands it is generally true that increase in flow is directly under

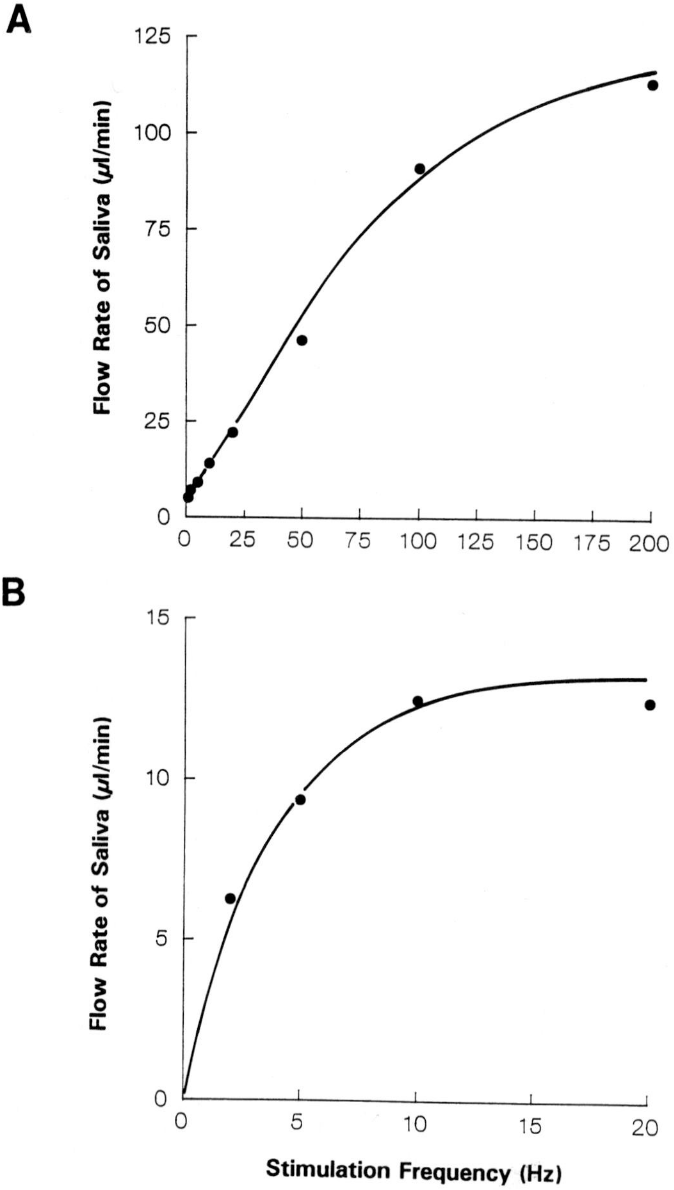

FIG. 9-5
Effects of varying frequencies of electrical stimulation of parasympathetic (*A*) and sympathetic (*B*) nerve parotid gland on salivary flow rate. (From Garrett JR, Thulin A: *Cell and Tissue Research* 159:179-193, 1975.)

the control of the autonomic nervous system. In particular, parasympathetic stimulation is very effective in producing the highest flow of saliva, whereas sympathetic activation is generally less effective (Fig. 9-5 A, B).

The data in Tables 9-1 to 9-3 and Fig. 9-4 were derived from analysis of saliva collected at the main excretory ducts of the gland, and the flow was manipulated reflexively by stimulation of either mechanoreceptors or gustatory receptors to mimic normal physiologic mechanisms of secretion. However, this method of producing saliva results from activation of either or both divisions of the autonomic nervous system. To study the influence of the parasympathetic and sympathetic nerve supplies on salivary flow and composition, increases in flow are usually induced by drugs that activate parasympathetic or sympathetic receptors on the acinar cell. In animal experiments it is possible to stimulate electrically either the parasympathetic or sympathetic innervation of a gland and to control precisely the mode by which secretion is evoked.

Secretion of Water and Electrolytes

Using a parasympathomimetic drug to alter salivary flow in the human parotid gland, the changes in concentration of Na^+, K^+, Cl^-, and HCO_3^- can be studied systematically (Fig. 9-6). The changes in concentration for Na^+, K^+, Cl^-, and HCO_3^- resulting from parasympathetic stimulation are similar to those resulting from reflex-

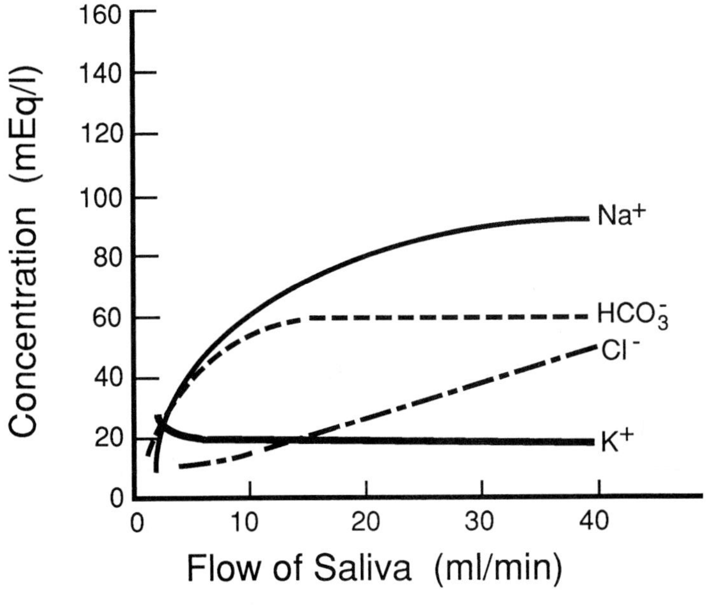

FIG. 9-6
Variations in concentrations of ions in human parotid gland saliva as flow rate is increased by parasympathetomimetic stimulation. (From Thaysen JH, Thorn, NA, Schwartx IL: *American Journal of Physiology* 178:155-159, 1954.)

TABLE 9-4
Ionic concentration in mEq/L of primary secretions in rat submaxillary gland compared with plasma

	Control	Carbachol*	Isoproterenol†	Plasma
Na	136	139	136	147
K	8.5	4	5.5	4.4

Data from Young JA, Martin CJ: Electrolyte transport in the excurrent duct system of the submandibular gland. In Emmelin N, Zotterman Y, editors: *Oral Physiology*, Oxford, 1972, Pergamon Press.
* Parasympathetomimetic drug
† β-Sympathetomimetic drug

ively induced salivary flow. It is now known that the changes in ionic concentration with flow can be explained by a two-stage secretory mechanism.

In the first stage saliva is formed initially in the lumen of the acinar cells. By analyzing samples of this saliva, called primary saliva, it has been shown to be plasma-like in concentrations of Na^+, Cl^-, and HCO_3^-. The concentrations of ions in primary saliva are relatively unaffected by changes in flow rate or the source of stimulation (Table 9-4). The concentration of K^++ ions in primary saliva is greater than in plasma.

In the second stage of secretion the primary saliva is modified as it flows down the duct system. The ducts seem to be impermeable to water, but sodium is

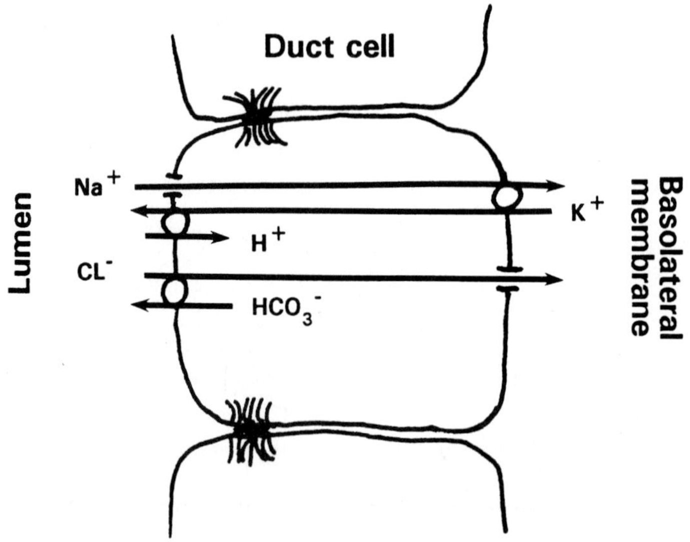

FIG. 9-7
Ionic fluxes across a salivary duct cell. An energy dependent Na^+/K^+ pump maintains a low intracellular Na^+ and a high K^+ concentration. Sodium enters the cell from the lumen via a Na^+ channel and is then pumped out via the Na^+/K^+ pump. Chloride enters and leaves the cell via Cl^- channels on the luminal and basolateral membranes. Potassium enters the cell via the basolateral Na^+/K^+ pump and passes into the lumen through a K-H exchanger. Other exchangers transport bicarbonate, sodium, and chloride.

actively reabsorbed and potassium secreted across the duct wall (Fig. 9-7). At low flow rates the sodium reabsorption mechanism is sufficient to remove all the sodium from the saliva before it enters the oral cavity. At high flow rates the reabsorption mechanism is insufficient to remove all the sodium so that increasing amounts of sodium appear in the final saliva. In contrast, at low flow rates potassium is secreted at a sufficient rate to increase the concentration of potassium above the levels found in primary saliva. At high flow rates the secreted potassium is diluted considerably so that the concentration in final saliva is lower, but still higher than plasma concentration.

During nerve stimulation the rate at which ions are transported across the ducts changes. When parasympathetic nerves are stimulated or cholinergic agonists are applied to ducts, sodium reabsorption and potassium secretion are inhibited, whereas bicarbonate secretion is stimulated. β-Adrenergic agonists and a high level of sympathetic nerve stimulation mimic all the actions of cholinergic stimulation. On the other hand, β-adrenergic stimulation enhances sodium adsorption.

Secretions of Proteins

Protein secretion by salivary glands consists of the initial uptake of amino acids, peptide synthesis and glycosylation, condensation, and exocytosis. Several amino acid uptake systems have been described: one for basic amino acids, one for acidic amino acids, and two for neutral amino acids. Peptide synthesis and glycosylation take place in the rough endoplasmic reticulum and Golgi cisternae. Condensation of the secretory proteins begins in the Golgi apparatus and continues in the condensing vacuoles and immature secretion granules. The secretory granules pass through several morphologic changes and often have inclusions which remain undissolved even when discharged into the duct lumen. Finally the secretory granules merge with the luminal membrane when exocytosis occurs (Fig. 9-8).

Protein can also be secreted without any apparent degranulation. Although stimulation of the parasympathetic nerve supply to the rat parotid gland usually results in saliva with a low protein concentration, prolonged stimulation can lead to a substantial output of protein without any apparent loss of secretory granules. These results suggest that the protein content of parasympathetically evoked saliva production results from a secretory mechanism that is different from exocytosis usually seen when the sympathetic nervous system is stimulated.

Although most of the organic components of saliva are secreted by the acinar cells, some proteins are synthesized and secreted by ductal cells. These include the growth factors (nerve growth factor, epidermal growth factor) and digestive enzymes such as ribonuclease and proteinases. Of the various proteinases and peptidases found in the ductal cells, renin, kallikrein, and tonin are the most highly concentrated. These various organic components do not exist in all salivary glands, and, in the case of nerve growth factor, there is a considerable sexual difference in

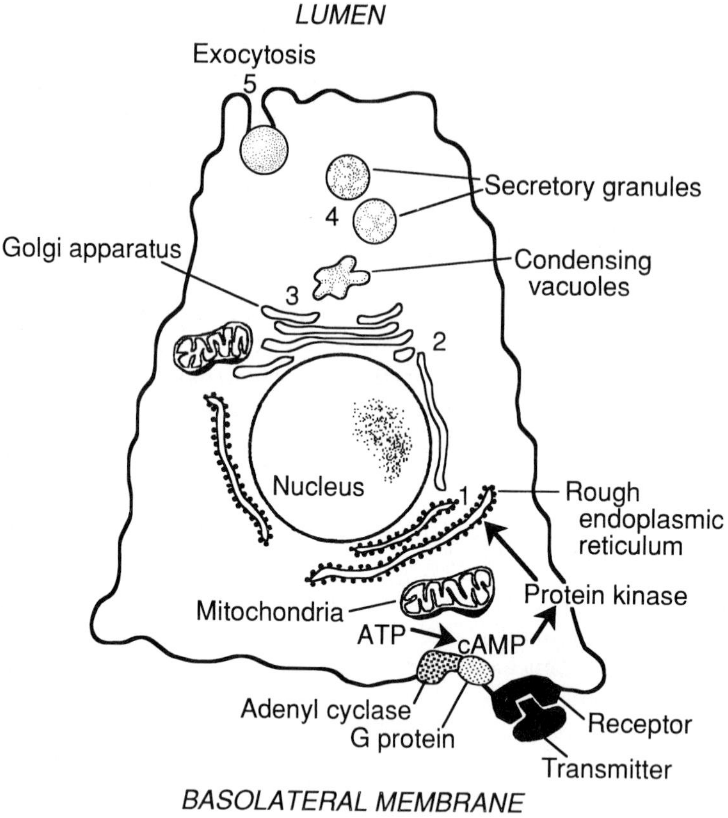

FIG. 9-8
Excitation-secretion coupling involved in protein secretion by salivary acinar cells. Secretion is initiated when a neural transmitter (usually norepinephrine) is released from a nerve terminal. The transmitter binds to a receptor on the basolateral membrane, which is coupled by a G protein to adenyl cyclase. Activation of adenyl cyclase catalyzes conversion of ATP to cAMP, which activates protein kinases and protein synthesis in the rough endoplasmic reticulum (*1*). Synthesized proteins are pinched off to form Golgi vesicles (2), where they are modified and concentrated in condensing vacuoles (*3*) to form secretory granules (*4*). Increased production of cAMP also activate release of the secretory granules in a process called exocytosis (*5*).

the amount secreted. Some of the peptides are released by α-adrenergic stimulation while others are controlled hormonally. To be effective many of these substances need to enter the circulation. However, secretion into saliva with subsequent swallowing and reabsorption has been shown to lead to insignificant increases in plasma levels of these components. Therefore, despite relatively abundant levels of these biologically active compounds in the ductal cells, their precise role is still uncertain.

CONTROL OF SALIVARY SECRETION

Parasympathetic control

The parasympathetic secretomotor neurons controlling the salivary glands lie in a long column of cells, the salivatory nucleus, which extends from the rostral pole of the dorsal motor nucleus of the vagus nerve to the genu of the facial nerve in the medulla (Fig. 9-9). Electrical stimulation of these neurons results in secretion of saliva. The most rostral and caudal parts of this dorsal cell column are called the superior and inferior salivatory nuclei respectively, although there is no distinct anatomic boundary. By injecting neural tracers into the salivary glands, and by electrical stimulation of various regions of the salivatory nuclei, it has been demonstrated that the submandibular and sublingual glands are controlled by the superior salivatory nucleus whereas the parotid and lingual (von Ebner's) salivary glands are controlled by the inferior salivatory nucleus.

However, these neural tracing experiments also demonstrate considerable overlap between the parasympathetic neurons with efferent fibers distributed in the

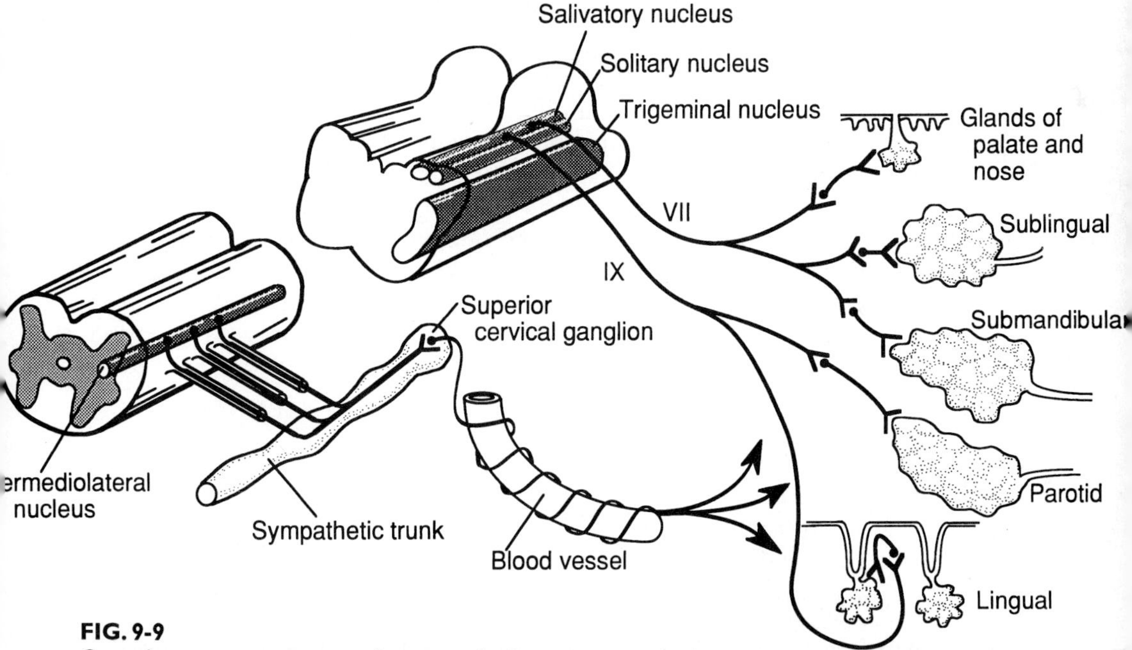

FIG. 9-9
Central nervous system control centers of salivary secretion. In the medulla the parasympathetic salivatory nucleus contains cell bodies of efferent preganglionic secretomotor fibers that are distributed to salivary glands with the facial (VII) and glossopharyngeal (IX) nerves. These efferent fibers synapse in peripheral parasympathetic ganglia. Postganglionic fibers distribute to salivary glands. Cell bodies of preganglionic sympathetic neurons are situated in intermediolateral nucleus of thoracic spinal cord. Preganglionic fibers are distributed to superior cervical ganglion of sympathetic trunk, where they synapse with cell bodies of postganglionic neurons. Postganglionic symapthetic secretomotor fibers are distributed to the various salivary glands with blood vessels.

glossopharyngeal nerve and those with efferent fibers in the facial nerve. So referring to these cell groups as the inferior and superior salivatory nuclei is somewhat questionable. At the caudal extent the salivatory nuclei merge into the dorsal motor nucleus of the vagus nerve, a column of parasympathetic cells that control a number of vital functions including gut secretions. The entire extent of the combined salivatory and dorsal motor nucleus of the vagus is closely related to the medial border of the nucleus of the solitary tract.

The parasympathetic neurons of the salivatory nuclei have spindle-shaped cell bodies with two major dendrites that divide into a number of secondary dendrites. The dendrites travel long distances and terminate in the trigeminal and solitary nuclei. Little is known regarding the connections made by the parasympathetic neurons. However, the dendritic terminations in the trigeminal and solitary (gustatory) nuclei indicate possible connections between the sensory and secretomotor nuclei that might underlie reflex mechanisms of salivary secretion (see Fig. 9-9).

Efferent parasympathetic fibers originating in the salivatory nuclei travel in cranial nerves and are distributed to all the salivary glands. Parasympathetic fibers to the submandibular and sublingual glands exit the brain stem in the nervus intermedius (facial, cranial nerve VII, nerve sensory branch), and join the chorda tympani which then merges with the lingual nerve (a branch of the trigeminal nerve). The parasympathetic fibers then connect in the submandibular ganglion, and the postganglionic fibers distribute to the two glands. The efferent supply to parotid and lingual (von Ebner's) salivary glands travel in the glossopharyngeal nerve (IX). Parasympathetic fibers to the parotid gland travel in the tympanic plexus, lesser superficial petrosal nerve and synapse in the otic ganglion. Postganglionic fibers travel to the parotid gland in the auriculotemporal nerve. Lingual salivary glands receive their efferent parasympathetic supply through the lingual-tonsilar branch of the glossopharyngeal nerve. The fibers synapse in Remak's ganglion, which consists of a series of dispersed ganglion cells located in the posterior tongue (see Fig. 9-9).

Sympathetic Control

The sympathetic nerve supply to the salivary glands is derived from the superior cervical ganglion. Preganglionic fibers to the superior cervical ganglion have cell bodies located in the intermediolateral nucleus situated in the upper thoracic segments of the spinal cord. The preganglionic fibers ascend in the paravertebral sympathetic trunk to the superior cervic ganglion. After a synapse in the ganglion the postganglionic fibers travel to the glands as a plexus of nerves associated with blood vessels (see Fig. 9-9).

Distribution of Nerve Fibers in Glands

Once the secretomotor fibers reach the gland they distribute and connect with acinar cells, myoepithelial cells, and blood vessels. Two types of neuroeffector relationship have been shown between nerve endings and acinar cell basement membranes. In the first, termed epilemmal, the axon is separated from the acinar cells by a basal lamina. In the second, called hypolemmal, the axon is closely apposed to the acinar cell beneath the basal lamina. The second type is usually but not always associated with parasympathetic, cholinergic innervation, whereas the first is often related to sympathetic innervation. Fibers innervating acinar cells may also innervate other structures in the gland because a single axon may contact, in passing, both acinar cells, myoepithelial cells, and perhaps blood vessels. Because nerve terminals can contain different neurotransmitters, stimulation of a particular axon could result in very complex actions at effector sites within the gland.

Excitation Secretion Coupling

Salivary secretion is initiated when neural transmitter substances bind to cell surface receptors, and, through the generation of various intracellular second messenger, activate the cellular mechanisms responsible for protein or fluid secretion. Salivary acinar cells possess a number of different receptors capable of interacting specifically with various neurotransmitters. Parasympathetic synapses interact with cholinergic or muscarinic receptors and the neural transmitter is acetylcholine. Norepinephrine is the postganglionic sympathetic transmitter. Experiments with various sympathetomimetic agonists and antagonists have revealed that both α-adrenoreceptors and β-adrenoreceptors may be at work in coupling neural and secretory activity of salivary glands.

Until recently it was thought that salivary secretion could result only from excitation of cholinergic and adrenergic receptors. However, it has been shown that after blockage of the muscarinic response by atropine, stimulation of the parasympathetic supply to the rat parotid gland still causes salivary secretion. This "atropine-resistant" secretion results from noncholinergic transmitter release, originating in nerve fibers containing neuropeptides such as substance P, vasoactive intestinal peptide (VIP), and calcitonin-gene-related peptide (CGRP). These neuropeptides do not seem to act on their own, but probably play a complementary role, interacting with acetylcholine to enhance salivary secretion.

TABLE 9-5
Relative volumes of fluid secretion induced by sympathetic stimulation*

	Dog	Cat	Rabbit	Rat	Sheep
Parotid	−	+	+	++	+
Submandibular	++	+++	(+)	++	(+)
Sublingual	(+)	++		−	
Types of adrenoreceptors responsible for secretion of fluid					
Parotid	(β)	β(α)	α(β)	αβ	β
Submandibular	β	α(β)	(β)	αβ	
Sublingual	?	α(β)			

From Emmelin N: Nervous control of mammalian salivary glands, *Philosophical Transactions of the Royal Society of London* B296:27-35, 1981.

* Relative flow rates indicated by +,-; parentheses in upper portion indicate flow is minimal and in the lower portion indicate that stimulation of this receptor is less effective in initiating flow of saliva; blank entries indicate that data are not available.

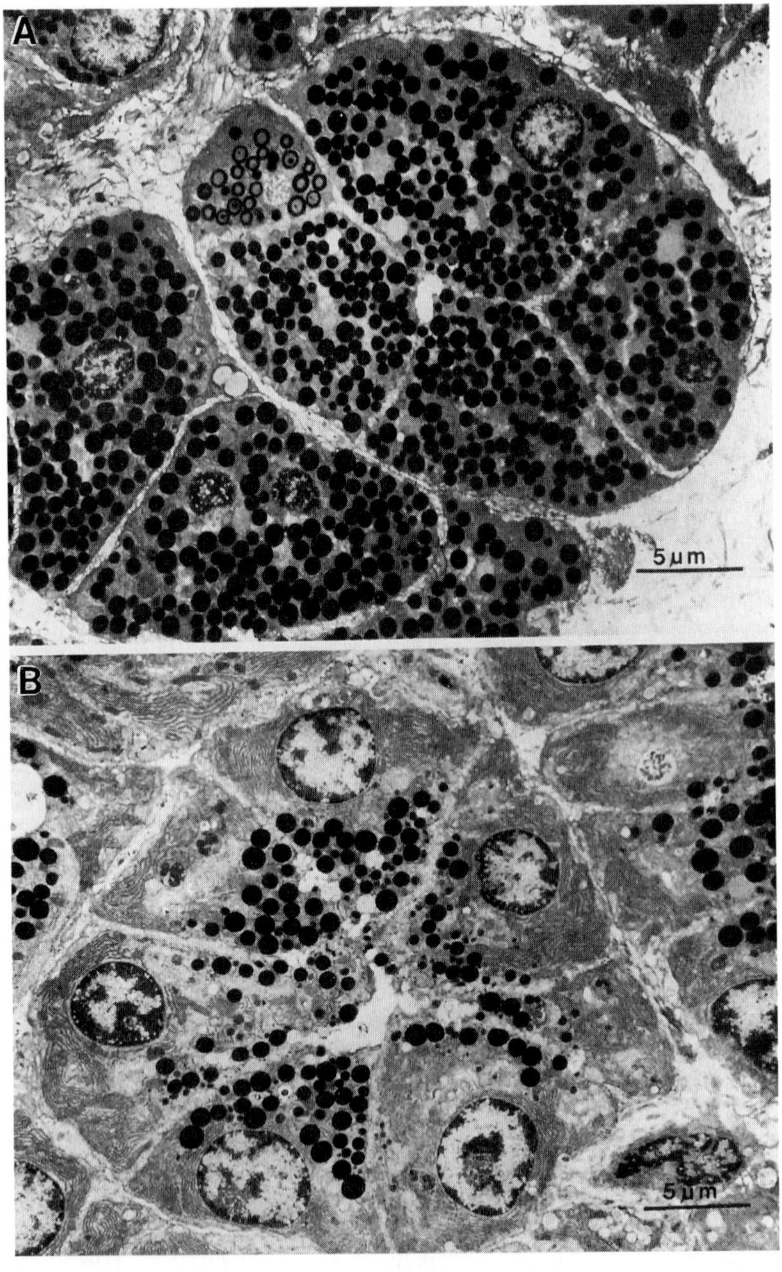

FIG. 9-10
Low power electron micrographs of the parotid gland of a rat. **A**, Acini from the unstimulated gland, packed with dark staining secretory granules. **B**, Acini from the contralateral parotid gland after stimulation of the sympathetic nerve supply, resulting in almost total depletion of the secretory granules. (From Garrett JR, Thulin A: *Cell and Tissue Research* 159:179-193, 1975.)

TABLE 9-6

Effect of autonomic nervous system stimulation on salivary secretion*

Stimulation	Duration (min)	Flow (ml/30 min)	Amylase (mg/ml)	Degranulation
Sympathetic, 10/sec	30	0.065 ± 0.025	30.63 ± 2.22	++++
Parasympathetic, 10/sec	30	0.850 ± 0.25	0.043 ± 0.08	?

Adapted from Proctor GB, Asking B, Garrett JR: Differences in the protein composition of rat parotid salivas evoked by sympathetic and parasympathetic nerve stimulation, *Comparative Biochemistry and Physiology* 92A:589-592, 1989.

*Values are mean ± S.D of 5 observations.

Although all salivary acinar cells seem to possess cholinergic (muscarinic) receptors on the basolateral membrane, there is considerable variability in the sympathetic innervation. For some glands sympathetic stimulation is ineffective in producing saliva. For other glands sympathetic stimulation produces a relatively low flow of saliva high in protein, while in other glands secretion is abundant (Table 9-5). There is also considerable variability in the type of adrenoreceptor present. Therefore, some glands possess only α receptors while activation of β receptors is effective for other glands. In another group of glands both receptors are present but are not equally effective when stimulated. In general, however, parasympathetic activation provides the main drive for the secretion of fluid by salivary glands, and sympathetic stimulation leads to secretion of protein. For example, electrical stimulation of the sympathetic nerve to the rat parotid gland causes a small flow of saliva with a high concentration of amylase associated with extensive degranulation of the acinar cells (Fig. 9-10). If the same level of stimulation is applied to the parasympathetic nerve supply to the rat parotid gland a considerable volume of saliva is produced, low in amylase content associated with insignificant degranulation (Table 9-6).

β-receptors are coupled by activation of a G protein to the formation of cyclic adenosine 3'5'-monophosphate (cAMP), activation of cAMP-dependent protein kinases, phosphorylation of specific target proteins, and ultimately mobilization and exfoliation of secretory granules (see Fig. 9-8). Cholinergic and α-adrenergic receptors are coupled to phospholipase C. Activation of receptors linked to phospholipase C generate diacylglycerol and inositol triphosphate (IP_3) which releases Ca^{2+} from the endoplasmic reticulum and this evokes the opening of the Ca^{2+}-activated K^+ channels in the basolateral membrane of the acinar cell. Opening this channel cause Cl^- to leave the cell through Cl^- channels on the luminal membrane of the acinar cell. This increases the lumen negativity which allows Na+ to move between the cells into the narrow intracellular spaces though leaky intercellular junctions at the luminal ends (Fig. 9-11). The net result of these transport events is the transcellular NaCl transport, followed by water. Because of this loss of water the acinar cells actually shrink during stimulation and regain their resting volume when stimulation ceases. Moreover, the cell shrinkage is accompanied by an increase in free intracellular Ca^{2+} concentration, which returns to basal levels once the cell volume returns to initial levels.

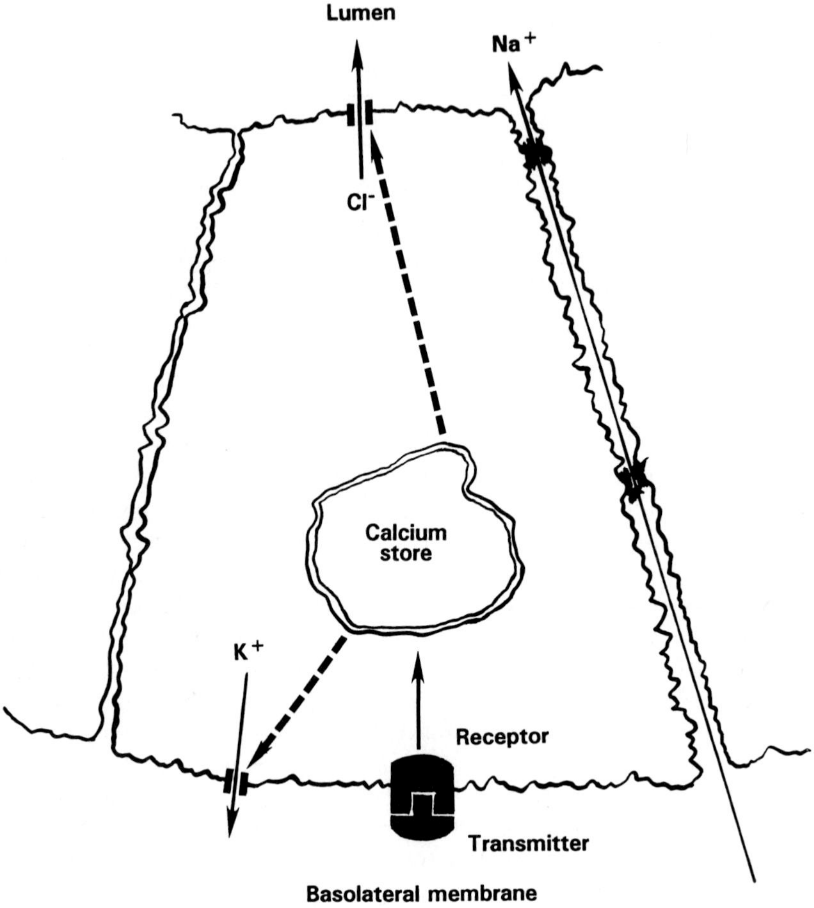

FIG. 9-11
Excitation-secretion coupling involved in electrolyte secretion by salivary acinar cells. Secretion is initiated when a neural transmitter (usually acetylcholine) is released from a nerve terminal. The transmitter binds to receptor on the basolateral membrane (muscarinic-receptor), which initiates the release of calcium from cellular calcium stores; this, in turn, evokes the opening of the calcium-activated potassium channels in the basolateral membrane of the acinar cell. Opening of this channel causes chloride to leave the cell by chloride channels on the luminal membrane of the acinar cell. This increases the lumen negativity, which allows sodium to move between the cells into the narrow intracellular spaces and through the tight junctions at the luminal ends. The net result of the transport events is the transcellular NaCl transport, with water following.

Myoepithelial Cells

Myoepithelial cells are innervated by both parasympathetic and sympathetic nerve fibers, and activation of either branch of the autonomic nervous system causes myoepithelial cells to contract. Because myoepithelial cell stimulation increases ductal pressure, myoepithelial cells actively expel saliva from the glands.

Parasympathetic contraction of myoepithelial cells involves cholinergic receptors, whereas sympathetic activation has been found to be exclusively under the control of α-adrenergic receptors. Therefore during salivary secretion there is an active cooperation between secretory and motor nerves. Once secretion is initiated, contraction of the myoepithelial cells facilitates expulsion of the saliva from the gland. This may be especially important for glands in which the secretion is particularly viscous.

Salivary Reflexes

Salivary secretion normally occurs when foods are placed in the mouth and occurs in anesthetized and even decerebrate animals. This reflex secretion results from stimulation of oral mechanoreceptors, especially periodontal ligament mech-anoreceptors, as well as taste buds. Afferent impulses travel along sensory fibers in the trigeminal, facial, and glossopharyngeal nerves, synapsing on second-order neurons in the trigeminal and solitary tract nuclei. Efferent activity to the salivary glands originates in the parasympathetic salivatory nuclei and the sympathetic nuclei in the spinal cord. The interconnections between the second-order sensory nuclei and the secretomotor nuclei are not well understood, but more than one synapse is in-volved. The location of the parasympathetic salivatory nuclei closely associated with the medial border of the solitary nucleus would facilitate interconnections (Fig. 9-9). The afferent projections to the sympathetic preganglionic neurons in the spinal cord travel in the intermediolateral column, which receives input from a number of brain nuclei including the solitary tract nucleus. Both the parasympathetic and sympathetic systems are therefore connected to brain stem nuclei and relay sensory information from the oral cavity.

Salivary secretion can be initiated by electrical stimulation of more rostral brain areas including motor cortex and the hypothalamus. Recent neural tracing experiments have revealed descending pathways from the hypothalamus to the parasympathetic salivatory nuclei and the sympathetic preganglionic neurons in the spinal cord; because the hypothalamus is associated with the control of feeding, these descending pathways could underlie mechanisms of salivation during feeding. In fact electrical stimulation of the lateral hypothalamus enhances the effectiveness of reflex salivary secretion initiated by oral gustatory stimulation.

Reflex salivation initiated by chewing has a significant unilateral component because salivary flow is highest on the chewing side of the mouth. Application of anesthetics to block sensory input from periodontal ligament mechanoreceptors results in a marked reduction in reflex salivation induced by chewing, implicating the significant role of these receptors in the trigeminal component of salivatory reflex activity.

Not all taste stimuli or foods are equally effective in promoting salivary flow. It has been known for many years that acids, particularly citric acid, initiate copious flow rates of saliva. Other taste stimuli are less effective in promoting salivary flow

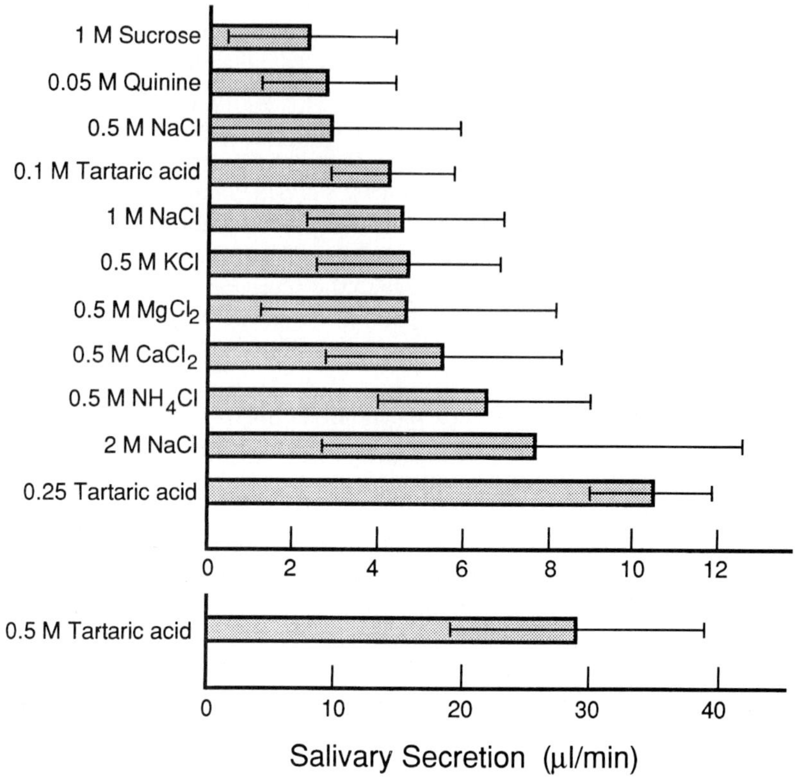

FIG. 9-12
Salivary secretion induced by different gustatory stimuli applied to the anterior tongue in rats. (From Kawamura Y, Yamamoto T: *Journal of Physiology (London.)*: 285:35-47, 1987.)

(Fig. 9-12). However, sucrose, although promoting only a small increase in flow, results in a significant production of salivary amylase. Since high flow rates of saliva usually result from parasympathetic stimulation and amylase secretion results from sympathetic nerve activity, it is possible that the connections between sensory nuclei and the autonomic nuclei are modality specific. Therefore the reflex activation of the salivary glands during feeding is complex and involves integration of sensory input from oral receptors and descending information derived from rostral brain structures on both parasympathetic and sympathetic secretomotor nuclei in the brain stem and spinal cord.

BUFFERING ACTION OF SALIVA

Reduction in salivary flow often results in a marked increase in dental caries and other oral pathologies. From this and other observations it is clear that one of the

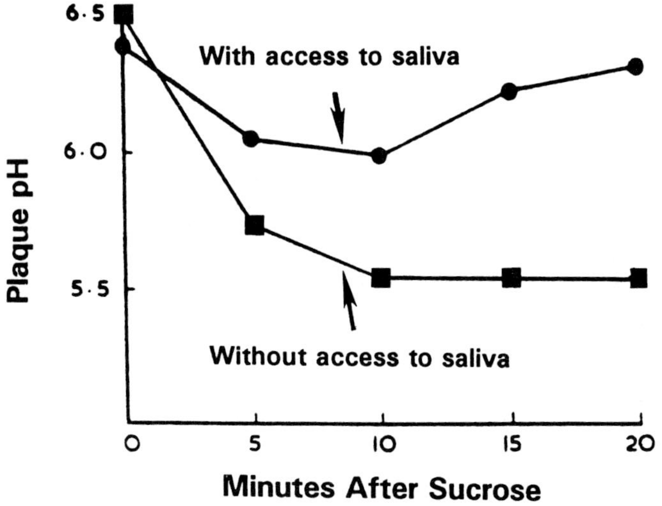

FIG. 9-13
Changes in plaque pH measured from humans after a suger rinse in the presence or abscence of saliva. (Adapted from Englander HR, Shklair IL, Fosdick LS, *Journal of Dental Research* 38:848-853, 1959.)

major functions of saliva is the maintenance of oral health by limiting the formation of acid from bacterial fermentation. The production of acid is believed to etch enamel, which is the initial stage in the development of dental caries.

An important role of saliva in maintaining the integrity of the oral and dental tissues is the control of oral pH. It is possible to measure the pH of plaque after an oral rinse with a sucrose solution. If access of saliva to the plaque is prevented there is a dramatic fall in plaque pH, whereas unrestricted salivary flow to plaque results in little alteration of plaque pH (Fig. 9-13). Saliva is, therefore, able to prevent the acidifi-

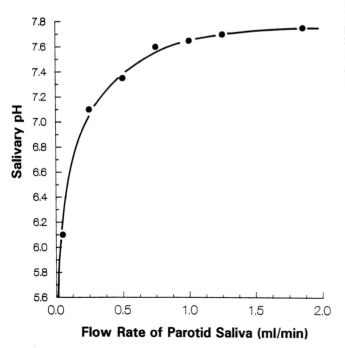

FIG. 9-14
Effect of salivary flow rate on the pH of parotid saliva. (Data from Shannon IL, Suddick RP, Dowd FJ: *Saliva, Composition and Secretion, Monographs in Oral Science*, vol 2, Basel, 1974, Karger.)

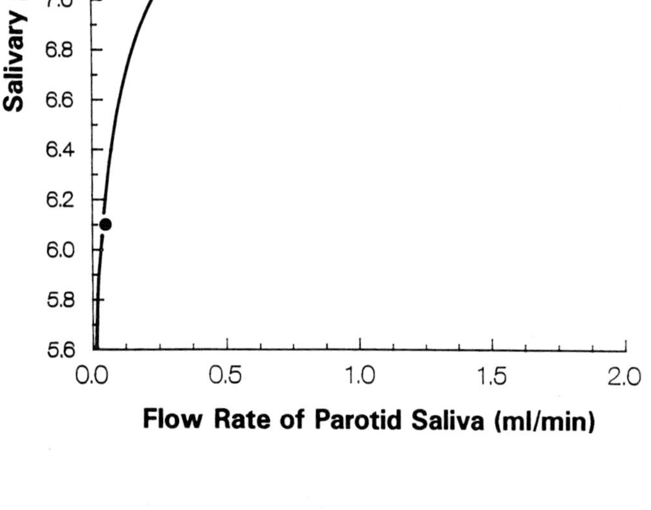

cation of the plaque.

A number of salivary constituents may contribute to the ability of saliva to control mouth pH, but the most important is bicarbonate. The concentration of bicarbonate in saliva increases with a rise in flow and the pH of saliva changes with flow (Fig. 9-14). Resting parotid saliva has a pH of 5.82 and a bicarbonate concentration of 0.6 mEq/L, whereas at high flow rates the pH rises to 7.67 and bicarbonate concentration increases to almost 30 mEq/L (see Table 9-2). Although other salivary components may help control mouth pH, bicarbonate is by far the major factor, because removal of the bicarbonate reduces the buffering capacity of saliva to a very low level. It can be concluded that to increase the buffering power of saliva it is necessary to increase saliva flow. This takes place under normal circumstances during feeding, when oral microorganisms are provided with substrates to ferment and lower mouth pH. When salivary flow is minimal, such as during sleep, the buffering action of saliva is limited. It is therefore important to remove food debris from the mouth to limit the supply of substrate for microorganisms and minimize the fall in mouth pH.

EFFECTS OF AGING ON SALIVARY SECRETION

Older individuals often report a prevalence of oral dryness and difficulty in swallowing and suffer tooth loss. It was assumed that these conditions resulted from altered salivary function, and several studies supported the concept that salivary flow is lowered with increasing age. Recent studies of salivary gland function, however, have suggested that the earlier conclusions were unfounded and that there is no generalized change in salivary gland function during aging. The underlying problem with the earlier studies related to subject selection (pathologic conditions were not adequately controlled) and methods of measurement which were not standardized as to time of day and flow rate all of which could alter composition. Moreover, many studies simply collected whole saliva which can be derived from many sources in the oral cavity. Recent studies have used saliva collected from the parotid and subman-dibular glands on a series of age groups (so-called cross-sectional data). There are no reported data from the same group of individuals at different ages (so-called longitudinal data), nor have data been collected on other salivary glands. But based on carefully controlled cross-sectional studies on human parotid and submandibular gland function it can be concluded that there are no generalized reductions in salivary secretion in healthy older individuals.

SUMMARY

The fluid bathing the oral cavity, saliva, is secreted by glands that drain by a duct system into the mouth. Saliva has many functions and is important for maintenance of oral health. Salivary glands comprise a large number of secretory units that consist of blind ending tubes lined with cells that secrete and modify saliva. Secretion is under the control of the autonomic nervous system, has a high flow during feeding, a low flow between meals, and a minimal flow during sleep.

Saliva is mostly water containing a low percentage of organic and inorganic components. Many of the components of saliva are derived from blood plasma, but other are synthesized within the gland. The composition of saliva changes with flow, some components increasing in concentration and others decreasing. Saliva is secreted in two stages. Primary saliva is the initial secretion, which is modified during passage down the ducts. Proteins are secreted by synthesis and formation of secretory granules, which are then discharged into the duct lumen by exocytosis.

All salivary gland secretory cells possess cholinergic receptors, but there is considerable variability in the sympathetic innervation. For some glands sympathetic stimulation is ineffective in producing saliva. For other glands sympathetic stimulation produces a relatively low flow of saliva high in protein, but in other glands secretion is abundant. There is also considerable variability in the type of sympathetic receptor and some glands possess only α receptors whereas other glands have β receptors. In general, parasympathetic stimulation of salivary glands is very effective in producing the highest flow of saliva, whereas sympathetic activation is generally less effective. In contrast sympathetic stimulation results in gland degranulation and a saliva high in protein.

At the level of the gland, sympathetic stimulation activates β-receptors that are coupled by activation of a G protein to the formation of cAMP and activation of cAMP-dependent protein kinases, the phosphorylation of specific target proteins, and ultimately mobilization and exfoliation of secretory granules. Cholinergic and α-adrenergic receptors are coupled to phospholipase C. Activation releases intracellular Ca^{2+}, which opens Ca^{2+}-activated K^+ channels in the basolateral membrane of the secretory cell. This causes Cl^- to leave the cell by Cl^- channels. Secretion of Cl^- causes an increase in lumenal negativity which allows Na^+ to move between the cells into the narrow intracellular spaces by way of leaky intercellular junctions. The net result of these transport events is the transcellular NaCl transport, with water following.

Salivary glands are controlled by parasympathetic and sympathetic nuclei in the medulla and spinal cord. The interconnections of these nuclei with sensory nuclei probably account for salivary reflexes in which flow and salivary composition are altered by chewing and taste stimuli.

The bicarbonate contained in saliva is the principal buffer of oral acidity. The concentration of bicarbonate and the pH of saliva rise with flow. Because the flow of saliva is minimal at night, oral pH is generally lower during sleep.

Although older individuals often complain of a dry mouth, careful study of aging populations free of pathology indicates that reduction in salivary flow is not a normal occurrence of the aging process.

SELECTED READINGS

Baum BJ: Changes in salivary function in older subjects. In Ferguson DB, editor: *Frontiers of oral physiology*, vol 6, *The aging mouth,* Basel, 1987, Karger.

Baum BJ: Principles of saliva secretion, *Annals of the New York Academy of Sciences* 694:17-23, 1993.

Garrett JR: The proper role of nerves in salivary secretion: a review, *Journal of Dental Research* 66:387-397, 1987.

Kleinberg I, Ellison SA, Mandel ID: *Saliva and dental caries*, New York, 1979, Information Retrieval.

Petersen OH, Gallacher DV: Electrophysiology of pancreatic and salivary acinar cells, *Annals and Review of Physiology* 50:65-80, 1988.

Petersen OH: Electrophysiology of exocrine gland cells. In Johnson LR, editor: *Physiology of the gastrointestinal tract*, New York, 1987, Raven Press.

Young JA and others: Secretion by the major salivary glands. In Johnson LR, editor: *Physiology of the gastrointestinal tract*, New York, 1987, Raven Press.

10

Mastication

LEARNING OBJECTIVES

At the end of this chapter you should be able to:

1. Describe the general characteristics of mastication.
2. Describe the basic pattern of jaw movements during mastication.
3. Describe the timing of a masticatory cycle.
4. Describe the pattern of muscle activity during a masticatory cycle.
5. Describe the anatomic and functional organization of the trigeminal sensory and motor nuclei.
6. Describe other motor nuclei involved in mastication.
7. Describe the influence of afferent sensory input on development of the trigeminal system.
8. Describe the reflex activity of orofacial musculature.
9. Describe the role of higher brain centers on masticatory activity.
10. Describe the influence of afferent sensory input on masticatory activity.
11. Describe the role of the brain stem pattern generator on rhythmical masticatory movement.

Controlled movement of the mandible is used in biting, chewing, and swallowing of food and fluids, and in the production of speech sounds. The integrated activity of the jaw muscles in response to efferent neural activity in the motor nerves results in mandibular movements which control the relationship between lower and upper teeth. Concurrent with the jaw movements are integrated movements of the tongue and other muscles controlling the perioral areas, pharynx and larynx. This chapter emphasizes the neuromuscular activities associated with mastication, in particular the cyclical movements produced by the elevation and depression of the mandible as food is sheared and formed into a bolus in preparation for swallowing.

Mastication of food is the initial stage in the process of digestion. Large pieces of food are reduced for swallowing, the food is broken apart, and the surface area increased, for the efficient action of digestive enzymes and to facilitate solubilization of food substances in saliva to stimulate taste receptors. In mammals mastication is characterized by large vertical movements of the lower jaw usually on one side of the dentition and in most species is accompanied by some transverse movements of the mandible, and protrusion and retrusion of the tongue.

Movements of the mandible and tongue begin in utero but coordinated masticatory movements occur late in gestation in precocious mammals and postnatally in altricial mammals. Even though most mammals are capable of masticatory movements early in life, most newborn mammals feed by suckling. There is a gradual transition from the motor patterns associated with suckling to those of mastication. The mechanisms controlling this transition are not known, but probably are multifactorial with maturation of anatomic and neural structures.

Bilateral sets of muscles move the jaw, that is linked across the midline. Control of the jaw muscles is not reciprocal as in limb movement, but bilaterally organized. It could, therefore, be concluded that the opening and closing of the jaw during chewing is a relatively simple movement compared with control of the limbs in locomotion. However, movements of mastication are quite complex and do not consist of simple mechanical grinding movements in which food is randomly reduced in size. During mastication food is efficiently reduced and mixed with saliva as the first stage of preparation for digestion.

MASTICATORY MOVEMENTS

An understanding of jaw movement patterns has been of great interest in clinical dentistry, particularly in the areas of orthodontics and prosthodontics. One of the goals of restoring occlusal form is to ensure tooth contact is integrated with jaw movement patterns. Therefore, numerous studies have been conducted to describe the path taken by the mandible during chewing, and to define the position of the mandible at rest (Box 10-1). Dentists have sought stable reference positions of the mandible to facilitate study of jaw relations on a simulator, or "articulator."

BOX 10-1
Recording Jaw Movement

Investigators studying mastication have used a variety of techniques to track excursion of the jaw during chewing. These techniques must be noninvasive and produce an accurate recording of jaw position and rate of movement over time in three dimensions.

Noninvasive techniques employ cinephotography or cinefluorography to record jaw movements. Disadvantages of these techniques are that the recordings are not continuous, not always in three planes, and require laborious tracings of movie frames to perform quantitative analysis.

All other techniques involve fixing a device to the jaw. Perhaps the simplest is a light source whose movement can be easily tracked in three planes and interfaced to a computer system for analysis. Other systems such as strain gauges record movement in only one plane.

Movement of the cranium is an important component of mastication, yet many investigators recording jaw movement fix the head, and therefore do not reflect true masticatory movements.

When jaw movements are recorded in combination with records of muscle activity, information can be obtained on the muscles responsible for making the movements. However, the placement of the electrodes to record muscle activity further interferes with normal jaw movements. Recently the use of high-speed video recording combined with continuous tracking of selected reference points has opened the way to record freely behaving animals.

Movements

During chewing the jaw moves rhythmically, opening and closing in a series of cyclical movements. The rate and pattern of jaw movement and jaw muscle activity are typical for a particular species of animal. Patterns of jaw movement and jaw muscle activity have been studied in a number of animals including humans. The pattern of jaw movements in various mammals is often characteristic of the animals' diet. Carnivores have specialized dentitions and temporomandibular joints for seizing and shearing food with a limited chopping movement of the mandible. Herbivorous animals make vertical, lateral, and anterior-posterior movements of the mandible to grind or mill fibrous plant foods. Animals that gnaw food have a masticatory pattern characterized by long anterior-posterior movements of the mandible and vertical and lateral movements. Primates have evolved a masticatory system that is relatively nonspecialized and is therefore adapted to chewing almost any kind of food material. Despite these major species differences, a single chewing cycle is usually divided into four phases. Beginning at the point of minimum opening, the jaw moves downward slowly followed by a faster opening phase. Next the

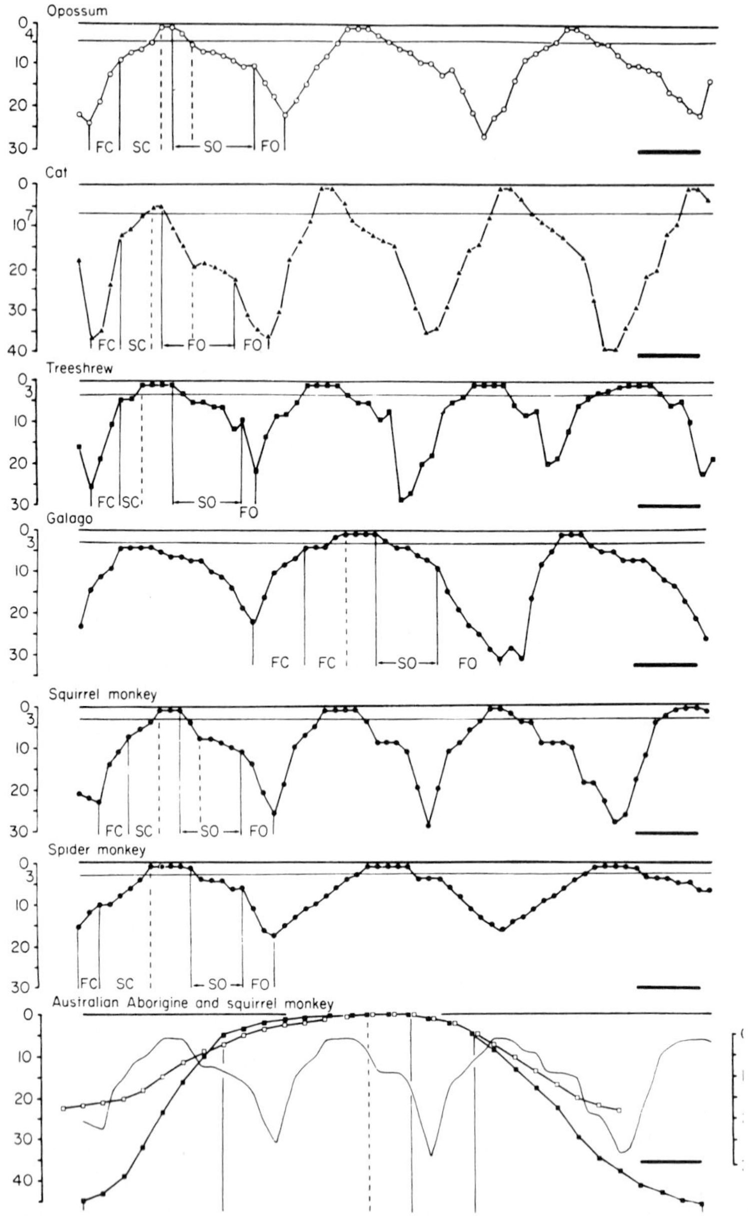

FIG. 10-1
Chewing cycles from a number of different species. All these recordings are in one plane and based on tracings of cinefluorographs, except for the human recording in which cinephotography was used. The jaw opening, called gape, is the angle between the upper and lower occlusal profiles. For the human recording gape is measured as the opening in millimeters from the horizontal plane of occlusion. The horizontal line is the level at which intercuspation first occurs. *FC*, Fast closing; *SC*, slow closing; *SO*, slow opening; *FO*, fast opening. (From Hiiemae, KM: Mammalian Mastication. In Butler PM, Joysey KA, editors: *Development, Function and Evolution of Teeth*. London, 1978, Academic Press, pp. 359-398.)

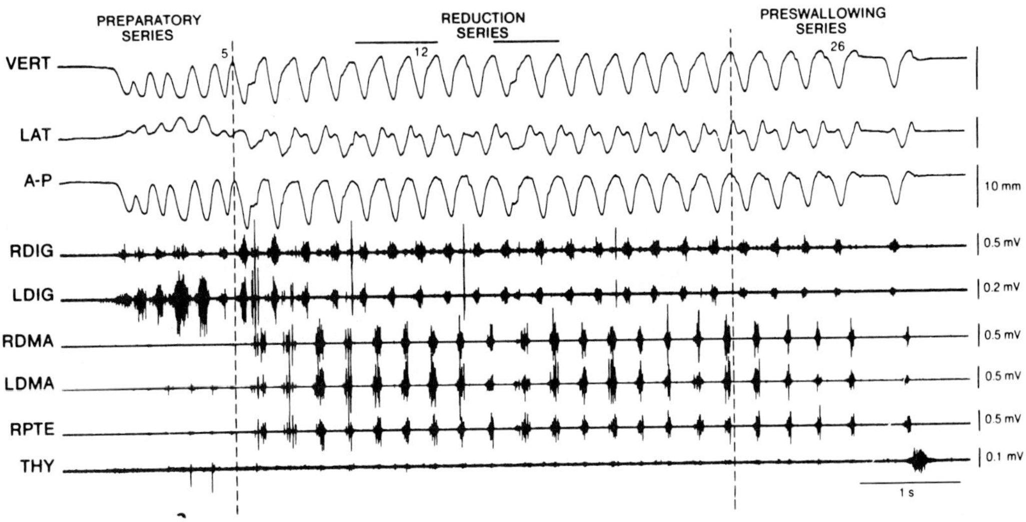

FIG. 10-2
Masticatory sequence recorded in three planes from a rabbit (*VERT*, vertical; *LAT*, lateral; *A-P*, anterior-posterior). A pellet of rabbit chow was placed into the mouth, transported to the molar teeth (preparatory cycles), chewed (reduction cycles) and prepared for swallowing (preswallowing cycles). EMG recordings were made simultaneously from the right and left digastric muscles (*RDIG*, *LDIG*), right and left deep masseter muscles (*RDMA*, *LDMA*), right pterygoid muscle (*RPTE*), and thyrohyoid muscle (*THY*). Swallowing is indicated by activity in the thyrohyoid muscle. (From Schwartz G, Enomoto S, Valiquette C, Lund, JP: *Journal of Neurophysiology* 62:273-287, 1989.)

jaw moves upward in a fast closing phase. The final phase is a slow closing during which the food is crushed between the teeth (Fig. 10-1).

A masticatory sequence consists of a number of chewing cycles and extends from ingestion to swallowing. During mastication the characteristics of the individual cycle vary depending on the state of breakdown of the food. The masticatory sequence can be divided into three consecutive periods. In the initial or preparatory period, food is transported back to the posterior teeth where it is ground during a reduction period. The bolus is then formed during the final, preswallowing, period. Movement of the jaws in these three periods differs depending on the type of foodstuff and the species of animal. For example, in a rabbit, only opening and fast-closing phases of a masticatory cycle are present during the preparatory period of a masticatory sequence. During the reduction period the cycle consists of opening, fast-closing, and slow-closing phases. In the preswallowing period, the cycle is made up of five phases, three taking place during jaw opening and two during jaw closing (Fig. 10-2).

During chewing the tongue plays an essential role in controlling the movement of the food and forming the bolus. For food to be broken down, it is positioned by the tongue in conjunction with the buccinator muscles of the cheek between the occlusal

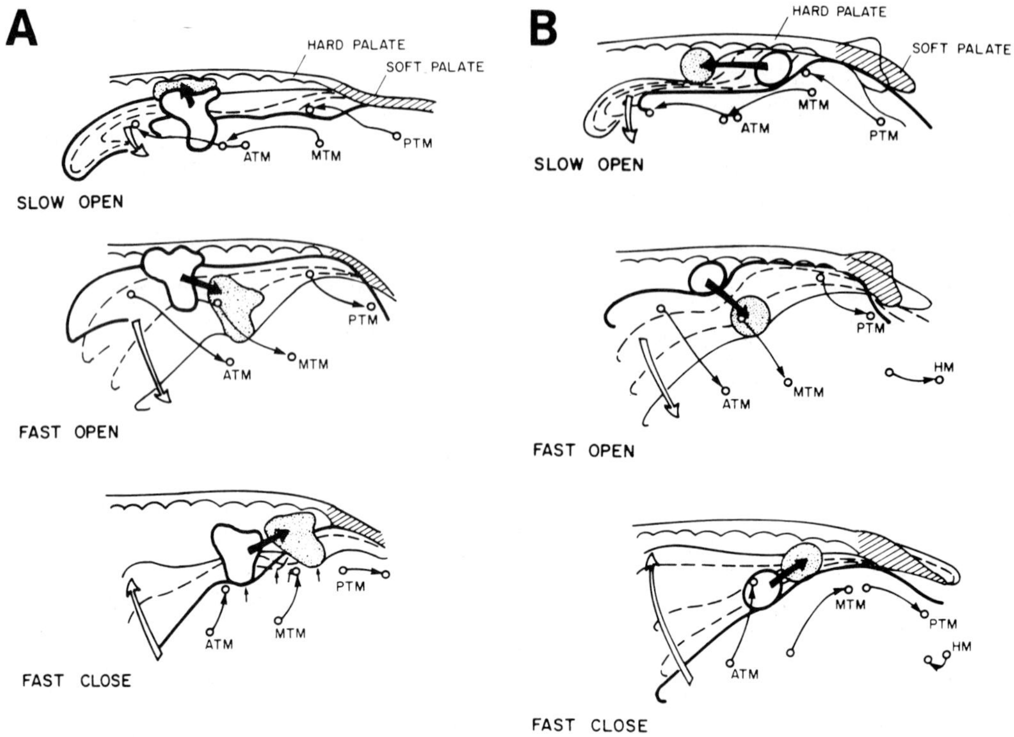

FIG. 10-3
Lateral tracings from cinefluorography of manipulation of a food bolus during mastication in opossum. **A**, Transport of food from anterior to posterior oral cavity. **B**, Distal movement of the food to the oropharynx. Large open arrows show direction and amplitude of jaw movement. Solid black arrows show movement of food through each phase. Heavy solid line shows position and shape of tongue and food bolus at the beginning and thin solid line their position at the end of each phase. Intermediate positions are indicated by dashed lines. Position of anterior (*ATM*), middle (*MTM*), and posterior (*PTM*) tongue and the hyoid (*HM*) markers is shown at the beginning and end of each phase. Their movement during each phase is indicated by thin black arrows. (Adapted from Hiiemae KJ, Crompton AW: Mastication, food transport, and swallowing. In Hildebrand M and others: *Functional Vertebrate Morphology*. Cambridge, 1985, Belnap Press, pp. 262-290.)

surfaces of the teeth. Solid and liquid food are transported within the oral cavity by the tongue. During the slow-opening phase of the chewing cycle, the tongue moves forward and expands beneath the food. The hyoid bone and the body of the tongue retract during the fast-opening and fast-closing phases, forming a trough that moves the food to the posterior oral cavity (Fig. 10-3, *A*,*B*). Once the food reaches the posterior oral cavity it is moved backwards below the soft palate by a squeezing action of the tongue. The tongue is important in collecting and sorting food that is suitable for swallowing, while returning larger pieces of food to the occlusal table for further reduction. Little is known of the underlying mechanism controlling the tongue during this activity.

Muscle activity

Contraction of the muscles that control the jaw during mastication consists of an asynchronous pattern of activity with wide variability in time of onset, time of peak activity, rate at which the peak is reached, and the rate of decline in activity (Box 10-2). The pattern of activity is determined by a number of factors such as species, type of food, degree of food breakdown, and individual factors. However, for most mammals there is a general pattern of muscle activity during a chewing cycle.

BOX 10-2
Electromyography

The cellular unit of contraction in a muscle is a muscle cell or fiber. During muscle contraction small groups of muscle fibers contract together because they are supplied by a single α motorneuron. The α motorneuron, its efferent fiber and terminal branches, and all the muscle fibers supplied by these branches make up a motor unit. Activation of the α motorneuron causes all the muscle fibers of the motor unit to contract. The number of muscle fibers in a motor unit is quite variable. Muscles controlling fine movements of the eye, middle ear, and larynx have the smallest number of muscle fibers in a motor unit, whereas motor units in limb and back muscles have up to 2000 muscle fibers. Contraction of the motor units in a muscle produces tension in the muscle.

During contraction, potential changes occur in each active muscle fiber. The sum of these potentials can be recorded by appropriately placed electrodes and is called electromyography, or EMG. The amplitude of the potential change depends on the size of the motor unit and the number of active motor units, but is influenced by electrode position, type of electrode, and the electronic equipment used to amplify and record the potential. Surface electrodes record from a large number of motor units. Implanted needle electrodes are necessary to record from individual motor units and muscles that are inaccessible to surface electrodes. Use of multiple electrodes permits recordings from groups of muscles active in controlling movements such as mastication. These simultaneous recordings from different muscles reveal the timing of muscle activity but cannot be used to compare the relative forces developed by individual muscles. Moreover, the EMG cannot be used to indicate whether a muscle is contracting isometrically (no change in muscle length) or isotonically (no change in muscle tension).

Despite these limitations EMG recordings of jaw muscle activity during chewing have revealed details of the pattern of activity of muscles that control the jaw. When combined with other manipulations such as stimulation of intraoral and perioral receptive fields, information on the role of sensory input on jaw muscle activity has been studied. When EMG and jaw movements are recorded simultaneously, sophisticated studies of masticatory movements can be performed.

Closing muscles are usually inactive during jaw opening, when the jaw-opening muscles are very active. Activity in jaw-closing muscles begins to be apparent at the beginning of the jaw closing. Activity of the jaw-closing muscles increases slowly as the teeth begin to interdigitate or as soon as food is encountered between the teeth. The closing muscles on the side where food is being crushed (so-called working

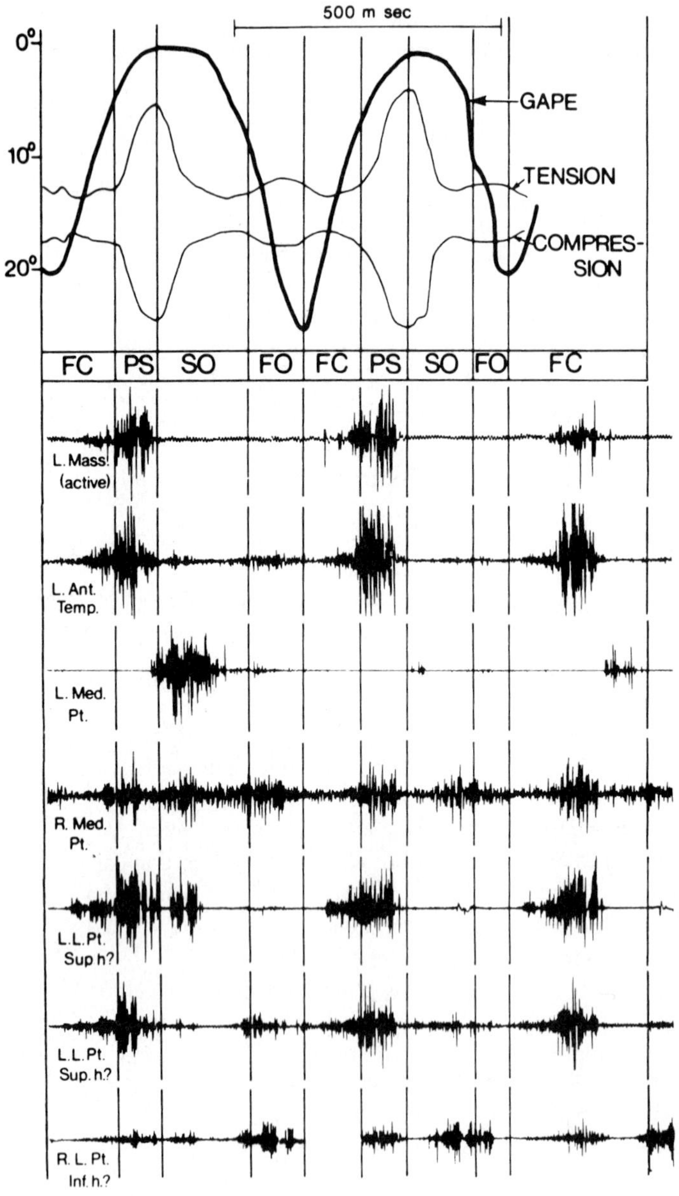

FIG. 10-4
EMG activity in a macaque monkey during two successive chewing cycles. The phases of the masticatory cycle are abbreviated as *FC*, fast closing; *PS*, power stroke; *SO*, slow opening; *FO*, fast opening. The muscle EMGs are recorded from: *L. Mass*, left masseter; *L. Ant. Temo.*, left anterior temporalis; *L. Med. Pt.*, left medial pterygoid; *R. Med. Pt.* right medial pterygoid. *L. L. Pt. Sup h?*, left lateral pterygoid with possible involvement of superior hyoid; *R. L. Pt. Sup h?*, right lateral pterygoid with possible involvement of superior hyoid. (Adapted from Hiiemae KJ, Crompton AW: Mastication, food transport, and swallowing. In Hildebrand M, and others: *Functional Vertebrate Morphology*, Cambridge, 1985, Belknap Press, pp. 262-290.)

side) are more active than the contralateral jaw-closing muscles. An example of jaw muscle activity during a masticatory cycle is shown in Fig. 10-4, which illustrates the pattern of muscle activity correlated with jaw movement pattern in a single species.

BRAIN STEM STRUCTURES IN CONTROL OF MASTICATION

The movements involved in mastication require the integrated activity of a number of muscles, controlled by trigeminal, hypoglossal, facial, and possibly other motor nuclei in the brain stem. The coordination of activity in these motor nuclei relies on sensory input from the oral cavity that terminates primarily in the trigeminal nucleus as well as the solitary tract nucleus. Other brain stem structures, such as the reticular formation, are also involved. An understanding of the mechanisms of mastication requires a detailed knowledge of these brain stem structures and the interconnections between them.

Trigeminal Sensory Nucleus

The trigeminal sensory nucleus is a column of neurons that extends along the lateral border of the brain stem from the pons to the spinal cord (Fig. 10-5). The most rostral portion of the nucleus is called the principal sensory nucleus (sometimes referred to as the main sensory nucleus) and the remainder is the spinal trigeminal nucleus. The spinal nucleus is subdivided, from rostral to caudal, into subnucleus oralis, interpolaris, and caudalis. Because the subnucleus caudalis is an extension of the dorsal horn of the spinal cord and has a similar histologic appearance, it is now often referred to as the medullary dorsal horn (see Chapter 2 for a detailed description of the medullary dorsal horn).

The peripheral innervation of this cell column arises from the trigeminal nerve. Central branches either bifurcate into ascending and descending limbs or simply descend on entering the brain stem to form the trigeminal tract. The rostral limb of the trigeminal tract wraps around the lateral aspect of the principal sensory nucleus, while caudally the descending limb comprises the spinal trigeminal tract along the lateral aspect of the spinal nucleus. Axonal collateral branches leave the trigeminal tract and enter the sensory nucleus forming terminal arbors at several different levels of the nucleus. The collaterals given off from the ascending branches enter the principal sensory nucleus and collaterals from the descending branches enter the spinal nucleus. Collaterals are topographically organized. Axons innervating the rostral mouth and face terminate medially and those that supply the caudal face terminate more laterally. The dorsal face is represented in the ventral part of the nucleus whereas axons innervating the ventral face and mouth terminate more dorsally. The morphology of the terminal arbors varies depending on the origin of the primary afferent fiber (Fig. 10-6).

The response properties, receptive fields, and morphology of trigeminal sensory nucleus neurons have been studied with combined intracellular recording and injec-

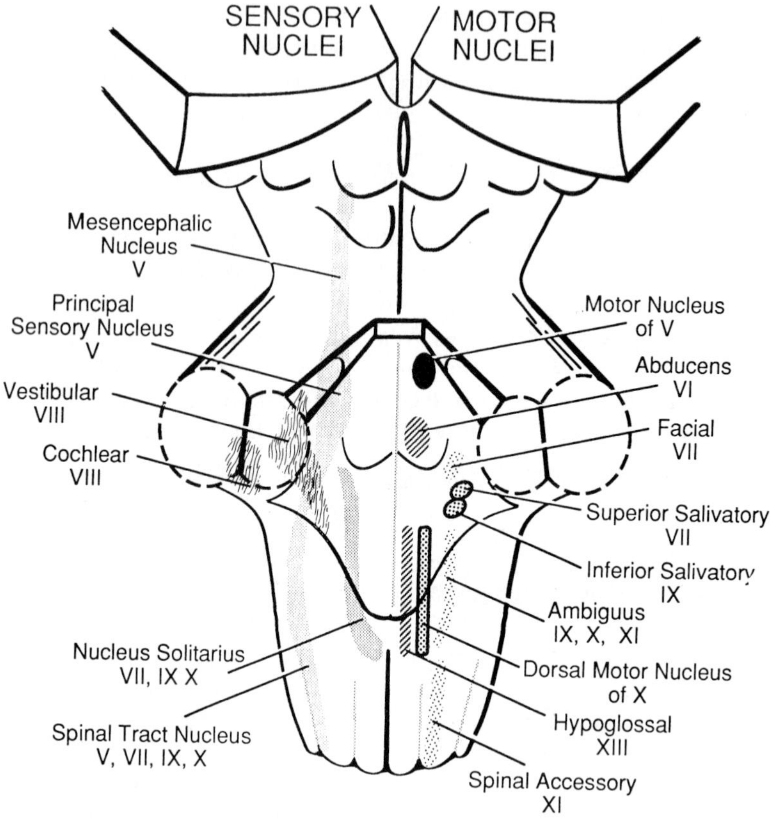

FIG. 10-5
Sensory and motor nuclei of the brainstem associated with cranial nerves III, V, VI, VII, VIII, IX, X, XI, XII. The nuclei occur bilaterally, but for ease of depiction, the sensory nuclei are shown at the left and the motor nuclei at the right.

tion of labels, so that direct comparisons can be made with neuron physiology and morphology. The nucleus contains different classes of neurons. Local circuit neurons have axons that are restricted to brain stem areas; projection neurons send axons to more rostral brain stem relay nuclei; and interneurons are involved with interconnections within the sensory nucleus. Within the subnucleus interpolaris, projection neurons have bigger receptive fields, cell bodies, dendritic trees, and axons than do local circuit neurons (Fig. 10-7). Based on differences in neuron morphology and projection patterns, subnucleus oralis consists of three major subdivisions: ventrolateral, dorsomedial, and the border zone. The ventrolateral division contains interneurons and two populations of projection neurons—one that projects to the spinal cord and another that sends axons to the medullary dorsal horn. Within the dorsomedial subdivision are a series of neurons projecting to the cerebellar cortex. Neuron groups in the border zone project to the cerebellum and medullary dorsal horn.

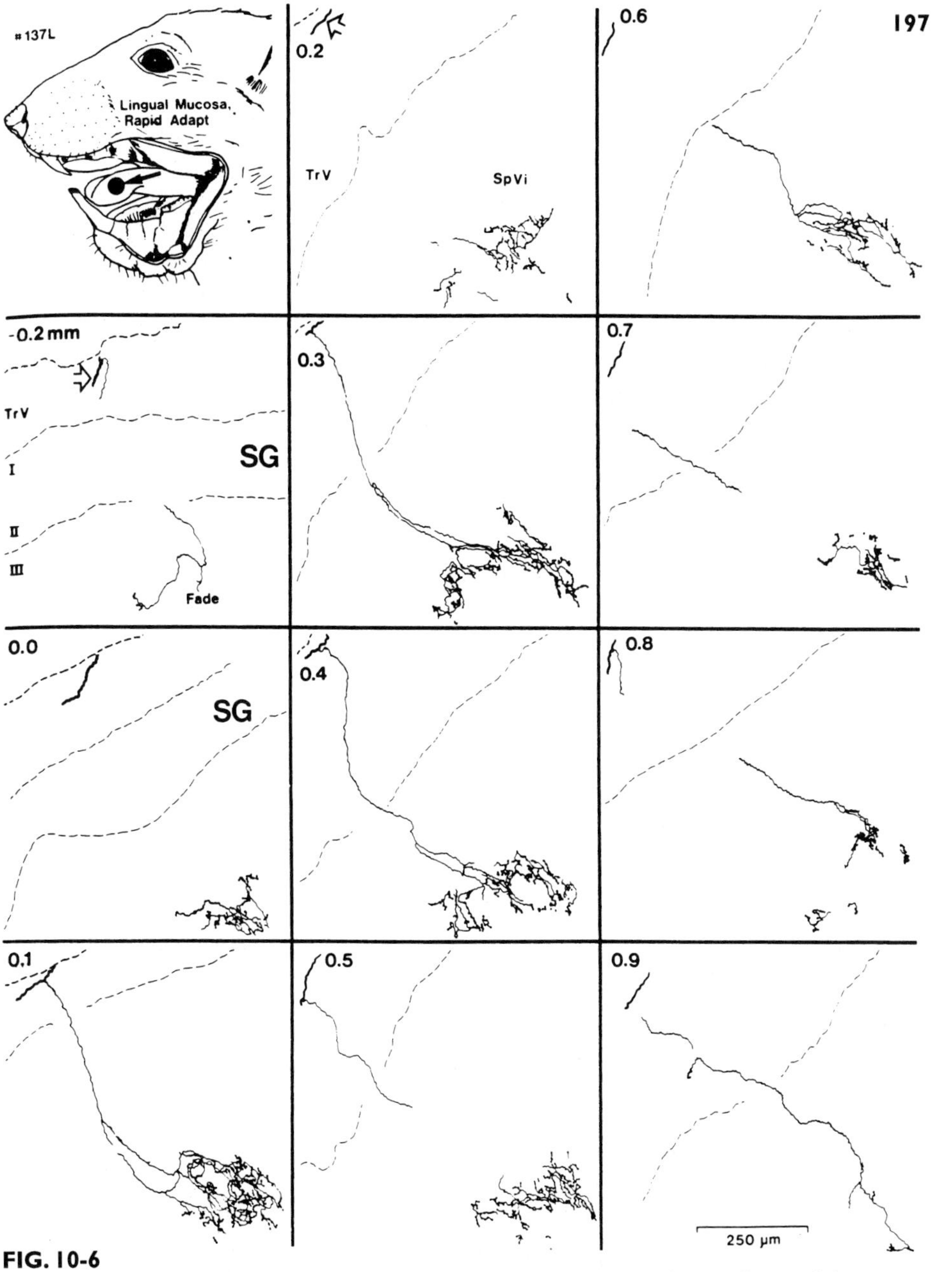

FIG. 10-6

Axon collateral termination of an afferent fiber that responded to tactile stimulation of the tongue. For an explanation of the technique used to obtain these data see Box 2-2. numbers refer to the rostrocaudal location of the collaterals referenced to the obex. Collaterals caudal to the obex have minus numbers, while those rostral to the obex are positive. This particular axon gave rise to 11 axon collaterals, 2 in trigeminal subnucleus caudalis and remainder in subnucleus interpolaris. *TrV*, spinal tract of trigeminal nerve; *SpVi*, subnucleus interpolaris of the trigeminal spinal nucleus; *SG*, substantia gelatinosa; I, II, III, laminae of subnucleus caudalis. (From Jacquin MF, Stennett RA, Renehan WE, Rhoades RW: *Journal of Comparative Neurology* 267:107-130, 1988. Reprinted by permission of Wiley-Liss, a division of John Wiley & Sons, Inc.)

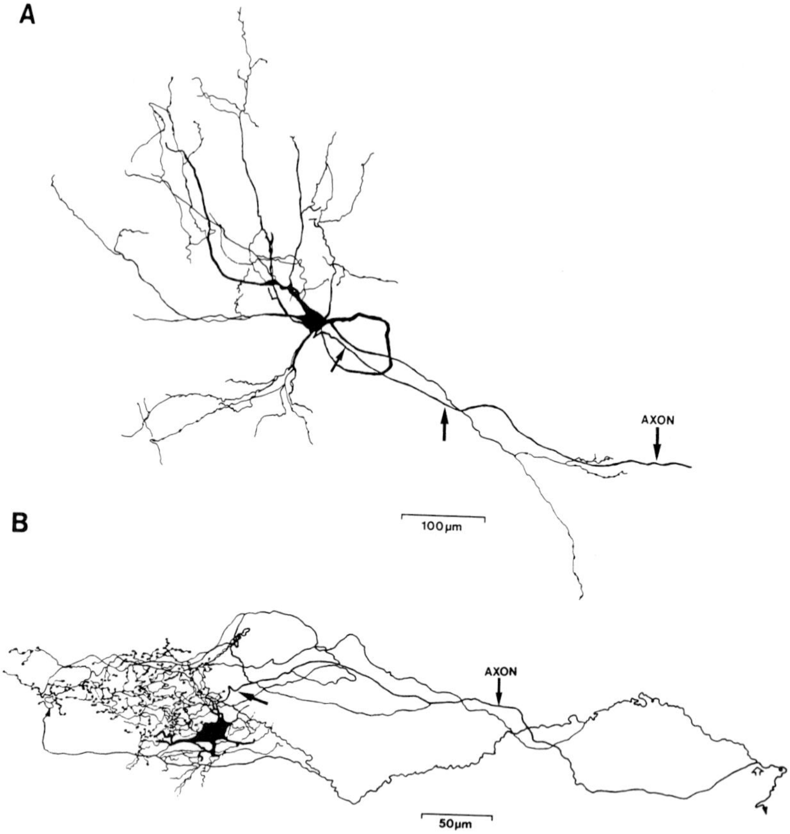

FIG. 10-7
Reconstruction of projection neuron (**A**) and a local circuit neuron (**B**) in the trigeminal subnucleus interpolaris of a rat. Both these neurons responded when a vibrissa was deflected. Note the different scale bars. (From Jacquin MF, Stennett RA, Renehan WE, Rhoades RW: *Journal of Comparative Neurology* 282:24-62, 1989. Reprinted by permission of Wiley-Liss, a division of John Wiley & Sons, Inc.)

The principal sensory nucleus is situated at the level of the trigeminal motor nucleus, and is bounded medially by the trigeminal motor root and laterally by the trigeminal sensory root. The principal sensory nucleus can be distinguished from the spinal nucleus by a lower density of neurons, and its lack of a population of large neurons with thick, long, straight, primary dendrites. A further difference between the principal and spinal nuclei is the presence of numerous rostrocaudally-directed myelinated axon bundles within the spinal nucleus. Light and electron microscopic examinations of neurons in the principal sensory nucleus has shown the presence of fusiform, triangular, and multipolar neurons. The branching pattern of the dendrites is relatively simple. Primary dendrites originate from either short extensions of the cell body or directly from the cell body. Secondary dendrites are long but do not seem to extend beyond the borders of the nucleus.

In the principal sensory nucleus, the subnucleus interpolaris, and medullary dorsal horn of rats and other rodents, clusters of afferent terminations called glomeruli or barrels can be demonstrated by use of histochemical staining techniques. The pattern of the glomeruli replicates the arrangement of mystacial vibrissae and sinus hairs on the face of the rat and dramatically demonstrates the topographical arrangement of the sensory nucleus (Fig. 10-8).

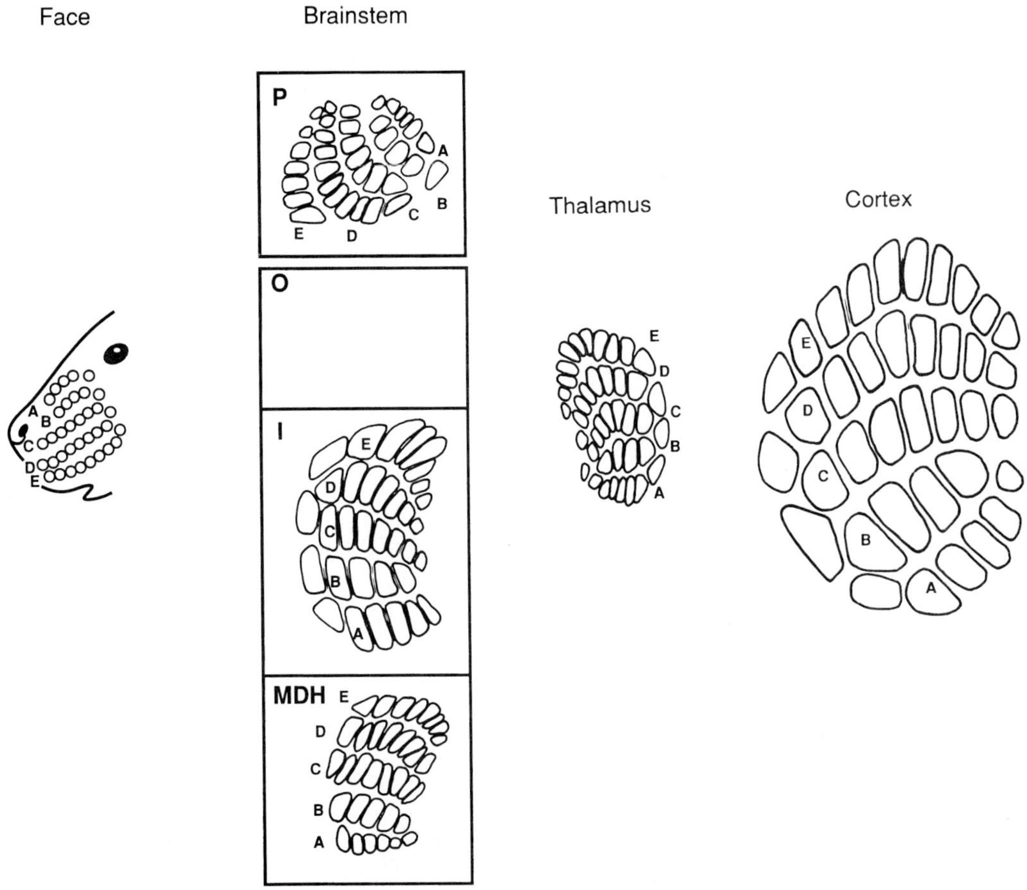

FIG. 10-8
Topographical projection of vibrissae system in rodent. Individual vibrissae are innervated by peripheral processes of trigeminal ganglion neurons. Each ganglion cell usually only innervates one whisker, although each whisker is innervated by many ganglion cells. Central procesess of these cells enter the brainstem and synapse in ipsilateral brainstem trigeminal nuclei in clusters of afferent termination called glomeruli. Pattern of glomeruli found in the principal sensory nucleus (*P*), subnucleus interpolaris (*I*) and medulllary dorsal horn (*MDH*) are direct representations of pattern of whiskers on face. Similar representations are found throughout ascending trigeminal system at level of thalamus and cortex. Individual rows of vibrissae are indicated by letters *A, B, C, D*, and *E*. O=subnucleus oralis (Adapted from Durham D, Woolsey TA: *Journal of Comparative Neurology* 223:424-447, 1984. Reprinted by permission of Wiley-Liss, a division of John Wiley & Sons, Inc.)

Trigeminal Mesencephalic Nucleus

The cell bodies of afferent fibers innervating muscle spindles of jaw-closing muscles and the cell bodies of periodontal ligament, gingival, and palatal mechanoreceptors are located within the mesencephalic nucleus, rather than in a peripheral sensory ganglion. This arrangement is unique within the central nervous system. Mesencephalic nucleus neurons are unipolar; the single axon bifurcates into peripheral and central branches. The central branch gives off numerous collateral branches which terminate in the motor nucleus, spinal cord, and other areas of the brain stem. The cell bodies of neurons innervating muscle spindles are found throughout the length of the nucleus and those from periodontal ligament receptors are restricted to the caudal half.

Trigeminal Motor Nucleus

Motoneurons controlling the muscles of mastication are contained in the trigeminal motor nucleus (see Fig. 10-5). Analysis of the distribution of motoneuron soma sizes indicates that the trigeminal motor nucleus contains both γ and α motoneurons. Numerous neural tracing studies have demonstrated that the alpha motoneurons innervating the muscles of mastication are anatomically separated within the nucleus (Fig. 10-9); the jaw-closing motoneurons are located in the dor-

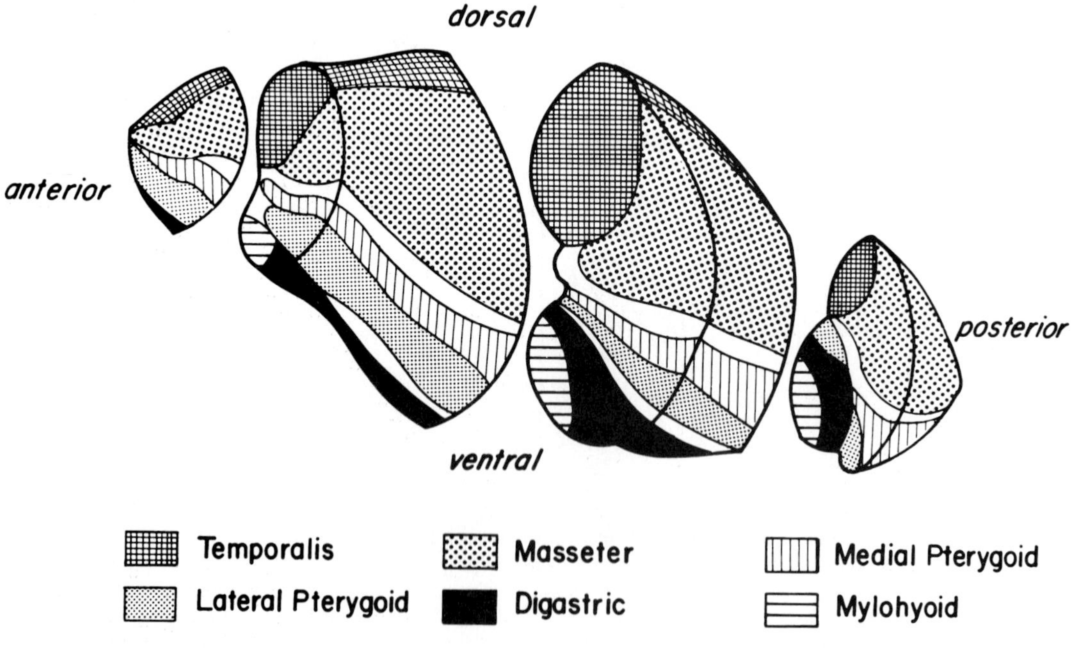

FIG. 10-9
Distribution of motoneurons in cat trigeminal motor nucleus. (From Batini C, and others: *Journal de Physiologie [Paris]* 72:301-309, 1976.)

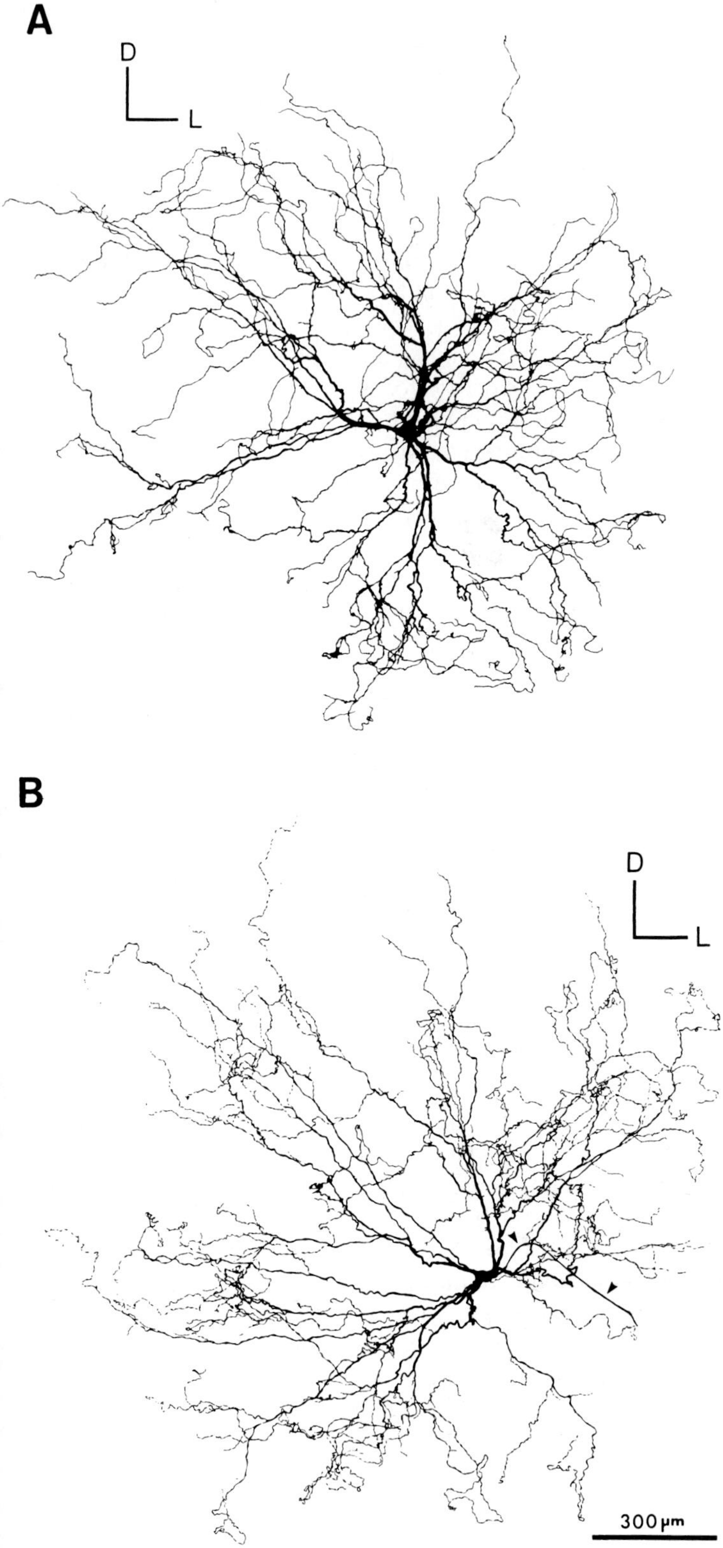

FIG. 10-10
Reconstruction of a masseter motoneuron (*A*) and a jaw-opening motoneuron (*B*) in the trigeminal motor nucleus of a cat. *D*, dorsal; *L*, lateral. (Adapted from Yoshida A and others: *Brain Research* 416:393-401, 1987.)

solateral, whereas the jaw-opening motoneurons are situated in the ventromedial division of the nucleus. Intracellular and extracellular recordings from masticatory moto-neurons have shown that synaptic inputs to jaw-opening and jaw-closing motoneurons are different. For example, activity orginating in the muscle spindles of jaw-closing muscles does not influence jaw-opening motoneurons, but neural activity originating in mechanoreceptors of oral and facial regions inhibits jaw-closing muscles and excites jaw-opening muscles. The technique of combining intracellular recordings with subsequent intracellular injection of dye or marker has been used to reveal the complex structure of trigeminal motoneurons. Masseter jaw-closing motoneurons can be grouped into different types, but jaw-opening motoneurons have similar morphologies (Fig. 10-10). As can be seen in Fig. 10-10, the dendritic tree of trigeminal motoneurons is extensive and complex. Dendrites from all the different motoneuron groups extend beyond the boundaries of the motor nucleus, but there is little overlap between the dendrites of motoneurons in the dorsolateral and ventromedial regions of the motor nucleus. This technique provides a detailed view of the microstructure of the trigeminal motor nucleus and is essential to an understanding of the reflex mechanisms underlying mastication.

Hypoglossal Motor Nucleus

The hypoglossal motor nucleus controlling the muscles of the tongue is more homogeneous than the trigeminal motor nucleus. It is composed of large, multipolar motoneurons and a population of small interneurons. The dendrites of the large motoneurons cross the midline to the contralateral hypoglossal nucleus or into the adjacent reticular formation. The small interneurons have only one or two dendrites that are totally contained within the nucleus.

Facial Motor Nucleus

The facial motor nucleus is made up of three longitudinal columns of motoneurons. The larger medial and lateral columns are separated by a smaller intermediate column. Neural tracing studies have shown that facial muscles (as well as one middle-ear muscle) are represented topographically within the nucleus. Muscles controlling the upper lip and nares have their motoneurons in the ventral and dorsal parts of the lateral cell column. Lower lip musculature is supplied by motoneurons in the intermediate cell column. Muscles associated with the ear are controlled by motoneurons in the medial cell column. Intracellular labeling has revealed major differences in the pattern of the dendritic trees between motoneurons in the three cell columns. The dendritic tree of facial motoneurons largely stays within the same subdivision that contains the soma, but sometimes extends beyond the border of the facial motor nucleus.

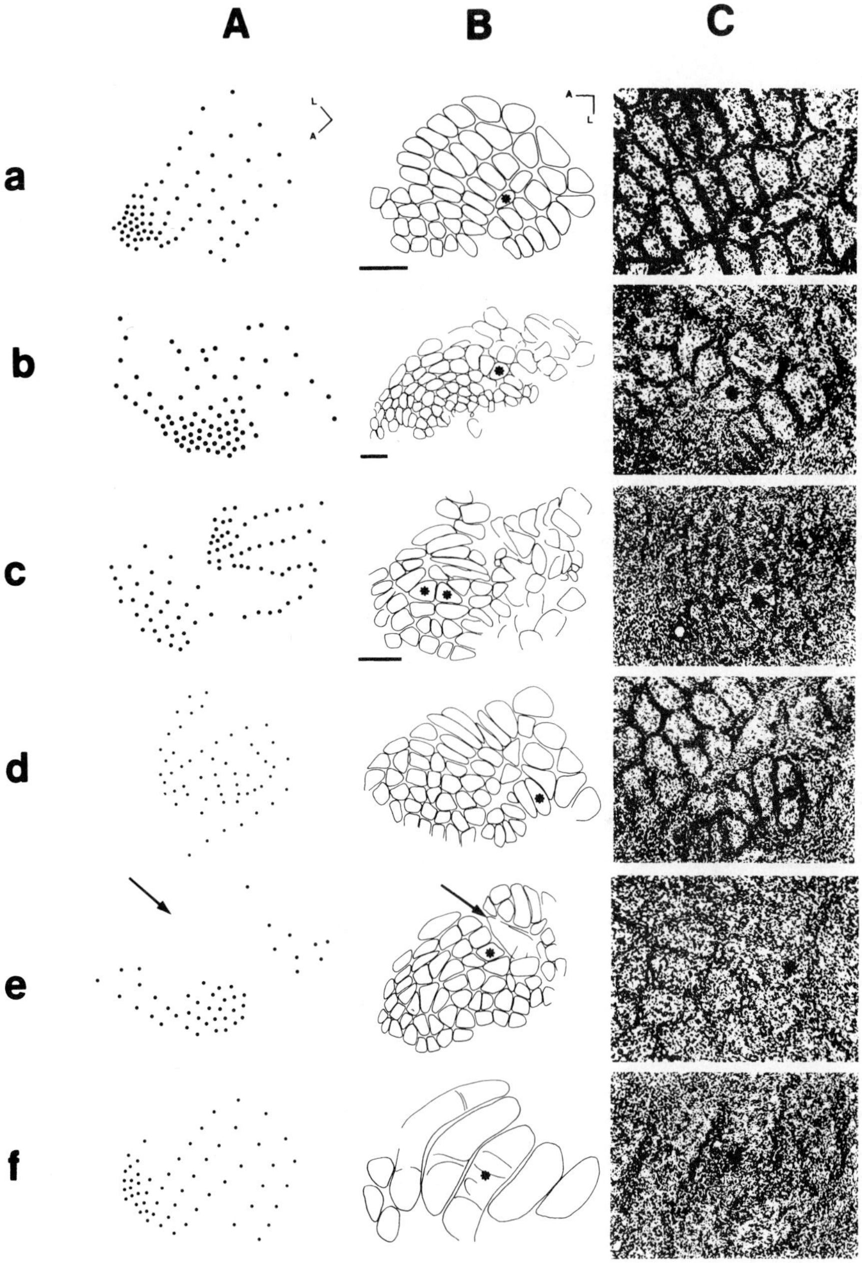

FIG. 10-11

Pattern of whiskers (*A*), cortical representation of the whisker pattern (*B*), and a histologic stain of the cortical "barrels" (*C*) in a mouse. Normal pattern is (*a*). In (*b-f*) various whiskers on the face have been experimentally manipulated during development, resulting in altered patterns of vibrissa representation in the cortex. Peripheral alterations in the whiskers have influenced development of normal pattern of "barrels" throughout the entire trigeminal ascending pathway as far as the cortex. In (*a*), *L*, lateral and *A*, anterior. Arrow in (e) indicates a wedge shaped region presumably representing the removed whisker pad. In column B, * indicates barrels in the photomicrographs in column C. Horizontal bar, 200μm. (From Andres KH, Van der Loos: *Anatomy and Embryology*, 172:11-20, 1985.)

Plasticity

If a row of mystacial vibrissae is removed in developing rats, major changes in the organization of the barrels in the trigeminal sensory nucleus occur. The discrete series of barrels is replaced by a single band (Fig. 10-11). Moreover, this change in pattern is reflected at each relay in the trigeminal pathway. Sectioning of the trigeminal nerve at birth results in a complete absence of any central pattern. There is a sensitive period during which damage to the vibrissae causes change in the barrel system. These results indicate that peripheral sensory input originating in the vibrissae is essential for the development of the characteristic topographical representation of the barrels. Because of the unique arrangement of the barrels, it is relatively easy to observe effects of altered afferent input on central nervous system development. However, this phenomenon may be more general, may apply to other aspects of the developing trigeminal system, and may be important in the development of neural circuits responsible for mastication and other orofacial functions.

CONTROL OF MASTICATION

Motor and sensory nuclei contained in the brain stem play a pivotal role in the control of mastication. In addition, a growing body of evidence suggests that the basic oscillatory pattern of masticatory movements originates in a neural pattern generator located in the brain stem. Afferent sensory input to these brain stem nuclei has a major influence on the form of a masticatory sequence. Finally higher brain centers influence the brain stem masticatory coordinating system. These three interconnected systems, the brain stem pattern generator, afferent input to the brain stem pattern generator, and higher brain centers' influence on the pattern generator, have been studied with regard to the control of mastication.

Brain Stem Activity During Mastication

Only the brain stem is essential to perform mastication. In animal experiments in which the brain stem was isolated from the higher brain centers, mastication and swallowing of food were possible. The basic rhythmical movements of mastication can also occur in the absence of any sensory input from the oral cavity, a fact indicating that the up and down movement of the mandible during mastication originates from within the brain stem. It is now believed that interconnected neural circuits form a neural oscillatory network that is capable of generating the pattern of masticatory movements. This neural oscillator is called a pattern generator or a masticatory center. The brain stem contains other pattern generators such as those responsible for respiratory movements and swallowing (see Chapter 11). The form of the rhythmical jaw movements produced by the pattern generator when central and peripheral inputs are eliminated is very regular and represents the basic pattern of masticatory movements. In normal mastication in which peripheral sensory input and input from higher brain centers is involved, the basic activity of the pattern generator is modified to produce the type of masticatory movements seen during chewing.

Although the presence of a pattern generator is well established, details of the neural circuits and precise anatomical location of the pattern generator have not been fully worked out. However, some of the neural circuitry involved in normal mastication has been revealed by the study of reflex muscle activity initiated by stimulation of orofacial structures.

A number of reflexes can be elicited from the orofacial area. These include tongue, facial, and various jaw reflexes. Since reflex activity of muscles in other body areas has proved useful in understanding neural connections, orofacial reflexes have been studied extensively and have revealed basic neural circuits that connect afferent sensory input with efferent motor output. These orofacial reflexes involve perhaps one motor nucleus and relatively few synapses, and are simple when compared to complex reflexes such as swallowing. It is sometimes assumed that the more complex reflexes are made up of a number of simple reflexes. However, the orofacial reflexes may not be the building blocks for more complex reflex activity, but they may serve protective functions and are only activated infrequently.

Perhaps the most studied orofacial reflex is the jaw-closing or jaw-jerk reflex, which can be elicited by tapping the point of the chin. The chin-tap stretches muscle spindles in the jaw-closing muscles and represents the sensory input that initiates the reflex. After a very short latency (about 6 msec) electromyograph (EMG) activity can be recorded in the masseter and temporalis muscles. EMG activity represents the motor output of the reflex arc to the jaw closing-muscles. Because of this short latency, this reflex can only involve one synapse (monosynaptic reflex) and therefore it is very similar to the knee-jerk reflex in which a tap on the patella of the knee joint initiates a short latency reflex kick of the lower leg. Study of synaptic activity with intracellular recordings from jaw-closing confirms that this is a monosynaptic reflex. Moreover, the neural circuit of the reflex is well understood and consists of the afferent fibers from the muscle spindles with their cell bodies in the mesencephalic nucleus. The neural circuit also involves axon collaterals from the central branch of the axon that synapses on motoneurons of the masseter and temporalis muscles (Fig. 10-12). This reflex, therefore, seems simple to understand and demonstrates the existence of monosynaptic connections between jaw elevator muscle spindle afferent fibers and alpha motoneurons that control the jaw elevator muscles. However, extensive study has shown this reflex to be much more complicated.

Although muscle spindles are a major source of input to the jaw-closing reflex, stimulation of periodontal ligament, temporomandibular joint, and other facial receptors by tapping the teeth, opening the jaw, or stroking the facial skin may result in a short latency jaw-closing reflex. The possibility that these other afferent inputs contribute to the jaw-jerk reflex is demonstrated by the fact that anesthesia applied to teeth or the lower jaw that would eliminate the periodontal ligament and facial

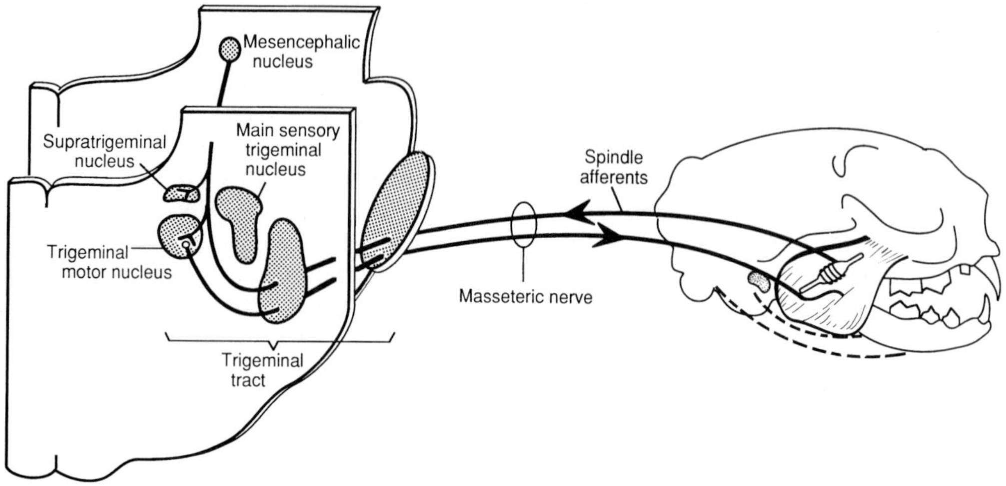

FIG. 10-12
Jaw-closing or jaw-jerk reflex. Tapping the chin stretches muscle spindles in a jaw-closing muscle. Excitation of muscle spindle afferent fibers with cell bodies in mesencephalic nucleus monosynaptically activates jaw-closing α motoneurons in the trigeminal motor nucleus, causing muscle to contract and close jaw.

input reduces but does not abolish the reflex. Jaw position can also have an influence on the reflex by inhibiting the response if the jaw is closed. The jaw-closing reflex can be increased by voluntary contraction of the jaw-closing muscles suggesting facilitatory activity.

The jaw-opening reflex is initiated by mechanical stimulation of the periodontal ligament and mucosal mechanoreceptors. The result is excitation of jaw-opening muscles and inhibition of jaw-closing muscles. This is not a monosynaptic reflex and at least one interneuron is involved in the reflex pathway (Fig. 10-13). Moreover, inhibitory interneurons may be at work in suppressing the activity of the jaw-closing muscles. A jaw-opening reflex can be initiated by stimulation of numerous other areas innervated by the trigeminal and other cranial nerves so that there may be a number of reflex pathways involved in this reflex.

Other simple reflexes involve the facial and hypoglossal motor nuclei. For example the eye-blink reflex is initiated by stimulation of corneal receptors innervated by the trigeminal nerve. Tongue reflexes result from stimulation of lingual (trigeminal) and laryngeal (vagus) receptors. The afferent fibers from these receptors terminate in the trigeminal and solitary nuclei respectively with interconnections to the hypoglossal nucleus.

Sensory stimulation of muscle spindles, teeth, tongue, eye, and other orofacial receptors results in a wide variety of reflex activities, illustrating the complexity of the neural connections. Intracellular recordings from motoneurons during stimulation of

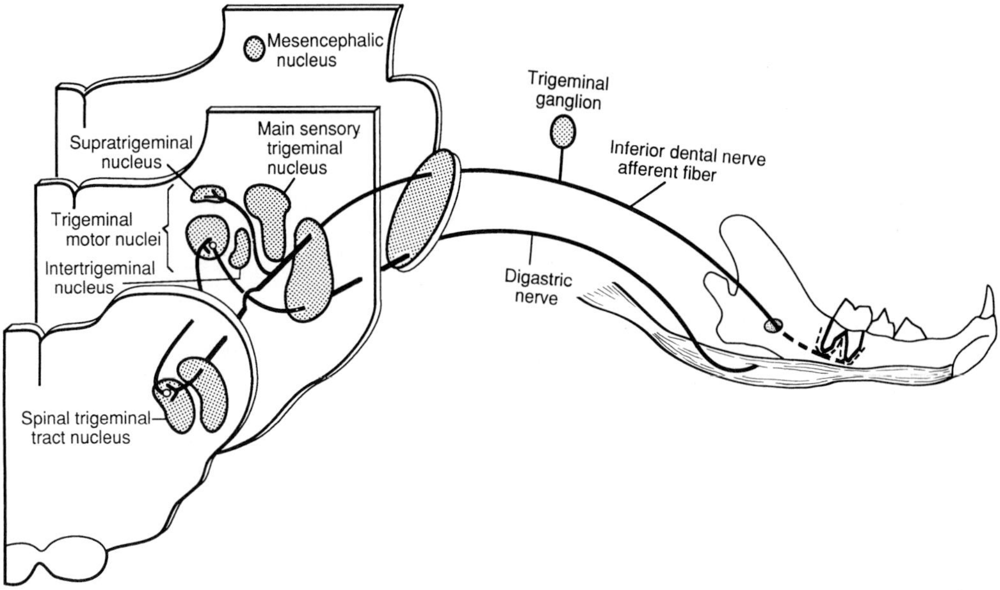

FIG. 10-13
Jaw-opening reflex. Stimulation of intraoral receptive fields excites mucosal receptors with afferent fibers terminating in the trigeminal spinal tract nucleus. Excitation of local circuit interneurons then activates jaw-opening α motoneurons in the trigeminal motor nucleus, causing muscle to contract and open jaw.

these same receptive fields reveal a complex series of changes in membrane potentials, illustrating the convergence and summation of inputs by the motoneuron. Moreover, the same sensory inputs can produce changes in other systems such as respiratory and cardiovascular activity. Study of these simple reflexes, while revealing basic details of brain stem neural interconnections, also discloses their complexity.

Mastication initiated by electrical stimulation of the cortex results in efferent discharge activity in the nerves that supply jaw-closing and jaw-opening muscles. The activity alternates rhythmically in bursts independent of the cortical stimulating frequency and occurs even when the animal is paralyzed. This rhythm is, therefore, independent of any muscle activity or resultant sensory feedback from muscle, joint, periodontal, or mucosal receptors. Based on these findings, it is generally accepted that masticatory rhythm is produced by a pattern generator in the brain stem which is activated by central as well as peripheral inputs and that the pattern generator produces rhythmical output at a set frequency independent of the input to the generator. On the basis of lesioning studies the pattern generator appears to be located in the reticular formation and in parts of the pons that contains the trigeminal nuclei. The major descending input to the pattern generator is the pyramidal tract, and electrical stimulation of the presumptive pattern generator results in rhythmical motoneuron firing.

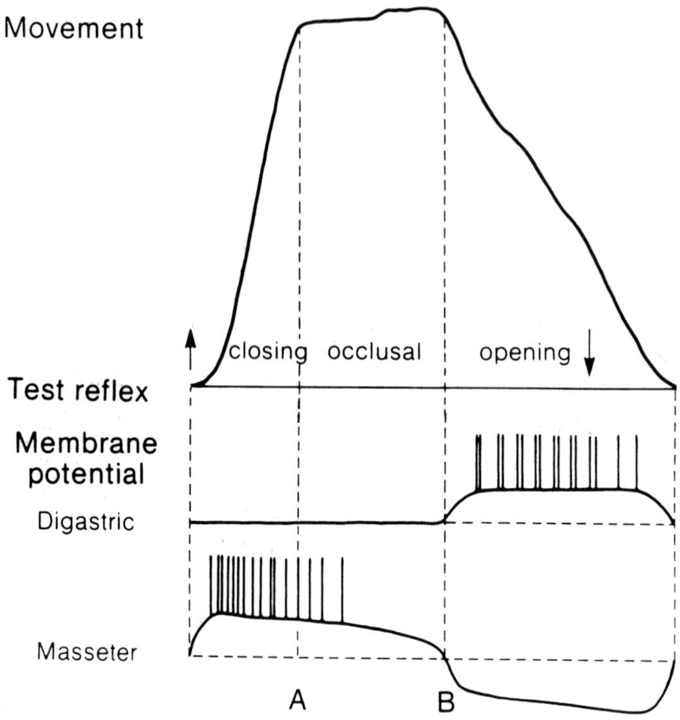

FIG. 10-14
Membrane potential changes of jaw-opening (digastric) and jaw-closing (masseter) motoneurons during a masticatory cycle. The dashed horizontal lines indicate the resting membrane potential. Upward deflection of the membrane potential indicates depolarization, while hyperpolarization causes a downward deflection. Not that action potentials occur during membrane depolarization. (From Lund JP, Olsson KÅ: *Trends in Neuroscience* 6:458-463, 1983.)

The activity of trigeminal motoneurons during chewing has been studied by using intracellular recordings from α motoneurons that control the masseter (jaw-closing) and digastric (jaw-opening) muscles. Changes in the resting membrane potential are related to different phases of the chewing cycle. The masseteric motoneurons are depolarized (excited) during the closing phase and hyperpolarized (inhibited) during opening. The digastric motoneurons are depolarized during opening but are not hyperpolarized during closing (Fig. 10-14).

Influence of Higher Centers

Electrical stimulation of the lateral part of the cortical motor area produces repetitive movements of the jaw and tongue. Although the connections between the cortex and the trigeminal motor nucleus are not direct, electrical stimulation of the sensorimotor cortex produces short latency changes in the excitability of masticatory motoneurons. Jaw-opening motoneurons are facilitated and jaw-closing motoneurons show reduced excitability. Ablation of the masticatory area of the cortex results in severe difficulty in eating. However, if the animals are carefully maintained they eventually regain the ability to feed. These experiments have lead to the hypothesis that the masticatory area of the cortex functions in the initiation of mastication. On the other hand, since animals in which this area has been removed eventually regain the ability to make voluntary masticatory movements, the cortex is not essential for the initiation of mastication.

Electrical stimulation close to the cortical masticatory area initiates tongue and other orofacial movements. Since tongue and jaw movements must be coordinated during chewing it has been suggested that besides initiation of mastication, the masticatory area of the cortex coordinates the activity of the various muscular systems involved in chewing and modulates their activity based on sensory feedback from orofacial receptors.

Influence of Afferent Input

The type, texture, and consistency of food in the mouth result in different chewing patterns. Presumably, the various chewing patterns result from the physi-

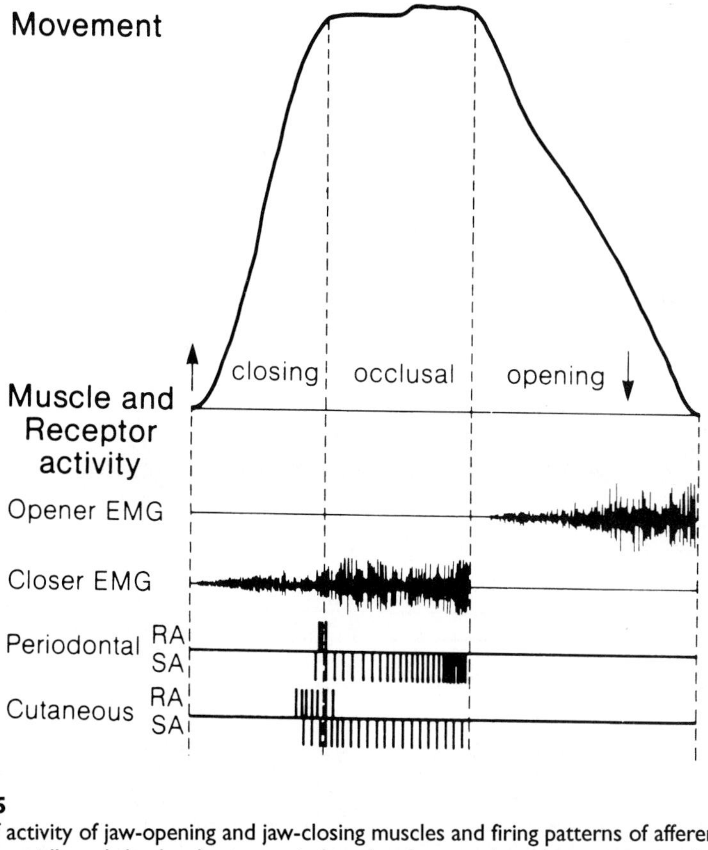

FIG. 10-15
Patterns of activity of jaw-opening and jaw-closing muscles and firing patterns of afferent fibers innervating rapidly and slowly adapting periodontal and mucosal mechanoreceptors during a masticatory cycle. (From Lund JP, Olsson KÅ: *Trends in Neuroscience* 6:458-463, 1983.)

cal properties of the foodstuff as well as sensory feedback to the brain stem masticatory integrating centers. In addition stimulation of different parts of the oral cavity and perioral areas in the absence of food in the mouth produces different chewing movements.

Neurophysiologic studies of activity in afferent nerve fibers has shown that once chewing begins, rhythmic firing of action potentials occurs with various phases of the chewing cycle. Because the cell bodies of jaw muscle spindles are situated within the central nervous system, it is possible to record the activity of jaw spindle afferent fibers during chewing in awake behaving animals. The frequency of action potentials in muscle spindle primary afferents is related to the degree of jaw opening and there is a brief burst of action potentials at the beginning and end of the opening phase of the chewing cycle (Fig. 10-15).

The activity of afferent fibers innervating periodontal mechanoreceptors has also been examined during chewing. The rapidly adapting mechanoreceptors fire a burst of action potentials as the teeth come into contact, and the slowly adapting mechanoreceptors become active as the teeth come in contact with or bite food material, but firing frequency increases as the biting pressure is increased (see Fig. 10-15).

Recordings made from human mechanoreceptors with receptive fields at the corners of the mouth showed two bursts of activity during a chewing cycle: one during jaw opening and one during closing (Fig. 10-16). Mechanoreceptor activity

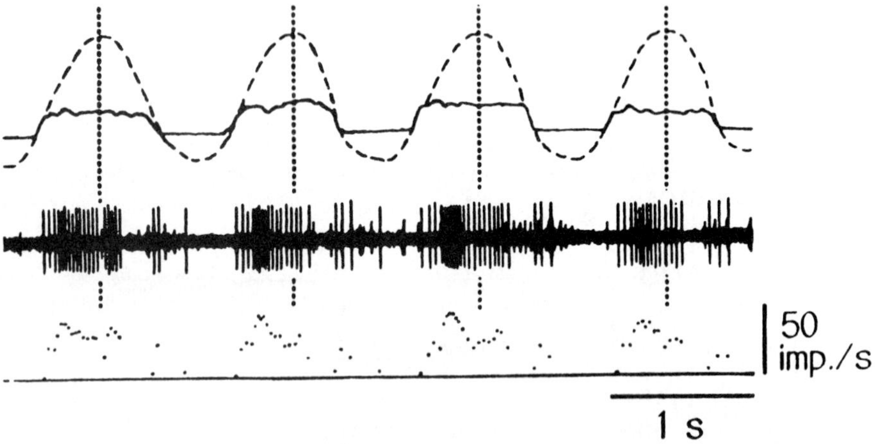

FIG. 10-16
Neural activity recorded from a human mechanoreceptor with a receptive field in the buccal mucosa 1 cm lateral to the corner of the mouth during chewing. Top trace is of chewing movement; middle trace is a neurophysiological recording from mechanoreceptive fiber in the infraorbital nerve; bottom trace is of instantaneous frequency of action potentials. (From Johansson and others: *Experimantal Brain Research* 72:209-214, 1988.)

was minimal at the reversal points of the chewing movements indicating that stretching of the perioral tissues was responsible for stimulating the receptors. The responses generated in these afferent fibers during chewing movements indicate that perioral mechanoreceptors provide proprioceptive information important in the feedback control of mastication.

SUMMARY

During chewing the jaw moves rhythmically. The pattern of movement and jaw muscle activity are typical for a particular species of animal. Despite these species differences descriptions of a single chewing cycle is usually divided into four phases. First the jaw moves downward slowly followed by a faster opening phase. Next the jaw moves upward in a fast closing phase. The final phase is a slow closing during which the food is crushed.

A masticatory sequence consists of a number of chewing cycles and extends from ingestion to swallowing. The sequence is divided into three consecutive periods. In the initial or preparatory period food is transported back to the posterior teeth where it is ground during a reduction period. The bolus is then formed during the final, preswallowing period.

There is a general pattern of muscle activity during a chewing cycle. Closing muscles are usually inactive during jaw opening, when the jaw-opening muscles are very active. Activity in jaw-closing muscles starts at the beginning of jaw closing. Activity of jaw-closing muscles increases slowly as the teeth begin to interdigitate. The closing muscles on the side where food is being crushed are more active than the contralateral jaw-closing muscles.

The coordination of activity of muscles used in mastication originates in complex interactions between several motor nuclei and sensory input from the oral cavity terminating primarily in the trigeminal sensory and mesencephalic nuclei, but also with the possible involvement of the solitary tract nucleus. Other brain stem structures, such as the reticular formation, also participate.

The cyclical movements of the jaw during mastication are generated and controlled at the level of the brain stem. The rhythmical activity is produced by a central pattern generator that influences the activity of several motor nuclei that control a large number of muscles that are active during chewing. Cortical output neurons connect both to the pattern generator and to the motor nuclei. Sensory input from perioral, intraoral, and muscle receptors terminating in the trigeminal nucleus also connects to the pattern generator and motor nuclei. Sensory input, reflecting intraoral conditions and muscle activity, can significantly modify chewing movements. Therefore, the final pattern of mastication is the result of interactions at the brain stem level of higher center influence and peripheral sensory feedback.

SELECTED READINGS

Bates JF, Stafford GD and Harrison A: Masticatory function: a review of the literature, *1*, The form of the masticatory cycle, *Journal of Oral Rehabilitation* 2:281-301, 1975.

Bates JF, Stafford GD, Harrison A: Masticatory function: a review of the literature, II, speed of movement of the mandible, rate of chewing and forces developed in chewing, *Journal of Oral Rehabilitation* 2:349-361, 1975.

Bates JF, Stafford GD, Harrison A: Masticatory function: a review of the literature, III, masticatory performance and efficiency, *Journal of Oral Rehabilitation* 3:57-67, 1976.

Herring SW: The ontogeny of mammalian mastication, *American Zoologist* 25:339-349, 1985.

Hiiemae KF: Mammalian mastication: a review of the activity of the jaw muscles and the movements they produce in chewing. In Butler PM and Joysey KA, editors: *Development, function and evolution of teeth*. London, 1978, Academic.

Hiiemae KJ, Crompton AW: Mastication, food transport, and swallowing. In Hildebrand M and others: *Functional vertebrate morphology*, Cambridge, Mass., 1985, Belknap Press, pp. 262-290.

Kawamura Y, ed.: *Frontiers of oral physiology*, vol 1, *Physiology of mastication*, Basel, 1974, Karger.

Lund JP and Enomoto S: The generation of mastication by the mammalian central nervous system. In Cohen AH, Rossignol S, Grillner S, editors: *Neural control of rhythmic movements in vertebrates*. New York, 1988, Wiley, pp. 41-72.

Lund JP: Mastication and its control by the brain stem, *Critical Reviews in Oral Biology and Medicine* 2:33-64, 1991.

Luschei ES, Goldberg LJ: Neural mechanisms of mandibular control: mastication and voluntary biting. In Brookhart JM, Mountcastle VB, editors: *Handbook of physiology*, section 1: *the nervous system*, vol II, part 2, *motor control*. Bethesda, 1981, American Physiological Society.

Taylor A: *Neurophysiology of the jaws and teeth*. Basingstoke, 1990, Macmillan.

11

Swallowing

LEARNING OBJECTIVES

At the end of this chapter you should be able to:

1. Describe the general characteristics of swallowing activity.
2. State the three phases of a swallow.
3. State the timing of a swallow.
4. Describe the sequence of events taking place during a swallow.
5. Describe the mechanisms that prevent aspiration of food during swallowing.
6. Describe the pressure changes recorded during a swallowing movement.
7. Describe the sequence of muscle contraction during a single swallow.
8. State the brain stem structures involved in the control of swallowing activity.
9. Describe the influence of afferent sensory input on swallowing activity.
10. Describe the mechanisms involved in the initiation of swallowing activity.
11. Describe the characteristics of suckling.
12. Describe the mechanisms of upper airway protective reflexes.
13. Describe the movements involved in vomiting.
14. Describe the brain stem control center responsible for initiating and programming vomiting movements.

Swallowing consists of a reflex sequence of muscle contractions that propels ingested materials and pooled saliva from the mouth to the stomach. The process occurs smoothly and effortlessly requiring the coordination of a large number of motoneurons typical of a complex reflex mechanism. Although swallowing can be initiated voluntarily, most swallows occur without any conscious effort. Over a 24-hour period, swallowing occurs as many as 1000 times. Swallowing frequency is highest during eating, least during sleep and occurs at a rate of about once per minute at other times. While sleeping swallowing occurs most often when falling asleep and awakening as well as during changes in sleep state between which there are long periods when swallowing is absent. Spontaneous swallowing is probably initiated to clear the mouth of saliva.

Swallowing not only serves to move nutrients from the mouth to the stomach, but also has important protective functions. In mammals the airway crosses the foodway at the level of the pharynx and larynx. It is imperative that solids and liquids do not enter the larynx. Interactions between the control systems of swallowing and breathing inhibit respiration during swallowing. Moreover, a vigorous set of reflexes such as coughing or choking are initiated if food or fluid invades the entrance to the trachea. As a consequence of one of these protective reflexes, swallowing is initiated to clear the airway of foreign material.

The essence then of the mechanism of swallowing is a timed series of events. Muscle contractions and relaxations must take place in a precisely ordered sequence if the smooth passage of a bolus from the mouth to the stomach is to take place. To accomplish this requires the integrated activity of a large area of the brain stem, six cranial nerves, and numerous receptors and muscles. Higher centers of the nervous system are also involved. The sequence is preprogrammed by neural circuitry in the brain stem called the "swallowing center," and once this center is triggered into action, the act of swallowing becomes entirely automatic.

SWALLOWING MOVEMENTS

Movements

Although swallowing is a continuous act, investigators have divided swallowing into preparatory, oral, pharyngeal, and esophageal phases. The preparatory phase merges into the terminal phase of mastication, involving formation of a food bolus. During the oral phase, the bolus is propelled from the oral cavity into the pharynx. In the pharyngeal phase the bolus is transported from the oropharynx into the esophagus and in the esophageal phase the bolus moves down the length of the esophagus to the stomach.

The oral and pharyngeal phases of swallowing take place very rapidly and last about 1 to 1.5 seconds. The oral phase lasts approximately 0.5 seconds and the pharyngeal phase 0.7 seconds. The esophageal phase is somewhat longer, liquids taking 3 seconds to pass from the pharynx to the gastroesophageal junction whereas solids usually take 9 seconds.

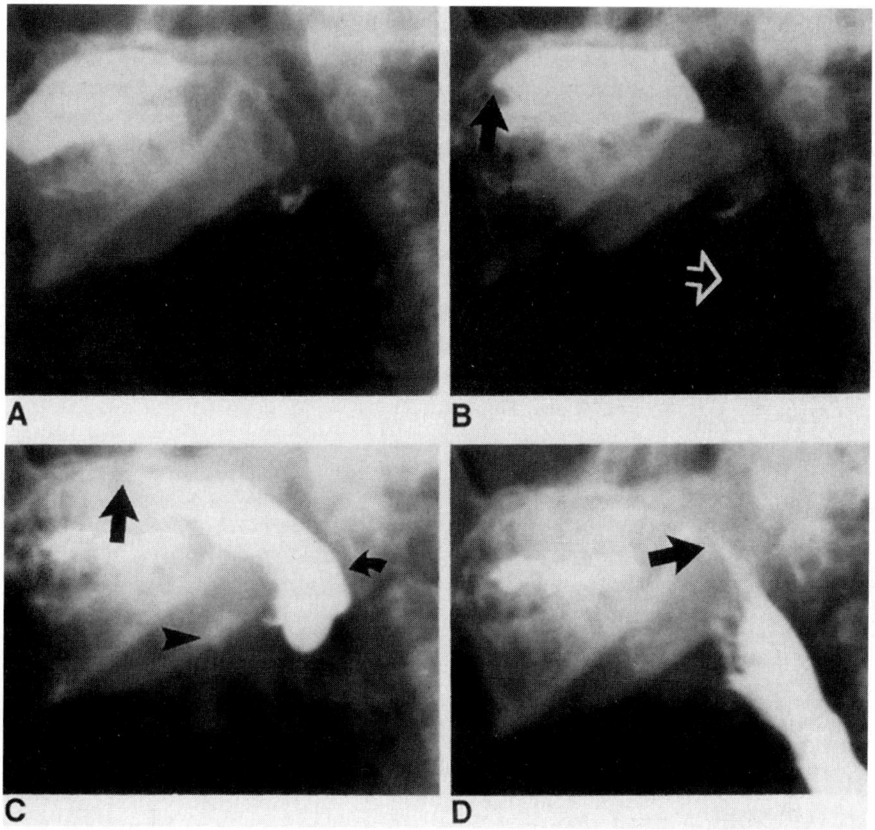

FIG. 11-1
Four frames taken at 30 msec intervals during lateral videofluorography of a swallowing sequence of a 10 ml barium bolus. **A**, Bolus is positioned on the tongue dorsum with tongue tip against the maxillary incisors. Posterior oral cavity is sealed off from oropharynx by approximation of posterior tongue and soft palate. **B**, With initiation of swallowing, tongue dorsum makes sequential contact (*solid arrow*) with a hard palate in a peristaltic sequence that begins to propel bolus into oropharynx. Air is present in laryngeal vestibule (*open arrow*). **C**, Small amount of air still present in laryngeal vestibule. As glossopalatal sphincter opens, tongue base moves froward and palate moves upward and backward to make contact with posterior pharyngeal wall (*curved arrow*) sealing off the nasopharynx. Hyoid (*arrowhead*) is well into its orad excursion and now overlaps posterior mandible. Leading edge of bolus fills valleculae. Tail of bolus (*straight arrow*). **D**, Bolus has left oral cavity and peristaltic stripping wave is seen at bolus tail (*arrow*) in oropharynx. Hyoid has moved further orad, and closed vestibule is empty of air. Upper esophageal sphincter is fully open and barium bolus flows into esophagus. (From Dodds WJ, Stewart ET, and Logemann JA: *American Journal of Radiology* 154:953-963, 1990.)

Before swallowing begins, a bolus is prepared and positioned on the dorsum of the tongue with the tongue tip pressed against the palatal aspect of the maxillary incisors or against the anterior hard palate. The bolus is located in a spoon-like depression of the tongue which is raised laterally against the buccal teeth and palatal mucosa. Posteriorly the pharyngeal part of the tongue arches up to meet the soft palate which pushes downward to keep the bolus from escaping into the pharynx (Figs. 11-1, *A*, and 11-2, *A*). This seal is referred to as the glossopalatal sphincter.

Once the bolus is positioned on the tongue dorsum, the oral phase of swallowing begins. The lips close and the maxillary and mandibular incisors come closer together. The anterior two thirds of the tongue elevates against the maxillary alveolar ridge and the anterior hard palate in sequential peristaltic contacts, propelling the bolus toward the pharynx. Several events now occur simultaneously. The base of the tongue moves downward and forward to expand the hypopharynx and provide a chute down which the bolus flows into the pharynx; the palate moves upward to open the glossopalatal sphincter to facilitate passage of the bolus; the palate contacts the posterior pharyngeal wall and the side walls of the nasopharynx are also opposed to seal off the nasopharynx and prevent penetration of the bolus into the nasal cavity (Fig. 11-1, *B* and *C*, and Fig. 11-2, *B*).

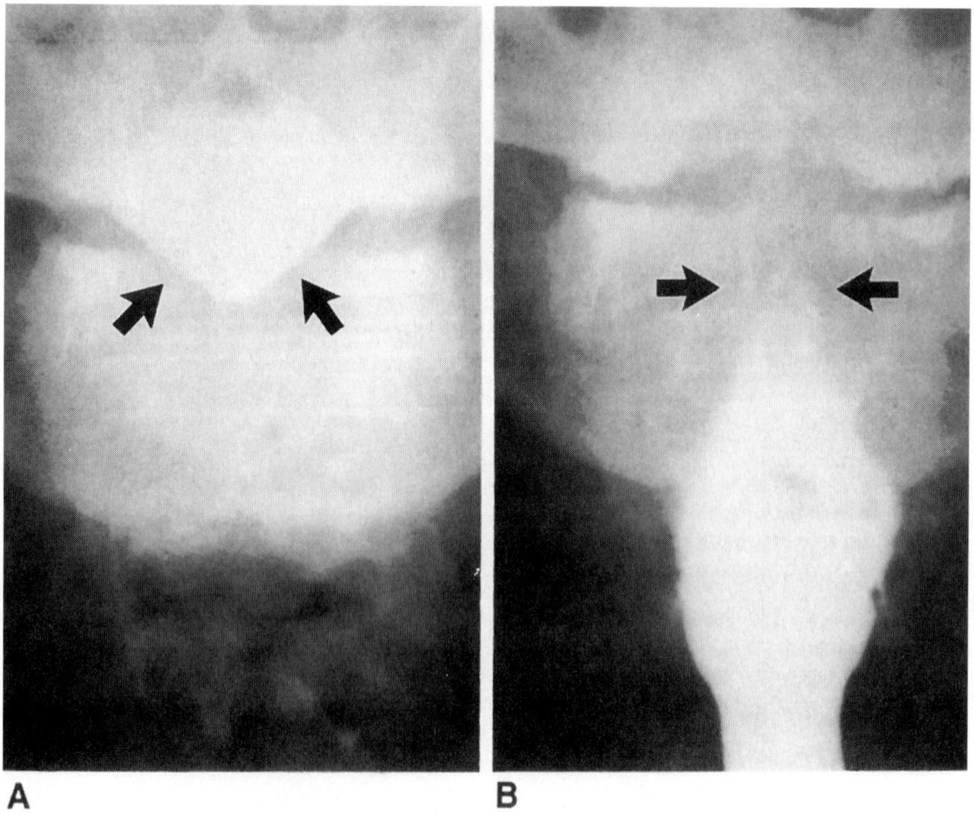

FIG. 11-2
Posterior videofluorography of a swallowing sequence of a 10 ml barium bolus. **A**, Just before swallowing begins, barium bolus is collected in a deep midline groove (*arrow*) on tongue dorsum. **B**, During early pharyngeal phase, barium has entered oropharynx. Superior constrictors approximate each other to seal off the nasal cavity. (From Dodds WJ, Stewart ET, and Logemann JA: *American Journal of Radiology* 154:953-963, 1990.)

Individual variations occur in the oral phase of swallowing. The upper and lower teeth usually come in contact during swallowing when the bolus passes into the pharynx. This tooth contact is thought to stabilize the mandible while the hyoid bone and larynx make superior and anterior movements. However, a significant number of individuals do not make tooth contact during swallowing. Moreover, in many of these persons the lips are also apart during swallowing and the tongue protrudes between the teeth to develop a peripheral seal to contain the bolus. These "tooth-apart swallowers" have been studied by orthodontists who hypothesize that the forward movement of the tongue contributes to the development of abnormal occlusions.

At the beginning of the pharyngeal phase, the posterior part of the tongue makes a rapid piston-like movement to propel the bolus through the oropharynx into the hypopharynx (see Fig. 11-1, *C*). The pharyngeal constrictors move upward and forward and begin propelling the bolus through the pharynx by sequential contractions. The leading edge of the bolus moves faster than its tail, so that the bolus elongates as it passes through the pharynx. The upper esophageal sphincter opens and the bolus enters the esophagus (Fig. 11-1, *D*). The diameter of the sphincter opening depends on the volume and viscosity of the bolus.

During the pharyngeal phase the laryngeal vestibule closes because of movement of the epiglottis. The epiglottis first moves from an upright to a horizontal position,

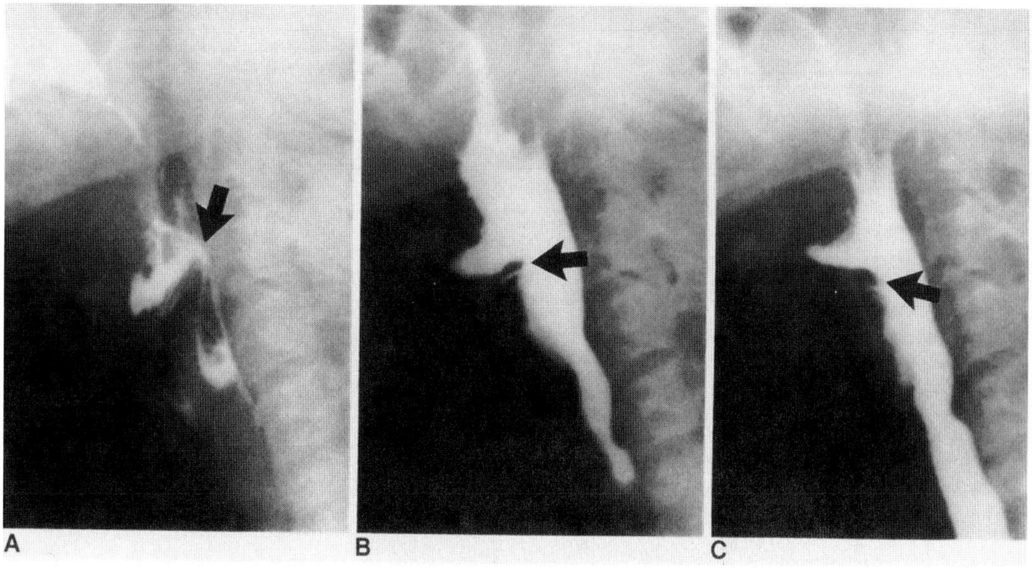

FIG. 11-3
Three frames taken at 30 msec intervals during lateral fluorography of a swallowing sequence of a 10 ml barium bolus to show movement of the epiglottis. **A,** Leading edge of bolus is just leaving mouth. Epiglottis (*arrow*) is horizontal. **B,** Leading edge of bolus has just entered region of upper esophageal sphincter. Epiglottis (*arrow*) is now horizontal. **C,** Upper esophageal sphincter is now fully open. Bolus flows into upper esophagus. Tip of epiglottis (*arrow*) has rotated caudally. (From Dodds WJ, Stewart ET, and Logemann JA: *American Journal of Radiology* 154:953-963, 1990.)

caused by elevation of the hyoid bone and larynx as well as by contraction of the thyrohyoid muscles. Further muscle contraction causes the tip of the epiglottis to rotate caudally over the laryngeal vestibule (Fig. 11-3). The epiglottis does not have to cover the laryngeal opening to prevent aspiration of food. Aspiration of food generally does not occur in individuals with an excised epiglottis. However, the epiglottis does direct the bolus into the piriform sinuses and, therefore, around the opening of the airway into the esophagus. It acts somewhat like a stick placed upright in a stream.

Several mechanisms operate to prevent aspiration of the bolus into the airway during the pharyngeal phase of swallowing. During this phase respiration is inhibited. Elevation of the larynx and upper esophageal sphincter shortens the distance the bolus must travel and, thereby, the time the bolus is present at the entry to the airway. Intrinsic muscles of the glottis forcefully approximate the true vocal cords. The piriform sinuses create lateral food channels so that the bolus generally deviates

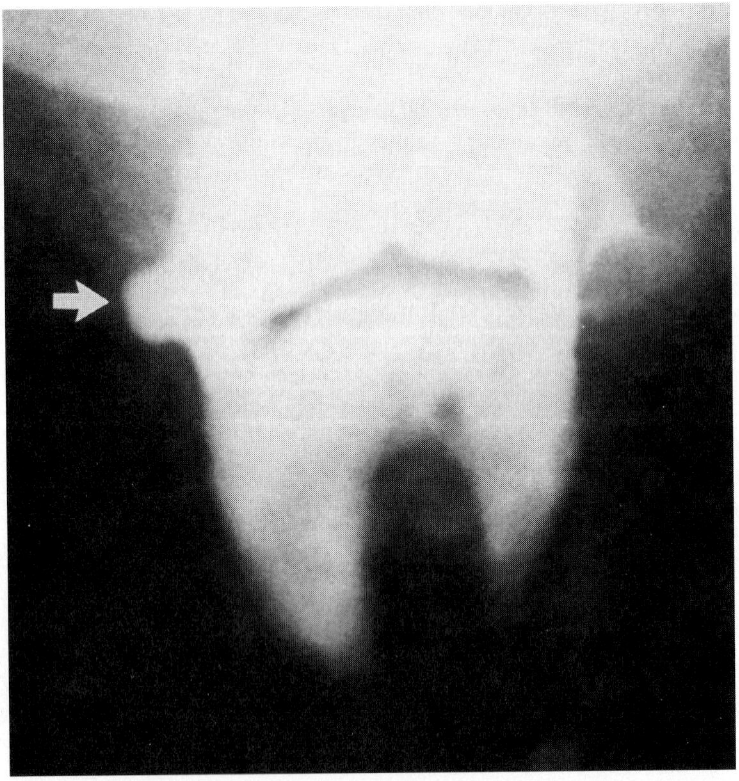

FIG. 11-4
Posteroanterior videofluorography of a swallowing sequence of a 10 ml barium bolus. Bolus is seen to split at horizontal free margin of epiglottis (horizontal filling defect in barium column) and flow mainly down lateral side channels of pahrynx. Smooth pharyngeal pouch on right side filled with bolus material is indicated by the arrow. (From Dodds WJ, Stewart ET, and Logemann JA: *American Journal of Radiology* 154:953-963, 1990.)

around the laryngeal opening (Fig. 11-4). Any residual bolus material trapped in the piriform sinus after the swallow is normally at a lower level than the laryngeal vestibule, making aspiration of residual material unlikely.

The last phase of swallowing, the esophageal phase, consists of peristaltic contractions; it begins as the bolus passes the upper esophageal sphincter. The contractions begin at the cervical level of the esophagus and take about 8 seconds to reach the lower esophageal sphincter which opens to admit the entry of the bolus into the stomach.

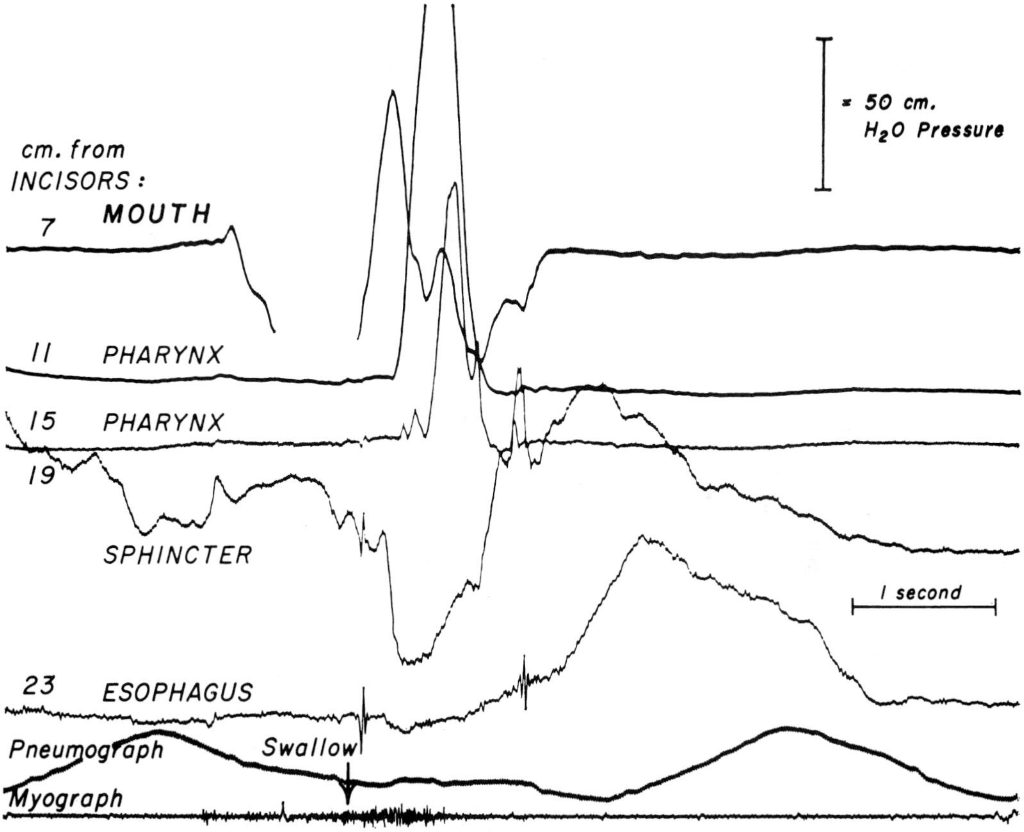

FIG. 11-5
Pressures in human pharynx and upper esophagus during a swallow. Pressure is measured at five distances from the incisors as indicated on left. Beginning of a swallow is indicated by the EMG recording (myograph) of jaw muscle activity. Respiration indicated by pneumograph recording is interrupted during swallow. Pressure in pharynx rises to a high level, and this increased pressure travels quickly down the pharynx. Pressure measurements in upper esophageal sphincter (19 cm trace) indicates that sphincter relaxes when pharyngeal pressure is high. As soon as pressure in the pharynx has fallen to baseline level, pressure in sphincter rises and remains high for more than 1 sec. While sphincter is tightly closed, peristaltic wave (23 cm trace) begins to move slowly down esophagus. (From Code CF, Schegel JF: Motor actions of the esophagus and its sphincters. In Code CF, editor: *Handbook of Physiology*, Section 6, *Alimentary Canal*, Vol. IV, *Motility*. Washington DC, 1968, American Physiological Society, pp. 1821, 1902.)

Pressure Changes

Food is moved through the mouth, pharynx, and esophagus by a positive-pressure wave. Pressure is developed by the piston-like action of the tongue and peristaltic muscle contractions. The sphincters between the oral and nasal cavities and at the upper and lower ends of the esophagus are important in directing the pressure wave in the right direction to guide the orderly passage of the bolus.

At the start of a swallowing sequence, the pressure in the mouth and pharynx is close to atmospheric, the upper esophageal sphincter is closed with a resting pressure between 16 and 60 cm H_2O, and the esophagus is at a subatmospheric pressure because of the negative pressure of the pleural cavity. The lower esophageal sphincter is also closed with a pressure of 10 cm H_2O.

The pressure changes produced by swallowing begin in the oral cavity. Once the mouth and nasopharyngeal sphincter are closed, pressure is built up by the piston-like activity of the tongue. Muscle contractions and relaxations produce an

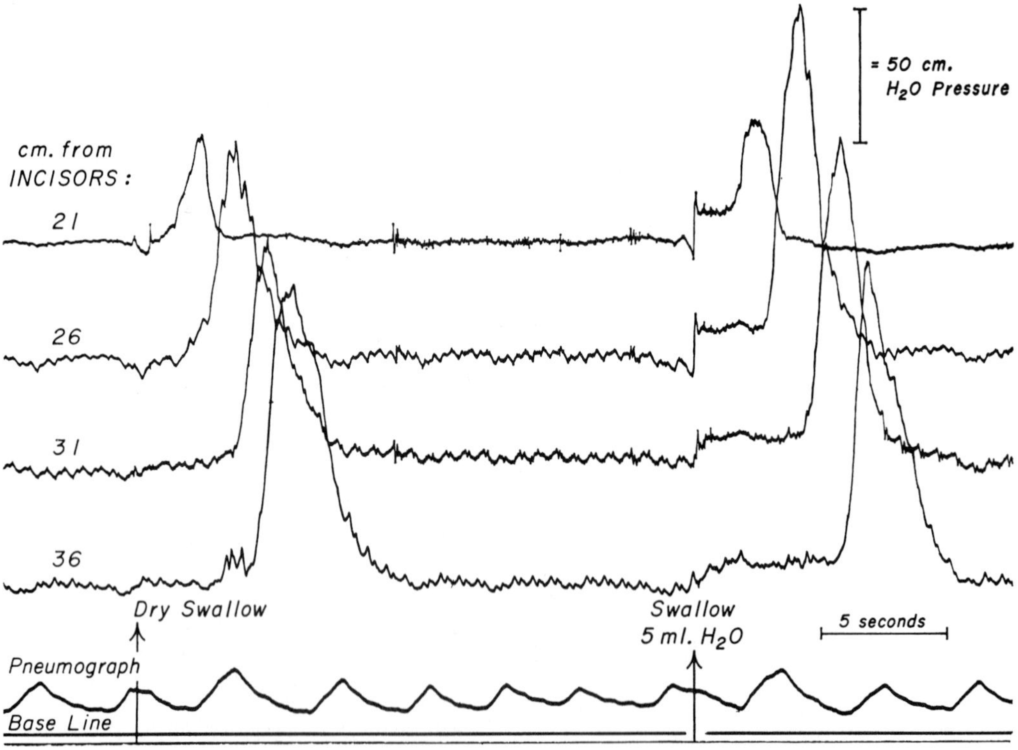

FIG. 11-6
Pressures in human esophagus during a dry (*left*) and wet (*right*) swallow. Pressure is measured at four distances from incisors as indicated on left. (From Code CF, Schegel JF: The physiological basis of some motor disorders of the esophagus. In *Surgical Physiology of the Gastrointestinal Tract*.. Rochester, Minn., 1963, Mayo Foundation, pp. 1-19.)

increase in pressure that starts at the tongue dorsum and travels through the oral cavity and pharynx toward the upper esophageal sphincter.

Relaxation of the upper esophageal sphincter occurs with, or just after, the contraction of the tongue and upper pharynx. The sphincter opens before the arrival of the pharyngeal sequential contraction wave. The bolus passes through the sphincter, which remains relaxed for about 1 second. The sphincter then closes and pressure rises abruptly to 70 to 100 cm H_2O for 2 to 4 seconds. As the contraction subsides, the sphincter pressure returns to resting level (Fig. 11-5).

Pressure changes in the esophagus during swallowing consist of pressure caused by the peristaltic wave and the added pressure of food forcefully expelled by the pharynx into the esophagus. Therefore, the pressure developed in the esophagus is less during a dry swallow and is produced by the peristaltic wave alone. When a bolus is swallowed the force of entry of the bolus is added to the pressure from peristalsis to give a larger resultant pressure wave (Fig. 11-6).

The lower esophageal sphincter relaxes for 3 seconds or more before the esophageal peristaltic wave reaches it, then contracts with a pressure of 20 to 35 cm H_2O once the bolus has passed into the stomach. With repetitive swallows, the sphincter relaxes with the first and remains relaxed until the last swallow has been completed.

Muscle Activity

A total of 31 paired muscles are involved in the preparatory, oral, and pharyngeal phases of swallowing. Electromyography (see Box 10-2) has been used to study the sequence of contractions of many of these muscles as well as muscle activity in the

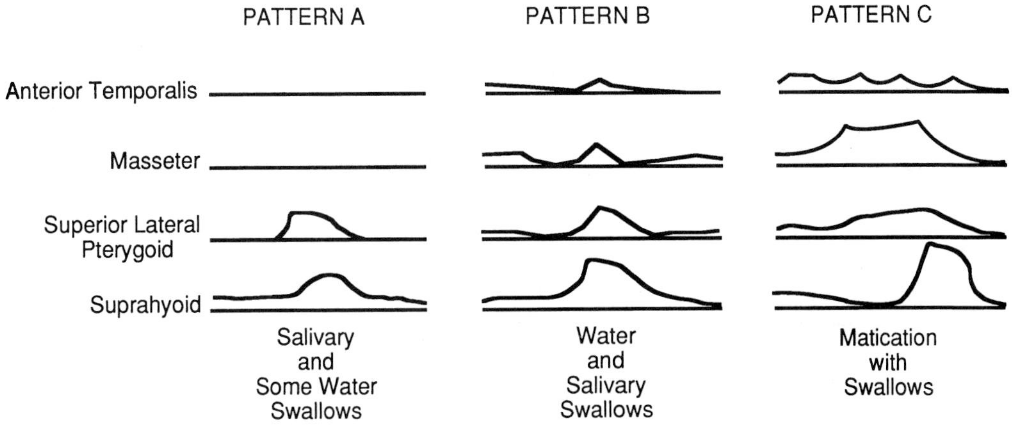

FIG. 11-7
During oral phase of swallowing intensity of activity in mandibular muscles varies depending on type of bolus and whether mastication is required to prepare ingested material for swallowing. (From Miller AJ: *Dysphagia* 1:91-100, 1986.)

esophagus during the esophageal phase. During the pharyngeal phase of swallowing, a set of muscles called the obligate muscles always participates. A contrasting muscle set, the facultative, has inconsistent muscle participation during the preparatory and oral phases of swallowing.

Muscle activity in the preparatory and oral phases is highly variable and involves various muscles controlling the face and mandible. Depending on the type of material being swallowed different muscle patterns occur. The medial pterygoid, masseter, and temporalis muscles that control the mandible are often active. Tension in the mandibular muscles serves to stabilize the base of the tongue during development of its piston-like movements. Facial muscles controlling the lips (labial muscles) and the cheeks (buccinator muscles) are also active during swallowing and contribute to development of an oral seal and stabilization of the mandible (Fig. 11-

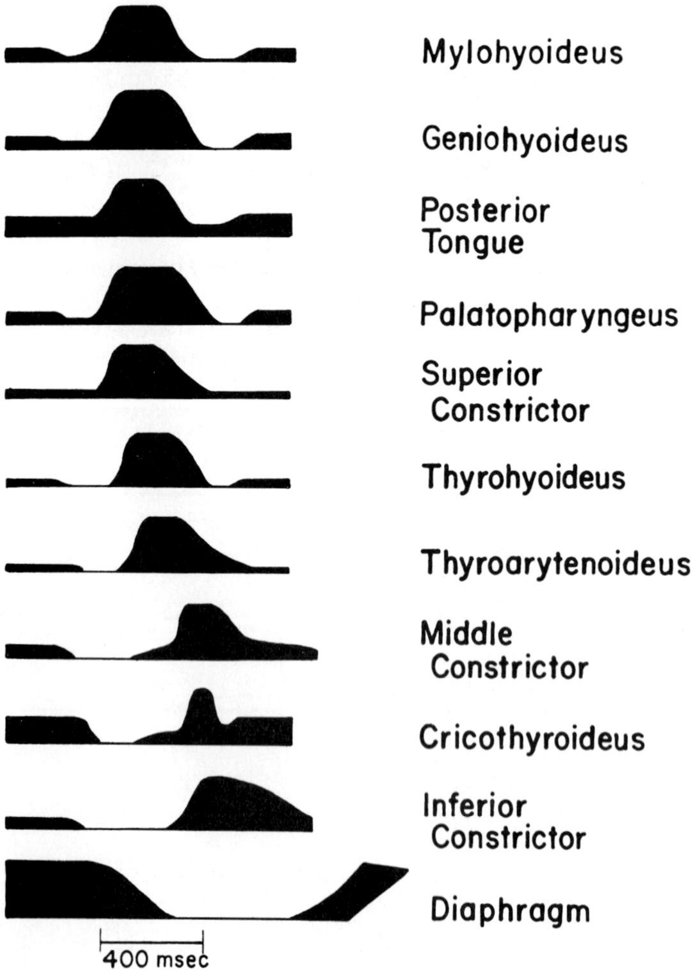

FIG. 11-8
Electromyographic recordings of muscle activity during a swallowing sequence. Increased amplitude represents increase in muscle activity, while decreases indicate inhibition of activity. (From Doty RW, Bosma JF: *Journal of Neurophysiology* 19:44-60, 1956.)

7).

The pharyngeal phase of swallowing is characterized by a complex pattern of muscle activity that, once initiated, produces activity in muscles controlling the hyoid bone, tongue, pharynx, and larynx in a stereotyped sequence of contractions, relaxations, and inhibitions. A set of muscles including the mylohyoid, geniohyoid, posterior tongue, palatopharyngeus, palatoglossus, superior constrictor, styloglossus, and stylohyoid are called the leading complex because they show activity at the beginning of a swallow (Fig. 11-8). The mylohyoid is the first muscle active in the leading complex preceding the other muscles by 30 to 40 msec. Maximal EMG activity takes place in the palatoglossus and palatopharyngeus muscles 80 msec later than the other muscles of the leading complex. Activity in the posterior part of the tongue usually ends 50 to 100 msec before the other muscles of the leading complex.

The pharyngeal constrictors fire in an overlapping sequence. The superior constrictor is part of the leading complex. Contraction in the middle constrictor begins about 125 to 135 msec after the start of activity in the leading complex. Within 300 msec after the onset of the leading complex, the inferior constrictor becomes active, sequentially following the middle constrictor.

The thyrohyoid and thyroarytenoid muscles begin to contract 45 to 1000 msec after the activity in the leading complex begins but cease to contract at about the same time as the leading complex. Activity in the cricothyroid muscle consists of a short burst as the contractions in the leading complex are subsiding.

The esophageal phase of swallowing begins 600 to 800 msec after the onset of activity in the mylohyoid muscle and consists of a caudally directed wave of EMG activity that lasts for 3 to 9 seconds. EMG recordings from the upper and lower esophageal sphincters show that they are continuously active. Before the arrival of the bolus this tonic activity ceases.

The timing and sequencing of the obligate muscles are programmed from before birth. However, activity of the facultative muscles undergoes developmental changes. Before the eruption of teeth, the facultative muscles used in swallowing are not the same as those participating after eruption. In the infantile swallow there is activity in the obicularis oris and buccinator muscle, active thrusting forward of the tongue, and an absence of activity in the levator muscles of the mandible. Once teeth have erupted, this pattern alters, with reduced activity in the labial and buccinator muscles, much reduced tongue thrust, and increased activity of the jaw elevator muscles. In some people the infantile pattern is retained and this is often accompanied by a malocclusion such as anterior open bite.

CONTROL OF SWALLOWING

Although the preparatory and oral phases of swallowing are under voluntary control the pharyngeal and esophageal phases are involuntary and take place in a temporally organized series of events. It is now well established that the organization of the swallowing motor sequence, including the motility of the smooth muscles of the esophagus, depends on the activity of brain stem neurons that belong to a functionally defined swallowing center. Interneurons in this center organize the whole sequence of muscle contractions of swallowing, so that the control of swallowing is a property of a precisely interconnected set of neurons.

Brain Stem Structures Involved in Swallowing

The swallowing center comprises three components (Fig. 11-9). Sensory input from the oral cavity, pharynx, larynx, and esophagus terminates in the nucleus trac-

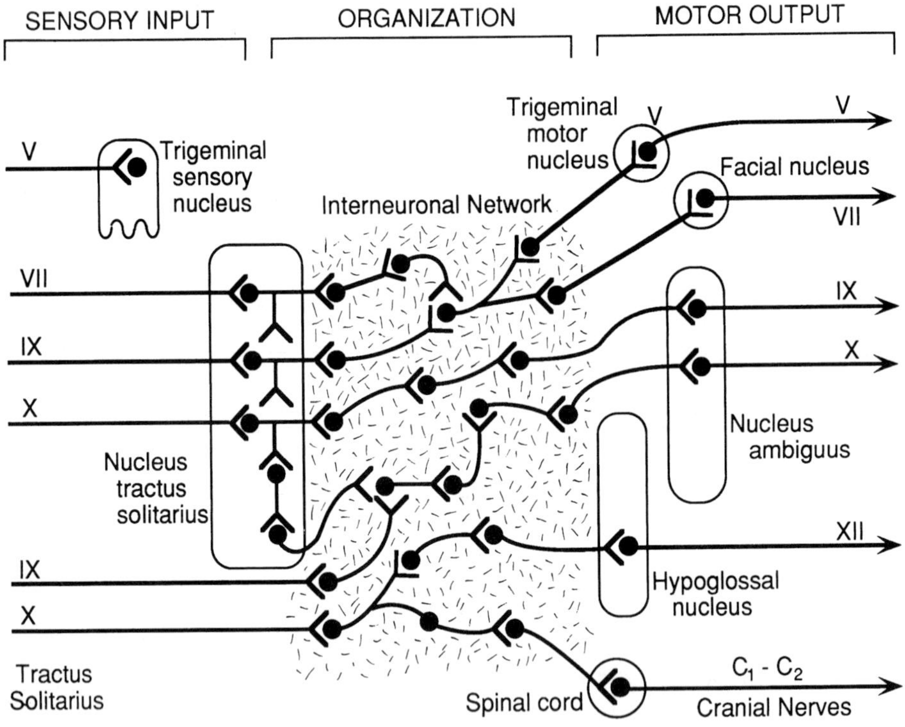

FIG. 11-9
Brainstem swallowing center. Sensory input from cranial nerves V, VII, IX, and X trigger and provide peripheral feedback to the swallowing center. Motor output to muscles involved in a swallowing sequence originates in several motor nuclei and is distributed to the muscles over cranial nerves. Nucleus tractus solitarius (*NTS*) and adjacent reticular formation situated dorsally, together with ventrally located reticular formation surrounding the nucleus ambiguus form, the swallowing center. The dorsally situated group is responsible for initiating swallowing and for programing the events of a swallowing sequence. Output of dorsal group is distributed by ventral group to appropriate motor nuclei. (From Dodds WJ, Stewart ET, Logemann JA: *American Journal of Radiology* 145:953-963, 1990)

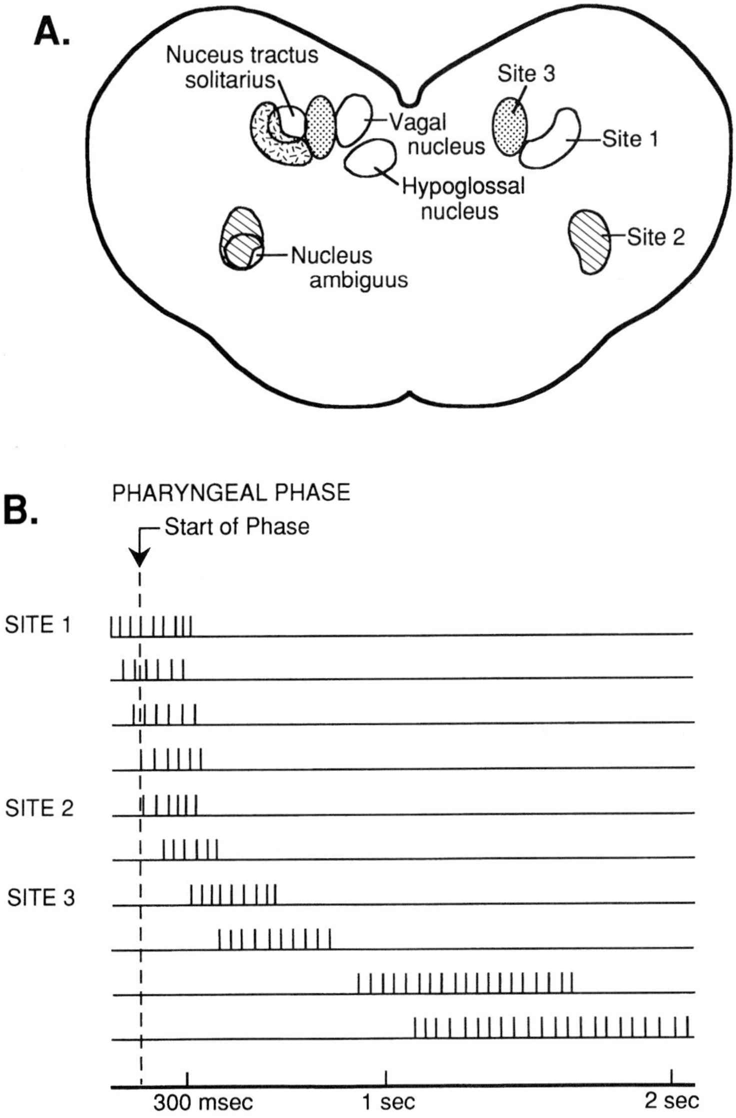

FIG. 11-10

A, Diagram of a coronal section through the caudal medulla indicating three regions where neurons are active during pharyngeal and esophageal phases of swallowing. Sites are indicated on right and anatomical landmarks on left. *Site 1*, situated close to the nucleus tractus solitarius includes neurons that are active early in swallowing. *Site 2*, near nucleus ambiguus, includes neurons active in late pharyngeal phase. *Site 3* indicates location of neurons that discharge late in pharyngeal phase or during all parts of the esophageal phase of swallowing. **B**, Action potential discharges recorded at the three sites, illustrating sequential activity in relation to start of pharyngeal phase of swallowing. (From Miller AJ: *Dysphagia* 1:91-100, 1986)

tus solitarius and trigeminal sensory nucleus that are involved in initiation of swallowing, especially the afferent activity in the glossopharyngeal and the superior laryngeal branch of the vagus nerves. Motor output of the center derives from motoneurons contained in nucleus ambiguus, facial, trigeminal, and hypoglossal motor nuclei as well as motoneurons contained in the cervical spinal cord. Between the sensory input and motor output of the center is an interneuronal network that programs, through excitatory and inhibitory connections, the entire sequence of events in a swallow. The center, therefore, is not a discrete anatomical entity, but consists of brain stem sensory and motor nuclei interconnected by a neuronal network.

Although the sensory input and motor output components of the swallowing center are well defined anatomical structures, the exact location of the interneuronal network is not a separate structure. However, as the result of lesioning experiments, stimulation of localized brain stem areas, and neurophysiological recordings, it has been established that the interneuronal network is situated in ventral and dorsal regions of the medulla. Recordings in these areas have identified neurons whose activity are closely linked to swallowing. The neurons become active at different times corresponding to the different phases of swallowing (Fig. 11-10). The neurons in the dorsal area are situated in the nucleus of the solitary tract and adjacent reticular formation, although the ventral neurons are located in the reticular formation that borders nucleus ambiguus.

The dorsal and ventral groups of neurons associated with swallowing have different functional roles. The dorsal group is responsible for initiation and organization of swallowing. Swallowing activity in these neurons is independent of any sensory feedback and destruction of this area results in suppression of swallowing whether initiated by stimulation of the superior laryngeal nerve or the cortical swallowing area. The role of the swallowing-related neurons in the ventral region is to distribute the swallowing excitation to the various motor nuclei that control swallowing muscles.

In summary, the sequence of muscle activity during swallowing depends on a dorsally and a ventrally situated network of interneurons located in the medulla. These two networks together with sensory input and motor output are called the swallowing center. The dorsally situated group of swallowing-related interneurons is responsible for initiating swallowing and programming the events of a swallowing sequence. The output of the dorsal group is distributed by the ventral group to the appropriate motor nuclei.

Influence of Afferent Input

Although swallowing can occur without any sensory input from peripheral receptors, the dorsal neurons associated with swallowing receive sensory input by way of the nucleus tractus solitarius. Recordings from these swallowing-associated neurons have demonstrated that they are activated when various areas of the pharynx, larynx, and esophagus are stimulated, and their discharge frequency is increased either when a bolus is swallowed or during distension of the pharynx and esophagus. Therefore, swallowing-associated neurons receive sensory information from pharyngeal and esophageal receptors and the central program may be modified by peripheral sensory feedback to alter the motor activity appropriate to the type of bolus being swallowed.

Afferent input from peripheral receptors can also exert inhibitory effects. All the neurons involved with control of the esophagus are inhibited during the oral and pharyngeal phases of swallowing. Therefore, although swallowing is a centrally programmed motor sequence, sensory feedback from peripheral receptors can exert an influence on the magnitude of the contractions and inhibit activity of the muscles as well.

Initiation of Swallowing

Swallowing can be initiated either voluntarily or by stimulation of various areas in the oropharynx, but it seems that some interactions occur between these two mechanisms. For example, repeated voluntary swallows with a dry mouth are difficult to maintain, and the task of swallowing becomes more difficult if the surface of the oral mucosa is anesthetized (Fig. 11-11). This is not because of fatigue of the neuromuscular system, because it is possible to produce repeated swallows in animals by electric stimulation of the superior laryngeal nerve without any signs of fatigue. It is also not possible to stimulate particular areas in the oropharynx and inevitably initiate a swallow. Some areas are more susceptible than others, with perhaps the epiglottis being the most sensitive area. It seems, then, that a swallow may be initiated voluntarily, but the presence of food or fluid in the oral cavity in contact with the mucosal receptors is required for continued swallowing.

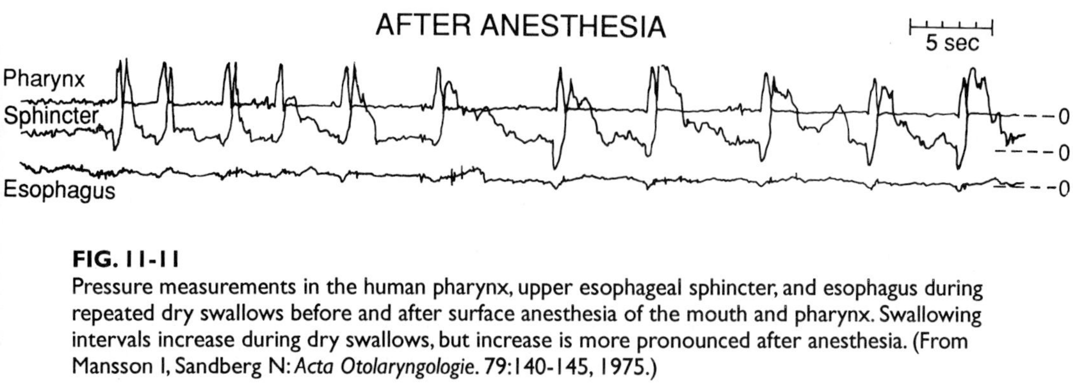

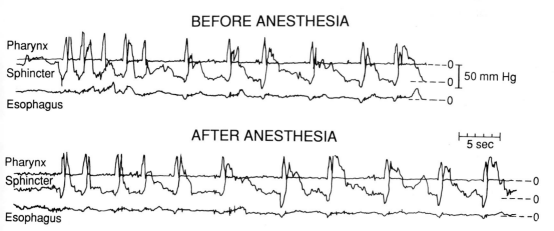

FIG. 11-11
Pressure measurements in the human pharynx, upper esophageal sphincter, and esophagus during repeated dry swallows before and after surface anesthesia of the mouth and pharynx. Swallowing intervals increase during dry swallows, but increase is more pronounced after anesthesia. (From Mansson I, Sandberg N: *Acta Otolaryngologie*. 79:140-145, 1975.)

Investigators of the mechanism of swallowing often electrically stimulate the superior laryngeal nerve to initiate a swallow. To initiate swallowing efficiently, a stimulation frequency of 30 to 50 Hz has been found to be optimal. Other characteristics of the stimulus parameters have also been found to influence the probability of initiating a swallow. These studies suggest that a pattern of sensory input is necessary for initiating a swallow and imply that the swallowing center is able to interpret patterns of afferent input to produce an appropriate motor response.

Influence of Higher Centers

Electrical stimulation of the motor cortex as well as other locations in the corticofugal pathway (internal capsule, subthalamus, amygdala, hypothalamus, substantia nigra, mesencephalic reticular formation) can produce swallowing, and the optimal stimulating conditions are similar to those used to initiate swallowing by stimulation of the superior laryngeal nerve. This suggests that the descending pathways from the cortex and the peripheral afferent pathway converge on the same area of the medulla responsible for decoding input to the swallowing center. Just as peripheral input is not necessary for swallowing, higher nervous centers are also not essential because swallowing occurs in anencephalic infants and in animals in which cortical ablation, or transection of the brain stem has been performed.

OTHER NEUROMUSCULAR ACTIVITY RELATED TO SWALLOWING

Suckling

Newborns and infants feed by a process called suckling in which the intake consists of fluids. Suckling is a complex process involving the development of negative pressure or suction in the oral cavity combined with jaw movements to express the milk from the nipple. Infants and small children usually produce suction by lowering of the jaw while the lips are sealed around the nipple to prevent entry of air into the oral cavity, whereas adults use inspiratory suction, a process similar to breathing through the mouth.

During suckling the infant first forms a teat from its mother's breast by sucking the nipple deep into the posterior part of the mouth to the junction of the hard and soft palates. By elevation of the jaw and tongue, the infant compresses, lengthens and shortens the teat, expressing milk which is swallowed. Negative pressures developed during suckling have been measured and vary over a wide range between 50 and 200 mm Hg, but much higher pressures have been reported. The pressure exerted depends on the infant's age, time of measurement during the feed, and since most of these measurements were made during bottle feeding, the type of nipple and bottle.

During suckling bursts of negative pressure are developed in between which there are periods when no sucking occurs (Fig. 11-12). Depending on the type of

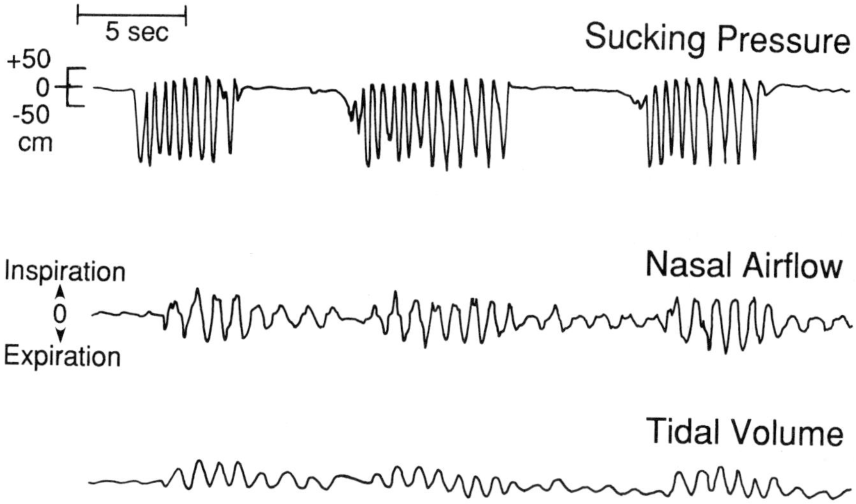

FIG. 11-12
Pattern of sucking pressure and respiration in a human term infant. (From Mathew OP: Regulation of breathing pattern during feeding. Role of suck, swallow, and nutrients. In Mathew OP, Sant'Ambrogio G, editors: *Respiratory Function of the Upper Airway*. New York, 1988, Marcel Dekker, Inc., pp. 535-560.)

nipple and bottle, infant sucking rate ranges between 40 and 90 sucks per minute while feeding. Respiration continues during the bursts of sucking.

The fetus is capable of sucking and swallowing aminiotic fluid in utero, indicating the motor program for these activities is developed long before birth. Fetal swallowing takes place in episodes 1 to 9 minutes in duration, occurring 20 to 7 times per day. The volume of amniotic fluid swallowed is similar to the volume of milk intake in the neonatal period.

Swallowing in the newborn is a liquid swallow and is related to suckling. No teeth are present, masticatory movements do not occur, and a semisolid bolus is not formed. The anatomies of the pharynx and larynx are also different from those of the adult. In the neonate the soft palate occupies much of the volume of the upper pharynx, which is more compact than in the adult. The epiglottis guides the larynx upward behind the soft palate and remains there during respiration. During development the epiglottis descends and assumes its mature functional role during swallowing.

Because of the anatomical relationships of the newborn pharynx and larynx, it has been suggested that infants can swallow without interruption of breathing. However when actual airflow is measured, swallowing was found always to interrupt airflow during suckling.

Upper Airway Protective Reflexes

A number of very powerful reflexes such as sneezing, coughing, gagging, and choking can be initiated by stimulating various areas of the pharynx and upper airway. These reflexes have protective functions and often are accompanied by altered respiration and cardiovascular changes as well as swallowing and other autonomic reflexes. Laryngeal protective reflexes are resistant to anesthesia, asphyxia, and various central depressant drugs. The area surrounding the entry to the airway is perhaps the most reflexogenic and serves to prevent aspiration of ingested material.

The major sensory innervation of the larynx is the superior laryngeal branch of the vagus nerve. Histologic examination of the laryngeal mucosa has revealed a number of sensory endings that range from intraepithelial "free nerve endings" to more complex receptors such as taste buds that are especially concentrated on the surface of the epiglottis opposite the laryngeal opening. Recordings from single afferent fibers of the superior laryngeal nerve during stimulation of the laryngeal surface have revealed two major groups of receptors: a group responding to mechanical stimulation of the mucosa and a group responding to chemical stimulation. Mechanoreceptors are important in feedback control of swallowing as well as initiation of upper airway reflexes. Chemoreceptors respond to a variety of stimuli including vapors such as ammonia as well as salt solutions. Taste buds are the most obvious receptor that initiates responses to chemical stimuli. These structures are called taste buds because they are anatomically similar to taste buds found throughout the oral cavity. However, because of their location it is unlikely that they result in conscious taste sensation, and central tracing and recording studies of the superior laryngeal nerve show no overlap between the termination of the superior laryngeal nerve in the nucleus tractus solitarius and the projection of the oral taste buds.

Carefully controlled studies of laryngeal chemosensitivity, in particular the epiglottis, have revealed that these receptors respond to chemical stimuli that differ from the saline-like environment of the larynx. In fact consistent results could only be obtained if the chemical stimuli were dissolved in saline. Therefore, responses are obtained when water is flowed over the epiglottis because the saline environment is removed; this explains the often reported presence of "water receptors" in the larynx. Therefore, laryngeal taste buds monitor their chemical environment and respond when this environment changes resulting in the initiation of protective reflexes.

Vomiting

Nausea and vomiting are biological protective mechanisms to rid the body of ingested toxins. They serve as an important defense mechanism, protecting the gut and the remainder of the body by triggering events that lead to the ejection of the toxins. As a protective reflex vomiting is more likely to be highly developed in animals that bolt their food with little time spent in sensory evaluation of food by the taste system. This may explain why carnivorous animals such as cat, dog, and ferret have been extensively used in investigations of vomiting and screening of antiemetic agents.

Although the protective nature of vomiting is important, vomiting occurs as a symptom of disease conditions ranging from pyloric stenosis and sudden raised intracranial pressure to cardiac infarction. Nausea and vomiting are also associated with a number of therapeutic regimens such as radiation therapy, surgical anesthesia, and levodopa administration for treatment of Parkinson's disease.

The vomiting reflex may also be evoked by a number of other causes such as pregnancy and motion sickness in which the vomiting is of no practical significance and may even lead to problems associated with dehydration and loss of ions.

It is apparent that the causes of vomiting have little in common yet they all result in the complex sequence of physiological events that precede or accompany the act of vomiting. These include nausea, a psychic experience which may or may not be associated with vomiting, usually accompanied by widespread autonomic reflexes such as salivation, dilation of the pupils, sweating, and pallor. Retching, consisting of labored rhythmic activity of the respiratory musculature, usually precedes or accompanies vomiting.

Events in vomiting are usually divided into preejection, ejection, and postejection phases (Fig. 11-13). The preejection phase is characterized by licking, salivation, pallor, and changes in visceral function such as tachycardia and the relaxation of the proximal stomach. The preejection phase may last for a few minutes,

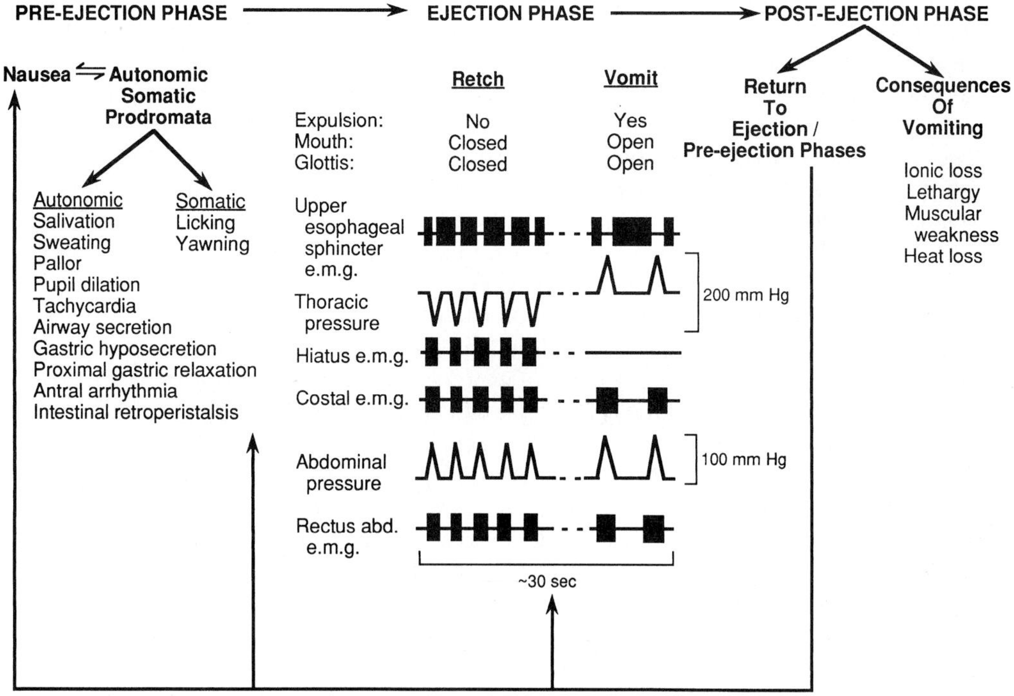

FIG. 11-13
Summary of events occurring during three phases of vomiting. (From Andrews PLR, Hawthorn J: *Balliere's Clinical Gastroenterology* 2:141-168, 1988.)

as in apomorphine induced emesis, hours, or even days as when accompanying chemotherapy, pregnancy, and motion sickness. The ejection phase, which usually ends with the ejection of the contents of the upper gut through the mouth, comprises retching followed by forceful expulsion of food during vomiting. Retching is characterized by rhythmic inspiratory movements against a closed glottis. During retching, all parts of the diaphragm, abdominal muscles, and external intercostal muscles contract simultaneously with the glottis closed. This activity, which occurs in bursts every one or two seconds, results in a rapid decrease in intrathoracic pressure coincident with increases in intraabdominal pressure. The upper esophageal sphincter relaxes during each retch, but contracts between retches. The reason gastric contents are not expelled during retching is probably the different patterns of thoracic, diaphragmatic, and abdominal muscle activity occurring in retching and vomiting. Up to 25 retches may precede a vomit but some stimuli such as apomorphine produce a considerable amount of retching and relatively little vomiting.

At the end of a series of retching movements vomiting usually occurs. The major driving force for the expulsion of gastric contents is contraction of the rectus abdominus and external oblique muscles that overlie the stomach. The stomach antrum relaxes to contain the contents of the proximal stomach. During expulsion the upper esophageal sphincter relaxes, the abdominal walls contract, and both the intrathoracic and intraabdominal pressures become positive at about 100 mm Hg.

Like swallowing, vomiting is programmed in the medulla by a group of nuclei capable of generating all components of the emetic response. These nuclei, when activated by afferent information, integrate the activity and synchronize all the outputs of the vomiting system. With electrical stimulation and lesioning experiments, an area has been localized in the reticular formation ventrolateral to the nucleus tractus solitarius that is essential for vomiting. This area is connected to a specialized chemoreceptor trigger zone in the area postrema that is responsive to emetic agents. The area postrema is located at the caudal end of the floor of the fourth ventricle and consists of a V shaped strip of vascularized tissue. The medullary area responsible for controlling vomiting is located close to other centers in the medulla that control salivation, respiration, and the cardiovascular system that facilitate interconnections between these centers.

Vomiting can be initiated in a number of ways. Sensory input to medullary vomiting nuclei originates in many parts of the body. Such stimuli as raised intracranial pressure, pain, distension or injury to the uterus, stomach, duodenum, and bladder, and events leading to unequal rotation of the vestibular organs can all produce vomiting presumably by way of afferent sensory connections. Substances that cause local irritation of the gut and peritoneum initiate vomiting by stimulating vagal nerve endings that project to the medulla. Emetic agents absorbed into the blood stimulate the medullary vomiting control system directly through the chemoreceptor trigger zone in the area postrema. Vomiting can also occur for psychogenic reasons, and children can often vomit voluntarily. Therefore, vomiting can be triggered by a widespread series of pathways.

SUMMARY

Swallowing consists of a reflex sequence of muscle contractions that moves food from the mouth to the stomach and also has important protective functions to clear the upper airway of foreign material. Swallowing is a timed series of muscle contractions and relaxations that takes place in a precisely ordered spatiotemporal sequence. Once swallowing is initiated it is an entirely automatic series of events.

Swallowing is divided into preparatory, oral, pharyngeal, and esophageal phases. In the preparatory phase a food bolus is formed. During the oral phase, the bolus is propelled from the oral cavity into the pharynx. The pharyngeal phase involves bolus transport from the oropharynx into the esophagus and the esophageal phase is the transport of the bolus through the esophagus to the stomach.

Food is moved through the mouth, pharynx, and esophagus by a positive-pressure wave. Pressure is developed by the piston-like action of the tongue and peristaltic muscle contractions. Sphincters are important in directing the pressure wave to guide the orderly passage of the bolus.

During the pharyngeal phase, a set of muscles called the obligate muscles always participates in swallowing. During the preparatory and oral phases muscle participation is inconsistent and this set is called the facultative muscles. The pharyngeal phase is characterized by a complex pattern of muscle activity that, once initiated, produces activity in muscles that control the hyoid bone, tongue, pharynx, and larynx in a stereotyped sequence of contractions, relaxations, and inhibitions. The esophageal phase of swallowing consists of a caudally directed wave of muscle activity.

Preparatory and oral phases of swallowing are under voluntary control and the pharyngeal and esophageal phases are involuntary. The organization of the swallowing motor sequence depends on the activity of the brain stem neurons belonging to a functionally defined swallowing center. Interneurons in this center organize the whole sequence of muscle contractions involved in swallowing.

In infants suckling consists of bursts of negative pressure interspersed with periods when no sucking occurs. Swallowing in the newborn is a liquid swallow, and is related to suckling.

A number of reflexes, including sneezing, coughing, gagging, and choking, can be initiated by stimulating areas of the pharynx and upper airway. These reflexes have protective functions and are accompanied by altered respiration and cardiovascular changes as well as by swallowing and other autonomic reflexes.

Nausea and vomiting are biological protective mechanisms to rid the body of ingested toxins. They serve as an important defense mechanism, protecting the gut and the remainder of the body by triggering events that lead to the ejection of the toxins. Vomiting is usually divided into preejection, ejection, and postejection phases. The preejection phase is characterized by licking, salivation, pallor, and changes in visceral function such as tachycardia and the relaxation of the proximal stomach. The ejection phase comprises retching and the forceful expulsion of food during vomiting.

Vomiting is programmed in the medulla by a group of nuclei capable of generating all components of the emetic response. These nuclei are connected to a specialized chemoreceptor trigger zone in the area postrema that is responsive to emetic agents.

SELECTED READINGS

Andrews PLR, Hawthorn J: The neurophysiology of vomiting, *Bailliere's Clinical Gastroenterology* 2:141-168, 1988.

Bartlett D Jr: Respiratory functions of the larynx, *Physiological Reviews* 69:33-57, 1989.

Borison HL: Area postrema: chemoreceptor circumventricular organ of the medulla oblongata, *Progress in Neurobiology* 32:351-390, 1989.

Davis CJ, Lake-Bakaar GV, Grahame-Smith DG: *Nausea and vomiting: mechanisms and treatments*. Berlin, 1986, Springer-Verlag.

Dodds WJ, Stewart ET, Logemann JA: Physiology and radiology of the normal oral and pharyngeal phases of swallowing, *American Journal of Radiology* 145:953-963, 1990.

Jean A: Control of central swallowing program by inputs from the peripheral receptors: a review, *Journal of the Autonomic Nervous System* 10:225-233, 1984.

Jean A: Brain stem control of swallowing: localization and organization of the central pattern generator for swallowing. In Taylor A, editor: *Neurophysiology of the jaws and teeth*, Basingstoke, 1990, Macmillan.

Kucharczyk J, Stewart DJ, Miller AD: *Nausea and vomiting: recent research and clinical advances*, Boca Raton, 1991, CRC Press.

Mathew OP: Regulation of breathing pattern during feeding. Role of suck, swallow, and nutrients. In Mathew OP, Sant'Ambrogio G, editors: *Respiratory function of the upper airway*. New York, 1988, Marcel Dekker, pp. 535-560.

Mathew OP, Sant'Ambrogio FB: Laryngeal reflexes. In Mathew OP, Sant'Ambrogio G, editors: *Respiratory function of the upper airway*. New York, 1988, Marcel Dekker, pp. 259-302.

Miller AJ: Deglutition, *Physiological Reviews* 62:129-184, 1982.

Miller AJ: Neurophysiological basis of swallowing, *Dysphagia* 1:91-100, 1986.

Miller AJ: Swallowing: neurophysiologic control of the esophageal stage, *Dysphagia* 2:72-82, 1987.

Miller AJ: The search for the central swallowing pathway: the quest for clarity, *Dysphagia* 8:185-194, 1993.

Widdicombe J: Nasal and pharyngeal reflexes. Protective and respiratory functions. In Mathew OP and Sant'Ambrogio G, editors: *Respiratory function of the upper airway*. New York, 1988, Marcel Dekker, pp. 233-258.

12

Speech

LEARNING OBJECTIVES

At the end of this chapter you should be able to:

1. Describe the basic characteristics of speech and language.
2. Describe the development of language.
3. Describe the adaptive characteristics of language.
4. Describe the anatomy of the vocal tract.
5. Describe the basic sounds produced by the vocal tract.
6. Describe how the voice is produced.
7. Describe the role of articulation in voice production.
8. Describe the role of resonance in voice production.
9. Describe the control of air pressure during voice production.
10. Describe the central nervous system centers controlling language.
11. Describe the aphasias.
12. Describe the asymmetry of the language production centers.
13. State current theories relating to language production.
14. Describe how changes and pathology of the oropharynx can result in alterations of speech production.

Although humans communicate by sign language and writing, by far the most common means of human communication is spoken language or speech. Speech is used to communicate between individuals and to communicate internally during thought processes and involves speech production and speech perception. The speed with which this all takes place is remarkable. During speech production, 12 to 14 speech sounds are produced each second and during speech perception, 50 to 60 segments of speech can be perceived each second. Given the necessary computational complexity and the precision of the muscle activity, this is an amazing accomplishment.

For speech to be understood both the speaker and listener must belong to the same language group, which is a group of individuals that have learned the symbolic meaning of the speech sounds used by that language. Intimately associated with the spoken language is the set of symbols representing the written form of the language. This ability to deal in complex symbolic systems such as written language is unique to humans. It has permitted humans to store knowledge and experience and has directly resulted in the evolution of the human race independent of genetic evolution. With a relatively small vocabulary and a basic set of rules we are able to form an unending set of original sentences never spoken before. Languages all use a similar basic set of rules but different sounds. For example in all languages sentences have a defined structure of words grouped into phrases and phrases combined to form sentences. Therefore, despite the large number of languages spoken around the world, human language may be a unitary phenomenon, with a common genetic basis underlying the neurobiologic process of language production.

Language is both innate and learned. Early infant speech perception does not rely on specific language experience. Therefore, from birth infants have the ability to discriminate sounds. Parts of the cerebral cortex important in speech and language are also developed at birth and show the typical asymmetry of the adult brain. This asymmetry suggests that phonetic experience is not essential for development of central

TABLE 12-1

Stages of Language Acquisition

Age	Language ability
12 weeks	Smiles, coos, vowel-like sounds
20 weeks	Consonantal sounds, labial fricatives, spirants, and nasals
6 months	Babbling. One-syllable utterances, 'ma,' 'da,' 'di.'
1 year	Beginning of language understanding. Definite single words, 'mamma,' 'dadda.'
$1\frac{1}{2}$ years	Words used singly; repertoire of 30 to 50 words.
2 years	Two-word phrases. 50 to several hundred words in the vocabulary.
$2\frac{1}{2}$ years	Three or more words in many combinations; functions begin to appear; many grammatical errors and idiosyncratic expressions; good understanding of language.
3 years	Full sentences; few errors; vocabulary of around 100 words.
4 years	Close to adult speech competence.

Based on Lenneberg EH: *Biological foundations of language*, New York, 1967, John Wiley.

nervous system speech areas. Moreover, despite the fact that language must be learned by mimicry, it is achieved in a series of regular steps common to most languages (Table 12-1). Within a short time span and with almost no direct instruction a child will analyze the language completely. In fact, although many subtle refinements are added between the ages of 5 and 10, most children have completed the greater part of the basic language acquisition process by the age of 5. By that time a child will have dissected the language into its minimal separable units of sound and meaning and will have discovered the rules for combining sounds into words, the meanings of individual words, and the rules for recombining words into meaningful sentences. Therefore, although each individual has to learn her or his native language, this takes place in the context of a genetically controlled neural substrate.

Language is an adaptation because all organs used in speech production were evolved for another function. The lips, teeth, tongue, and jaws are masticatory organs. The lungs, nasal cavity, soft palate, and glottal folds are part of the respiratory system (Fig. 12-1). In fact all mammals possess these structures but only humans can speak. At some point in evolution the speech system developed and was able to control these organs independently. Muscles commanding the speech organs are controlled by motor nuclei situated in the brain stem, which for speech production are activated by control centers in rostral parts of the brain rather than locally within the medulla.

The syllables, words, and sentences used in all human languages are formed from a set of speech sound called phones. Only a subset of the phones is used in any particular language. The phones that distinguish meaning in a particular language are called phonemes, defined as the smallest difference in sound that distinguishes different content, as, for example, the difference between the sounds *d* and *t*. The content of every known language can be described as a relatively small number of phonemes. In addition the construction of the alphabet is predicted on the assumption that a language consists of combinations of a limited number of distinctive sounds of phoneme size.

PHONATION

Vocal Tract

The human vocal tract is an acoustic tube of variable cross section about 17 cm long, extending from the vocal folds to the lips. The cross-sectional area of the vocal tract can be varied from zero (complete closure) to about 20 cm^2 by the placement of lips, jaw, tongue, and velum (the name used for the soft palate in speech science). The trap-door action of the velum couples the vocal tract proper to a secondary cavity involved in speech production—the nasal tract. The nasal cavity is about 12 cm long and has a volume of about 60 cm^3 (Fig. 12-1).

Voiced Sounds

Voiced sounds exemplified by vowels are produced by raising the air pressure in the lungs and forcing the air to flow through the glottis (the orifice between the

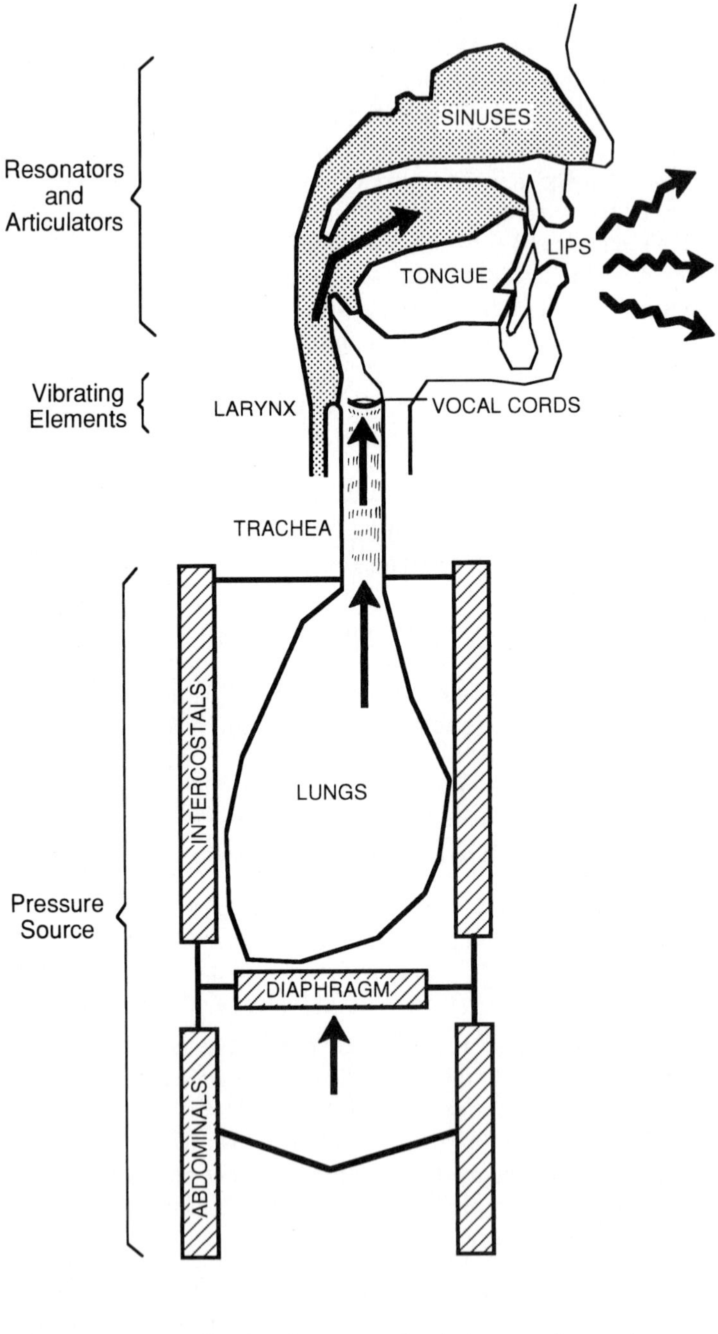

FIG. 12-1
Vocal tract with power source, vibrating elements, and articulators and resonators.

vocal cords), causing the vocal cords to vibrate. The vibrations interrupt the airflow and generate quasi-periodic broad spectrum pulses that excite the vocal tract. The vibrating ligaments of the vocal cords are 18 mm long and the glottal opening typically varies in area from about 0 to 20 mm^2. The laryngeal muscles controlling the vocal folds are divided into tensors, abductors, and adductors. Rises and falls in the pitch of the voice are controlled by the action of the tensors—the crico-thyroid and the vocalis muscles. Variations in subglottal pressure are also important in controlling the degree of laryngeal vibration.

Articulation and Resonation

Once the basic sounds are produced by the vocal tract they are modified to produce intelligible sounds by the processes of articulation and resonance. Articulation is the process of producing sounds in speech by means of movements of the lips, mandible, tongue, and the palatopharyngeal mechanisms in coordination with respiration and phonation (Fig. 12-2). The terms to describe sounds indicate the part of the mouth where the sound is articulated. For example, a bilabial sound is articulated by both lips; *m*, *p*, and *b* are three bilabial sounds. There are differences between these bilabials. *M* is articulated by both lips but the air escapes through the nose and *m* is, therefore, a nasal sound. *P* is a voiceless sound and *b* is a voiced sound. Therefore, the lips look similar during production of the words *mat*, *pat*, and *bat*. An individual relying on lip-reading as a substitute for hearing would have to guess the meaning of these three words based on the context in which they are used.

By use of the resonant properties of the vocal tract the basic voiced sounds are filtered. The final quality of the voice depends on the sizes and shapes of the various cavities associated with the nose and mouth. The form of some of these cavities can be changed by the various activities of the movable parts of the pharynx and oral cavity. The cavities associated with the nose are the nasal cavity, the sinuses, and the nasopharynx. Of these, only the nasopharynx is readily variable and its variation is produced by contractions of the pharyngeal muscles and movements of the soft palate. The cavities associated with the mouth are the oral cavity and the oropharynx. Both of these cavities can be varied considerably by contraction of appropriate muscles. All these cavities pick out and amplify the fundamental sound produced by vibration of the vocal cords. This function is known as resonance. It is by these movements of the soft palate, larynx, and pharynx that humans achieve the fine balance between oral and nasal resonance that is characteristic of the voice of that particular individual.

For voiced sounds the excitation source is the volume velocity of air as it passes the vocal cords. The flow is typically pulsive and periodic. The vocal tract acts on this source as a filter with favored frequencies, corresponding to the acoustic resonances of the vocal tract. These resonances are usually referred to as formants. These resonant frequencies are 500, 1500, and 2500 Hz. During speech these formants

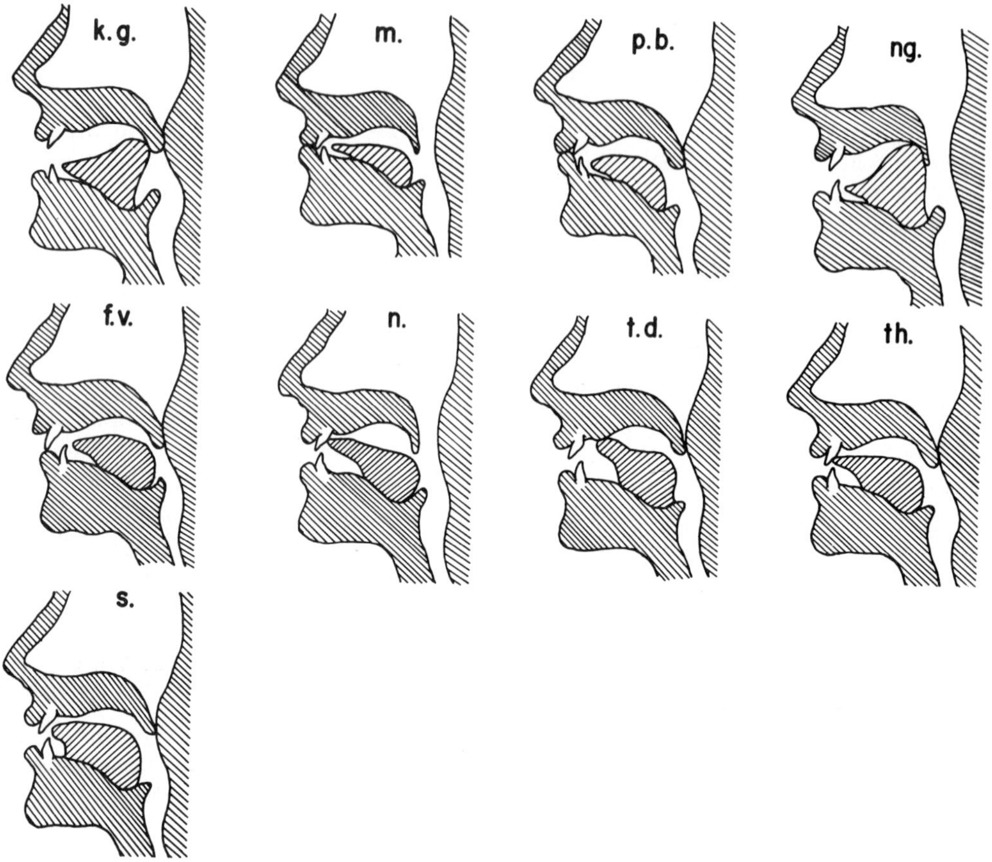

FIG. 12-2
Position of oral structures during production of various consonants. (From Jenkins GN: *The Physiology of the Mouth*, Oxford, 1970, Blackwell Scientific.)

change their frequency with time at relatively slow rates (Fig. 12-3).

All these vocal sources have a broad spectrum of frequencies that extend over the voice frequency range of 100 to 3000 Hz. The vocal system acts as a time-varying filter to impose its resonant characteristics on the sound waves generated by the broad spectrum sources.

Besides voiced sounds the vocal system can produce two other basic kinds of voiceless sounds: fricative sounds and plosive sounds. Fricative sounds, exemplified by the consonants *s*, *sh*, *f*, and *th*, are generated when the vocal tract is partly closed at some point and air is forced through the constriction at high enough velocity to produce turbulence. Fricative consonants require a very fine adjustment of the articulators, and they are sounds most frequently defective in cases of malocclusion or denture use.

Plosive sounds, typified by the consonants *p*, *t*, and *k*, are produced when the

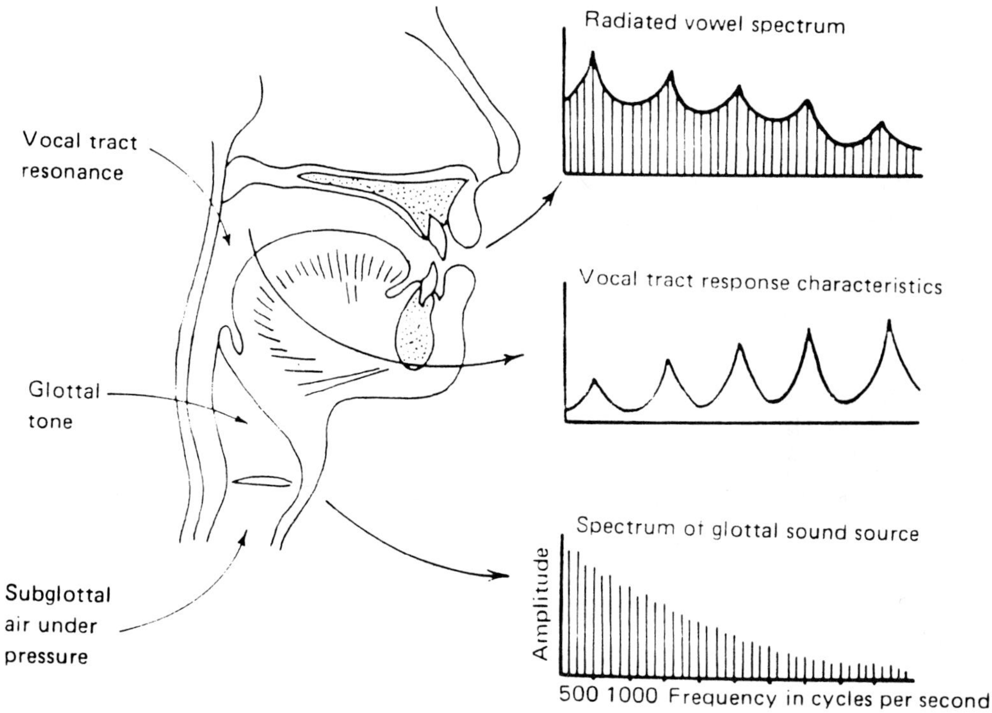

FIG 12-3
Production of a vowel. On the right is represented the radiated spectrum of glottal sound source together with vocal tract acoustical response and final radiated vowel spectrum. (From Zemlin WR: *Speech and Hearing Science: Anatomy and Physiology*, Englewood Cliffs, 1981, Prentice Hall.)

vocal tract is closed completely (usually with the lips or tongue), allowing air pressure to build up behind the closure, and is then abruptly opened. The sharp sound produced when the air is released is often followed by a fricative sound or aspiration (see Fig. 12-2). Operation of the voiced and voiceless sources is not mutually exclusive. For some sounds, such as the voiced fricative consonants *v* and *z*, two sound sources act in combination.

The generation of movements for speech involves the continuous utilization of sensory information from the muscle receptors and cutaneous mechanoreceptors that are distributed throughout the respiratory, laryngeal, and orofacial systems. Afferent information is used to refine certain parameters of motor programs in relation to varying states of the periphery, yielding a more specific and detailed set of motor commands for actual motor execution. For example, if a perturbation is introduced to the lower lip during the elevation for a bilabial sound, compensatory adjustments are observed in both the upper lip and jaw. These data imply that sensory information is used not only to correct errors in individual movements but also to make adjustments among multiple movements in speech and motor gestures.

Control of Pressure

The power source for the voice is derived from air pressure in the lungs. The release of this pressure through the vocal folds is carefully coordinated. Monitoring the EMGs (Box 10-2) of muscles controlling the thorax and diaphragm as well as measuring lung volume and intratracheal pressure reveals the controlled release of pressure (Fig. 12-4). During speech lung pressure is slowly released, normal respiration is halted, and there is a very precise sequence of activity in widely different groups of muscles. The diaphragm is relaxed through most of the expiration and

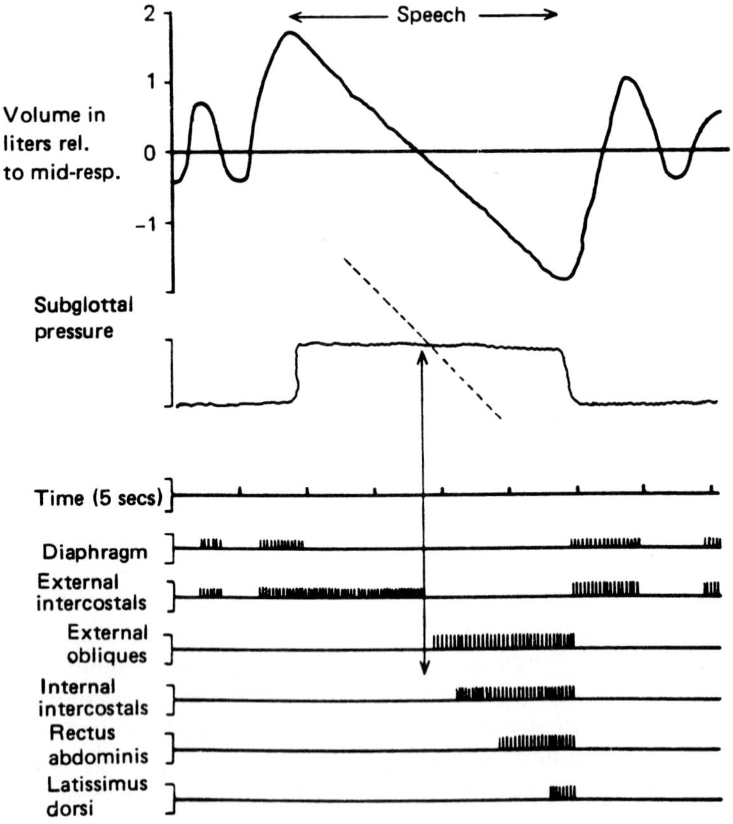

FIG. 12-4
Activity of respiratory muscles during speech production. The human subject took a deep breath and counted slowly from 1 to 32. Recordings show lung volume and intratracheal pressure as well as muscle EMG. (From Zemlin WR: *Speech and Hearing Science: Anatomy and Physiology* ed 2, 1981, p. 353. Reprinted by permission of Prentice-Hall, Inc., Englewood Cliffs, NJ.)

phonation, and the maintenance of the appropriate subglottal pressure is caused by activity in the intercostal, abdominal, and latissimus dorsi muscles.

NEURAL BASIS OF LANGUAGE

Localization of Language Control Centers

Mammalian vocalization requires the coordination of respiratory, laryngeal, and articulatory (supralaryngeal) movements. The motoneurons responsible for respiratory movement lie in the cervical, thoracic, and upper lumbar spinal chord; those controlling glottal closure are found in the nucleus ambiguus; and neurons responsible for control of articulatory movements are localized in the trigeminal motor nucleus, facial nucleus, rostral nucleus ambiguus, hypoglossal nucleus, and upper cervical spinal cord. Therefore, even at the level of the efferent control of muscle contraction (final common pathway), vocalization involves an extensive set of motoneuron pools extending from the pons to the spinal cord.

Transection of the brain axis above the trigeminal motor nucleus in animals renders these animals mute. Therefore, the neural information exchange between cranial motor nuclei, spinal respiratory motoneurons, and the somatosensory information entering the lower brain stem and spinal cord is not enough to initiate vocalization; a coordinating input from higher cerebral centers is required.

Until the middle of the 1960s, details of the location of these higher cerebral centers in humans were derived from just a few methods. The oldest is the neuropathologic studies of focal cerebral lesions in patients with defects or loss of the power of speech, called aphasias. A closely related method is the behavioral study of patients who have undergone surgical interventions such as the ablation of a cerebral lobe or even of an entire hemisphere. Other approaches that have been used are electric stimulation and recording of cerebral cortex in awake patients during surgical intervention, aimed at studying the effect of stimulation on language behaviors; established neuroradiologic techniques such as cerebral angiography and pneumoencephalography for indirect localization of lesions related to language disturbance; and study of language behavior after transient hemispheric inactivation induced by barbiturate injection into the carotid artery of one side (the Wada test). More recently, computerized tomography (CT) has been used in research on aphasias.

The study of aphasia has, therefore, played a major role in understanding the neural basis of language. The most common cause of aphasia is head trauma, which produces 200,000 cases in the United States each year. The next most frequent cause is stroke: 40% of major vascular events in the cerebral hemispheres produce language disorders. In the United States stroke results in 100,000 cases of aphasia per year. By careful behavioral study of language production neurologists have described several aphasias usually involving different areas of the cerebral hemispheres. One of the earliest aphasias to be described was *Wernicke's aphasia*—in which the patient may speak very rapidly, preserving rhythm, grammar, and articulation. The speech, if not listened to closely, may sound almost normal. However, it is abnormal in that it is remarkably devoid of content. The patient fails to use the correct word and instead uses circumlocutory phrases ("what you use to drink with" for "cup") and words devoid of content ("thing"). Another characteristic of Wernicke's aphasia is paraphrasia, in which one word or phrase is substituted for another, sometimes of related meaning ("spoon" for "knife") and sometimes unrelated ("hammer" for "paper"). Patients with Wernicke's aphasia have a severe loss of comprehension even though hearing of nonverbal sounds and music may be fully normal. The extent of the neural lesion is variable and parallels the presence or absence of associated linguistic disturbances such as inability to read (alexia) and write (agraphia). It also parallels the severity of the auditory comprehension and speech defects. The lesion extends into the parietal lobe, especially into the agranular gyrus (Fig. 12-5).

In *Broca's aphasia* speech is slow and labored, articulation is crude, and small grammatical words and endings of nouns and verbs are omitted so that speech has a telegraphic style. CT scans show the lesion is localized in the anterior language zone, and is not a combined lesion in Wernicke's and other motor areas (see Fig. 12-5). The anatomical and clinical correlations are not as consistent as those seen in Wernicke's aphasia.

Conduction aphasia resembles Wernicke's aphasia in the presence of mostly fluent normal speech and poor repetition, but relatively well preserved auditory compensation. CT scans show that conduction aphasia is commonly associated with

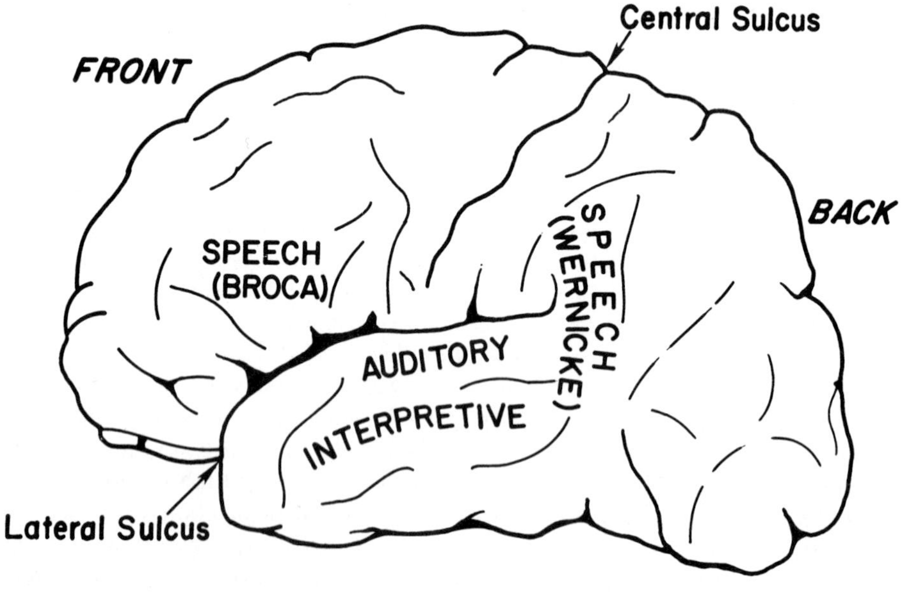

FIG. 12-5
Left (dominant) hemisphere of man, showing location of Broca's and Wernicke's areas. Note the relationship of these areas to the auditory cortex and the motor and sensory cortex in the area of the central sulcus.

a lesion located between the area frequently damaged in Wernicke's aphasia and the area in the frontal operculum commonly associated with Broca's aphasia. The lesion compromises structures that normally transfer auditory information to the motor system, a physiological step required for the act of repeating a sentence verbatim.

Patients with *global aphasia* are unable to speak or comprehend language; they cannot read, write, repeat, or name objects. Lesions are extensive and are those essentially supplied by cortical branches of the middle cerebral artery encompassing all of the perisylvian territory of the left hemisphere.

In *anomic aphasia* the only disturbance is in finding the correct words. This is an unusual form of aphasia that typically follows lesions in the posterior aspect of the left inferior temporal lobe, near the temporal-occipital border.

Transcortical motor aphasia results from a lesion that disconnects Broca's area from the supplementary motor cortex. The lesion gives rise to a nonfluent aphasia in which the patient will attempt conversation but can utter only a few syllables. In striking contrast, these patients are able to repeat words and phrases well. Comprehension of language is less disturbed.

Transcortical sensory aphasia follows disconnection of Wernicke's area from the posterior parietal temporal association area. This causes a fluent aphasia with defective comprehension, and a defect in thinking about or remembering the meaning of signs and words. The patient cannot read and write and has marked difficulty in finding words, but is able to repeat spoken language easily and fluently.

Lesions that do not affect the cerebral cortex, typically vascular lesions in the basal ganglia and thalamus, can also result in aphasia usually called *subcortical aphasia*. Often these aphasias are transient in nature.

Small lesions in the brain can selectively destroy the ability to read and/or write, without interfering with speech or other cognitive functions. Alexia with agraphia is associated with lesions of the association cortex that lies in the left parietal lobe, behind the auditory association cortex. Alexia without agraphia is associated with a left occipital lobe or with lesions that compromise the transmission of visual information from both the left and right visual cortices to the left language cortex.

Cerebral Dominance

It is essential for the neural defect to be confined to a specific area to produce the aphasia. Damage to the corresponding area on the other side of the brain leaves language abilities intact. Only rarely does damage to the right hemisphere of the brain lead to a language disorder. Of all patients with permanent language disorder caused by brain lesions, 97% have damage to the left side of the brain. The unilateral control of certain functions is called cerebral dominance. Moreover, not only is the left hemisphere dominant but specific cerebral areas, clearly related to language, are larger in the dominant hemisphere.

Sign language has also provided insight into language production. Unlike speech, signing consists of a series of hand gestures that are interpreted by means of the visual system rather than the auditory system. Despite these differences from vocal communication, signing is also localized in the left hemisphere. Therefore, lesions to the left hemisphere cause deaf individuals to become aphasic for sign language. Lesions in the right hemisphere do not produce these deficits.

Theories of Language Processing

Based on these extensive studies of language disorders and associated anatomic lesions, models of brain activity during language production have been constructed. The connectionist theory suggests that when a word is heard, the output from the primary auditory area of the cortex is received by Wernicke's area. If the word is to be spoken, the pattern is transmitted from Wernicke's area to Broca's area where the articulatory form is generated and sent to the motor area that controls the movement of the muscles of speech. If the spoken word is to be spelled, the auditory pattern is sent to the agranular cortex, where it elicits the visual pattern. When a word is read, the output from the primary visual areas passes to the angular gyrus, which in turn generates the corresponding auditory form of the word in Wernicke's area. Predictions can be made from this simple model. For example, if a lesion disconnects Wernicke's area from Broca's area, speech should be fluent—but abnormal—with good comprehension. Repetition of spoken language, however, should be grossly impaired. This in fact describes conduction aphasia. The underlying concept of the connectionist theory is, therefore, that language is processed serially from decoding in Wernicke's area to motor expression in Broca's and other areas of the cerebral cortex.

One of the problems with the classical descriptions of aphasia is that the analysis of the language deficit is crude: it is usually at the level of a deficit of naming objects, for example. However, language contains various types of linguistic information including information concerning the sound structure of the utterance (phonology), information about grammatical forms (syntax), and information concerning the meaning of the utterance (semantics). Careful behavioral analysis now indicates that the broad classifications of the aphasias commonly employed may in fact be inadequate. This has resulted in the suggestion that models of cortical language organization should include separate systems for different language functions. Evidence has accumulated that the cortical area involved with language is not singular, but rather is compartmentalized into separate areas for handling different languages, since there are lesions in multilingual persons that leave only one of their several languages intact. Separate areas have also been described that handle different aspects of grammar. Based on these and other studies the connectionist theory has been replaced by a modular theory in which language is processed in parallel with many different areas responsible for different cognitive tasks. Each distinct neural process is associated with different cognitive mechanisms, all of which may be selectively damaged.

CLINICAL CONSIDERATIONS

The shape of the vocal tract plays a key role in the resonant properties and articulation of speech production. If the form of the oral cavity is changed by orthodontic or prosthodontic treatment, patients will be compelled to change their methods of articulating a sound to some extent. Many patients are able to utilize a different phoneme and still produce good speech. However, in some cases of malocclusion, or before or after orthodontic treatment, it may be too difficult to produce one or more of the sounds, and the individual will consequently have a defect in speech production.

For a person to produce the same sounds before and after denture placement requires alterations in speech articulation. The form of the denture determines how much change is required. Generally speech changes after denture placement. Most listeners are tolerant and unaware of the change in sound or rapidly become accustomed to the slight difference. Consequently, most people wearing dentures are not considered to have a speech defect. The slight change of individual sounds that has taken place is still within the phoneme for each sound and is within the range of normal. The sounds most usually affected by dentures are those requiring a very fine adjustment of the tongue in coordination with other movements of the vocal tract. It is likely that sounds which are influenced most frequently by dentures are *s*, *r*, and *th*.

If the size of the nasopharynx is altered, there will be changes in nasal resonance. These changes are brought about by the lowering and raising of the velum during normal function. The velum must move rapidly to obtain a balance between oral and nasal resonance. Therefore, any interference with the neuromuscular structure of the palate can result in a disturbance of resonance. Lack of balance between oral and nasal resonance may cause excessive nasal tone that is frequently heard in postoperative cleft palate cases. Similarly, if the nose is blocked, for example with the common cold or by adenoidal growth, nasal resonance is lost and the voice sound is altered.

In general alterations in speech resulting from dental treatment are minor and may disappear with neuromuscular adaptation. Treatment of malocclusion and soft palate repair often result in distinct improvements in speech production.

SUMMARY

Languages all use a similar basic set of rules but different sounds so that human language is a unitary phenomenon with a common genetic basis. Language is both innate and learned. Individuals must learn their native language in the setting of a genetically controlled neural substrate. Language production is an adaptation because all organs used in speech were evolved for mastication and respiration.

The vocal tract is an acoustic tube of variable cross section, extending from the vocal folds to the lips. Movement of the velum (soft palate) couples the vocal tract to the nasal tract important in speech production. Raised air pressure in the lungs forces air past the vocal folds, causing them to vibrate and producing voiced sounds. The vibrations interrupt the airflow and generate pressure pulses that excite the vocal tract. Once the basic sounds are produced by the vocal tract they are modified by the processes of articulation and resonance to produce intelligible sounds. Besides voiced sounds the vocal system can produce voiceless sounds such as fricative sounds and plosive sounds. The vocal system acts as a time-varying filter to impose its resonant characteristics on the sound waves generated by the broad spectrum sources.

The study of aphasia or loss of the power of speech has played a major role in understanding the neural basis of language. By careful behavioral study of language production neurologists have described several aphasias that usually involve different areas of the cerebral hemispheres. In most individuals the neural defect in these aphasias is restricted to the left cerebral hemisphere. Damage to the corresponding area on the other side of the brain leaves language abilities intact. The unilateral control of certain functions is called cerebral dominance. Not only is the left hemisphere dominant but specific cerebral areas related to language are larger in the dominant hemisphere.

Based on studies of language disorders and associated anatomic lesions, models of the neural mechanisms of language production have been proposed. The connectionist theory suggests that language is processed serially from decoding in Wernicke's area to motor expression in Broca's and other areas of the cerebral cortex. Recently the connectionist theory has been replaced by a modular theory of language processed in parallel with various cortical areas that are responsible for different cognitive tasks.

SELECTED READINGS

Caramazza A: Some aspects of language processing revealed through the analysis of acquired aphasia: the lexical system, *Annual Review of Neuroscience* 11:395-421, 1988.

Damasio AR: The neural basis of language, *Annual Review of Neuroscience* 7:127-147, 1984.

Jürgens U, Ploog D: On the neural control of mammalian vocalization, *Trends in Neuroscience* 4:135-137, 1981.

Ojemann GA: Cortical organization of language, *The Journal of Neuroscience* 11:2281-2287, 1991.

Poizner H, Bellugi U, Klima ES: Biological foundations of language: clues from sign language, *Annual Review of Neuroscience* 13:283-307, 1990.

Werker JF, Tees RC: The organization and reorganization of human speech perception, *Annual Review of Neuroscience* 15:377-402, 1992.

Index

U